THE INTERNATIONAL YEARBOOK FOR CHILD PSYCHIATRY AND ALLIED DISCIPLINES

Volume 1

The Child in His Family

The Child in His Family

Edited by

E. JAMES ANTHONY, M.D.
St. Louis, Missouri, U.S.A.

and

CYRILLE KOUPERNIK, M.D.
Paris, France

ROBERT E. KRIEGER PUBLISHING COMPANY
HUNTINGTON, NEW YORK
1979

Original Edition 1970
Reprint Edition 1979

Printed and Published by
ROBERT E. KRIEGER PUBLISHING COMPANY, INC.
645 NEW YORK AVENUE
HUNTINGTON, NEW YORK 11743

Printed in the United States of America

Library of Congress Cataloging in Publication Data

Main entry under title:

The Child in his family [vol. 1]

Reprint of the edition published by Wiley, New York, as v. 1 of the International yearbook for child psychiatry and allied disciplines.
Bibliography: p.
Includes index.
1. Child psychiatry. 2. Parent and child.
I. Anthony, Elwyn James. II. Koupernik, Cyrille, 1917-
III. Series: International yearbook for child psychiatry and allied disciplines ; v. 1.
[RJ499.C484 1979] 618.9'28'9008 78-31654
ISBN 0-88275-863-2

Contributors

Nathan W. Ackerman (M.D.), Director of Professional Program, The Family Institute, New York, U.S.A.

E. James Anthony (M.D.), Ittleson Professor of Child Psychiatry, Division of Child Psychiatry, Washington University School of Medicine, St. Louis, Missouri, U.S.A.

C. Barat (L. ès L.), Psychologist, Laboratoire de Psychopathologie et Psychiatrie Sociales, Paris, France

John Bowlby (M.D.). Consultant Child Psychiatrist, Tavistock Clinic, Tavistock Centre, London, England

Hilde Bruch (M.D.), Professor of Psychiatry, Baylor College of Medicine, Houston, Texas, U.S.A.

Marianne Cederblad (M.D.), Director, Hökarängen's Child Guidance Clinic, Stockholm, Sweden

Stella Chess (M.D.), Associate Professor of Psychiatry, New York University Medical Center, New York, U.S.A.

Henri C. Collomb (M.D.), Professor de Psychiatrie, Faculte Mixte de Medecine et de Pharmacie de Dakar, Dakar, Senegal, West Africa

George Condominas (Ph. D.), Professor at L'Ecole Pratique des Hautes Etudes, Sorbonne (Section VI, Economic and Social Sciences), Paris, France

M. Girault (I.N.T.D.), Association L'Elan, Paris, France

Nahman H. Greenberg (M.D.), Associate Professor of Psychiatry and Director of Child Development Clinical and Research Unit, Department of Psychiatry, College of Medicine, University of Illinois at the Medical Center, Chicago, Illinois, U.S.A.

Ernest A. Haggard (Ph. D.), Professor of Psychology, Department of Psychiatry, University of Illinois at the Medical Center, Chicago, Illinois, U.S.A.

A.A. Khatri (M. Sc., M.A., LL.B), Senior Psychologist, B. M. Institute, Ahmedabad, Gujarat, India

Cyrille Koupernik (M.D.), Formerly Assistant des Hôpitaux de Paris, Paris, France

Serge Lebovici (M.D.), Director, Centre Alfred Binet, Paris, France

Theodore Lidz (M.D.), Professor of Psychiatry, Yale University School of Medicine, New Haven, Connecticut, U.S.A.

Anna von der Lippe (Ph. D.), Amanuensis in Psychology, University of Oslo, Oslo, Norway

Reginald S. Lourie (M.D., Med. Sc. D.), Professor, Pediatrics (Psychiatry), George Washington University School of Medicine, Director, Department of Psychiatry, Children's Hospital of D.C., and Medical Director, Hillcrest Children's Center, Washington, D.C., U.S.A.

Frances K. Millican (M.D.), Research Associate, Department of Psychiatry and Research Foundation, Children's Hospital of the District of Columbia, Washington, D.C., U.S.A.

Salvador Minuchin (M.D.), Professor of Child Psychiatry and Pediatrics, University of Pennsylvania, and Director, Philadelphia Child Guidance Clinic, Philadelphia, Pennsylvania, U.S.A.

Lois Barclay Murphy (Ph. D.), Consultant, Infant-Rearing Study, Children's Hospital of D.C., Washington, D.C., U.S.A.

Peggy Papp (M.S.W.), Family Therapist, Family Institute, New York, U.S.A.

Colin Murray Parkes (M.D., D.P.M.), Member, Research Staff, School of Family Psychiatry and Community Mental Health, Tavistock Institute of Human Relations, London, England

Phoebe Prosky (M.S.W.), Family Therapist, The Family Institute, New York, U.S.A.

Michael Rutter (M.D., M.R.C.P., D.P.M.), Reader in Psychiatry, Institute of Psychiatry, University of London, and Consultant Physician, Maudsley Hospital, London, England

K. Sablière (M.D.), Neuropsychiatrist, Laboratoire de Psychopathologie et Psychiatrie Sociales, Paris, France

Mara Selvini-Palazzoli (M.D., Lib. Doc.), Psychiatrist-Psychotherapist and Director, Centro per lo Studio della Famiglia, Milan, Italy

Emel Aktan Sumer (M.D.), Instructor in Child Psychiatry, Division of Child Psychiatry, School of Medicine, University of Istanbul, Istanbul, Turkey

Kai Tolstrup (M.D.), Medical Director Department of Child Psychiatry, University Hospital, Copenhagen, Denmark

Simone Valantin (Doct. Cand.), Maître Assistante, Faculte des Lettres et des Sciences Humaines de Dakar, Dakar, Senegal, West Africa

George Vassiliou (M.D.), Director, The Athenian Institute of Anthropos, Athens, Greece

Vasso G. Vassiliou (Ph. D.), Associate Director, The Athenian Institute of Anthropos, Athens, Greece

C. Veil (M.D.), Assistant Director of Studies, Practical School of High Studies (Economical and Social Sciences), Paris, France

Sula Wolff (M.A., M.R.C.P., D.P.M.), Consultant Child Psychiatrist, Royal Hospital for Sick Children, Edinburgh, Great Britain

Foreword

The International Association for Child Psychiatry and Allied Professions has not published reports on the proceedings of its International Congresses except for the Lisbon Conference of 1958 and the Hague Conference of 1962, which was under the direction of Dr. D. Arn van Krevelen, then President of the Association.[1] However, in a few other instances, the Congress stimulated the production of a subsequent book derived from leading presentations made at the Congress that focused on its dominant theme. This was the case at the Toronto Congress in 1954 on the Emotional Problems of Early Childhood,[2] and with the Hague Congress in 1962 on the Prevention of Mental Disorders in Children.[3]

The Sixth Congress took place in Edinburgh in 1966 and was devoted to the psychological and psychopathological study of the adolescent. A new departure in Congress procedure was inaugurated and was eminently successful. In the final months before the meeting, the participants received a bilingual volume (English and French) in which various invited specialists on both sides of the Atlantic discussed the psychiatric approach to the adolescent.[4] The novel idea behind the distribution of this pre-Congress book involved the *active* participation demanded of those attending the Congress. This implied transactions in working groups for which the members required some preparation. This concept of a *working Congress* has now taken root and was supplemented by a later volume that incorporated the most

[1] Krevelen, D. A. van, *Pédopsychiatrie et Prévention,* Hans Huber, Berne, 1964.

[2] Caplan, G., *Emotional Problems of Early Childhood,* Basic Books, New York, 1955.

[3] Caplan, G., *Prevention of Mental Disorders in Children,* Basic Books, New York, 1961.

[4] Caplan, G. and S. Lebovici, *Psychiatric Approach to Adolescence; L'Abord Psychiatrique de l'Adolescence* (bilingual), Excerpta Medica Foundation, Amsterdam, 1966.

pertinent and interesting productions at the Congress in a post-Congress book on the psychosocial perspectives of adolescence.[5] With this development, it seemed as if the Executive Committee of the International Association had committed itself to the production of two Congress books every four years. The success of these, however, oriented the Committee toward further developments. In planning for the 1970 Congress in Israel, the Committee concluded that the international scientific exchange in the field of child psychiatry and allied disciplines to which it was dedicated would be much enhanced by an annual publication summarizing the best that the young disciplines had to offer each year. The International Association, which had been a loosely connected body that came to life every four years, was now taking on a more vital role in the scientific organization of knowledge and its regular and wide dissemination.

The advantage of an international yearbook is evident to those who work on the international scene. We are often struck by the number of important contributions that fail to cross language barriers and are therefore lost, sometimes permanently, to national scientific efforts. To have an international yearbook tapping the resources of many different disciplines will also help to offset professional barriers that deny free access of one discipline to another. The Association, therefore, by virtue of its charter is international, multidisciplinary, and bilingual and it was therefore logical that its yearbook should manifest the same characteristics. This is one of the reasons why the Association has always sympathized with the effort made by our colleague, D. Arn van Krevelen, since he took over the direction of the *Acta Pedopsychiatrica* to publish articles in French, English, and German. For the same reason, it is fitting that the *Acta* also publishes the news bulletins of the International Association.

These several considerations culminated in the decision to have an annual series dealing with the psychology and psychopathology of childhood development of which this volume is the first. By scanning the contents and the list of contributors, it will be clear that the overall objective of tackling certain problems has been realized by means of the common effort of specialists coming from many disciplines, many schools of thought, and many countries. It would also seem to

[5]Caplan, G. and S. Lebovici, *Adolescence: Psychosocial Perspectives,* Basic Books, New York, 1969.

have achieved its other important purpose which is to familiarize the members of the Association with the familial approach to the child prior to their participation in the Jerusalem Congress. In this book, the working through of the prominent theme of "The Child in His Family," as delineated by the leading speakers and discussants, will be presented to the wider audience unable to attend the Seventh Congress.

I would like to express my gratitude and that of the Association to the two publishers who have undertaken to share the burden of the joint publication: John Wiley & Sons, Inc. in the United States and Masson & Cie in France. I would also like to thank Dr. E. James Anthony and Dr. Cyrille Koupernik who have spent much time and energy in commissioning, collecting, and co-editing the many articles included in this first volume. This is a new experience in international scientific cooperation and the Executive Committee of the International Association for Child Psychiatry and Allied Professions over which I have the honor to preside is proud and happy to submit to its members all over the world this collection of noteworthy studies that reflect the present stage of development in our discipline.

S. LEBOVICI
President of the International Association for Child Psychiatry and Allied Professions

February 1970
Paris, France

Preface

The family is one of the most studied institutions of mankind and yet our knowledge of it remains scrappy and unsystematized. There are several reasons for this. In the first place, it is difficult to span all its dimensions in time and space. It is as variable as man himself and closely reflects the physical, social, and cultural conditions that he creates for himself. Historically, its beginnings are lost in the first, unchronicled emergence of the human species in its evolutionary development and, since the dawn of recorded time it has been a feature of human life in every part of the world. So many men, so many families! It can also be discerned in rudimentary form among the more highly evolved animals. Yet, although it shows this wide variation across cultures and within cultures, it still remains fundamentally the same. This is largely because the structure and function of what is generally referred to as the nuclear family tends to remain unchanged in spite of the embellishments added at any particular time by any particular culture. The child in the family shares both in the sameness that helps to make him a human individual and in the difference that makes him a recognizable member of a special cultural or social group.

Another reason that makes a study of the family difficult is the fact that we can only do so from the inside. From the time of birth, we are submerged in the intimacies and intricacies of family living and it is therefore impossible for us to observe the family from the outside projectively and without bias. We cannot shed this encompassing, developmental experience which not only leads us to look at other families from the perspective of our own, but also propels us, in some mysterious way, to replicate the attitudes, feelings, and behavior deriving from the family of origin within the family of procreation. Impaired by this transference, the vision is only too likely to be distorted.

A third reason that limits the investigator has to do with the consequence of self-consciousness. Man, in his development, has become a being with a bifurcated outlook that allows him to look both inwardly and outwardly so that his total experience of phenomena in his environment is a subtle admixture of the subjective and objective. What he sees is inextricably bound up with what he feels and what he thinks so that all his studies, even the most mechanistic, are more or less contaminated by introspection.

The fourth complex reason that affects his perspective derives from the differential structure and function of the family. The individual in the making within the setting of the family models his observations on the more powerful observations of his father and mother. The child's observations become polarized around two almost separate experiences of reality. The father's reality, in general, is focused on what is outside the family and corrected by the realities that prevail in the external world. The mother's reality, on the other hand, is more concerned with intrafamilial and intra-individual matters. This intrafamilial reality is of the kind that Freud described as "psychic reality" and is suffused with feeling, fantasy, and familiarity. In many respects, it is as real to the family as extrafamilial reality and is altogether a more significant reality. It is difficult, if not impossible, for the outside observer, unless he lives intimately with the family, to appreciate the nature of this type of reality. Looking in from the outside, you will be often tempted to dismiss this intrafamilial reality as unrealistic, meaning unrelated to the world outside in a logical continuity.

The last difficulty besetting family research is a problem afflicting all scientific study to some extent. The observer changes the field of observation when he enters it and his findings, if fed back to the field, may also bring about drastic changes. Social scientists have pointed a warning finger in the direction of what has been referred to as the "centipede effect" (the centipede, when asked how it managed to put one foot in front of the other with all its hundred feet, became immobilized). A family that looks at its multiple functions – providing the most convenient and carefree setting for the sexual activity of the parents, a safe and predictable environment for all its members, the domestication and socialization of the young, at times the care of the aged, and the transmission through the generations of cultural values – might well get entangled in its own workings. One might expect that in highly literate societies anxiety might follow closely on the heels of self-knowledge. A modern commentator has spoken out about this problem:

> Society is in the process of making parenthood a highly self-conscious, self-regarding affair. In so doing, it is adding heavily to the sense of personal responsibility among parents. Their tasks are much harder and involve more risks of failure when children have to be brought up as individual successes in a supposedly mobile, individualistic society rather than in a traditional and repetitious society. Bringing up children becomes less a matter of rule of thumb, custom, and tradition, more a matter of acquired knowledge, of expert advice. More decisions have to be made because there is so much more that has to be decided, and as the margin of felt responsibility extends so does the scope of anxiety about one's children.[1]

It would seem therefore that not only are there difficulties in studying the family but also hazards in doing so, and this is especially true of intense clinical studies in which iatrogenic side effects of guilt and shame may make their appearance. To know one's family is a logical extension of the ancient prescription, Know Thyself, and is to be recommended for a richer life experience but, like all prescriptions, there is always danger in overdosage and the wise clinician will keep this fact in mind when assessing tolerance of a family for insight.

Social Change and Family Psychopathology

In the course of reading this book, readers will appreciate not only the variations in family life throughout the world, but also the effects of changing world conditions.

There is no doubt that the two major wars of our time and the more localized although no less protracted wars that occur from time to time have had a disturbing influence in human relationships even at the most intimate level of association. There is some evidence that family disruption tends to parallel world disruption and that wars bring an increase in divorce whereas peace restores family stability.

Another major turmoil had its onset in the last century but it is continuing to exercise profound effects in the developing countries. This is the factor of industrialization and its concomitants of urbanization, migration, mobile communication, and a very appreciable increase in the material standard of living. Industrialization brings

[1]Titmuss, R., *The Family. National Council of Social Service Publication,* The British National Conference on Social Work, National Council of Social Service, 1954.

about radical changes in society which, in turn, bring about agonizing reappraisals, rearrangements, and revolutions within and between individuals. This has caused, as is evident in some chapters, certain radical changes in family structure and process. One of the basic shifts has been from the consanguineous, authoritarian, patriarchal, multifunctional, and rural family type to a smaller, conjugal, democratic, and urban family type in which many of the traditional family functions have been taken over by outside agencies. This change predisposes to an increase in instability, especially during the period of transition. On the positive side, there are indications that family tyranny (with such ugly features as wife- and child-beating) has disappeared; employment, job satisfactions, and opportunities have become greater; and there is less aversion to work because it is no longer so mindless and monotonous. On the negative side, people can become intoxicated by the new freedoms and new facilities and new worlds of experience opened up to them and they can rush into novel situations largely unprepared and therefore very vulnerable to mishap and disappointment. All this is often accompanied by an ominous rise in psychopathology as documented in some of the articles. Such developing people would almost seem to require a moratorium, in the Eriksonian sense, to allow for some of the transitional disruption to be alleviated.

Apart from such transitional disturbances, urban families living in areas that have been long industrialized have gained considerably by the mutation. They have fewer children, less crowded and more comfortable quarters, less arduous employment, more money and, as a new departure for the lower classes, something that can be really called a home.

> For the first time in modern history, the lower class home, as well as the middle class home, has become a place that is warm, comfortable, and able to provide its own fireside entertainment – in fact, pleasant to live in. This means that the modern husband spends his evenings and weekends at home rather than with his mates in taverns, relaxing by a common fireside or puttering around the house retaining or improving its comfort and appearance.[2]

In short, this would seem to herald the emergence of a "home-centered society." With the current emphasis on ecology, as described by Minuchin in this book, there is no doubt that psychopathology, in

[2]Abrams, M., The Home-Centered Society, *The Listener*, 26 November 1959.

its widest sense, will soon need to include all the intra- and extra-familial appurtenances that belong to modern living. The brute realities of the material world as manifest in the culture of poverty can leave an indelible imprint on the psyche.

Family Deterioration and Psychopathology

Several articles in this book deal with the impact of a short-term crisis on family life, whether it be sickness, death, separation, or unemployment. A more general question is concerned with whether these more transient deteriorations are superimposed on a general decline of the family in contemporary life. There is some consensus that the family is in the process of changing although less agreement as to whether this is in the direction of improvement or eclipse. On the face of it, modern families certainly look healthier; they are smaller in size as a result of birth control, the children are more evenly spaced, they are more comfortably housed, more economically provided for, more independent of relatives, more mutually considerate of their members, more democratically managed, more oriented toward family life, more knowledgeable about children and how to bring them up, and much more in contact, through the mass media, with the world about them. On the whole, the families seem less encapsulated and the children less constricted. There is far more meaningful communication than ever before between the members.

There is no evidence, however, that children are mentally healthier in a child-centered than in a parent-centered home, although the psychopathology may take different form. Those who are pessimistic about the state of the world generally tend to be pessimistic about the modern family. They point to a sad diminution of the authority of the father, to the relative neglect by the working mother of her children, to the increasing use of surrogates in child care, and to the abdication of responsibility on the part of the parents for the behavior of their children. All this they see as a manifestation of a sick society spawning sick families and sick individuals. They feel that the loss of many of the "great permanences" ingrained through generations of tradition are being lost as the family is being gradually stripped of its functions. With the evolution of the small family, there is a danger of it becoming "a narrow, self-contained little den in which people suffocate each other with their possessive, stagnant, and petty emotions."[3] With the de-emphasis on kinship and tradition, the family is more inclined to see itself as a transient get-together. With their higher levels of aspiration, they egocentrically pursue their extrafamilial interests and concerns and may become relatively indifferent to and uncaring for one another

A British sociologist has denounced all this as "sheer, unfounded nonsense," insisting that not only has the family not declined but that it is as stable as ever and may even be much better off than at any other time in its history. What has evolved over the past century is a new type of family for a new age enjoying a measure of personal freedom, equality, mutuality, empathy for one another, and openness in relationships that can find no parallel in the past. Sex and love are becoming increasingly united and enjoyable. However, he does feel that there is perhaps a little too much emphasis on sex, love, and romanticism between the marital partners to the exclusion of other family interests and activities, meaning that there are subgroups in the family (parent-child, child-child) that deserve as much consideration. Despite the often drastic changes that have occurred with regard to structure and function in the family, the basic process of identification remains as strong as ever so that children continue to "inherit" their parents' occupations, their cultural attitudes and interests, their religious affiliations, and their political outlook. The members of a family still tend to disperse every morning (to work and school) and to reunite every evening at mealtime and after. This dispersal-reunion cycle, according to Zelditch, is a basic family experience that occurs under all conditions and leads to a primitive level of differentiation.[4] This is also true of the age and sex axis that structures every family irrespective of its cultural setting. Although differently organized than the compound families in less developed areas, the man and woman, when they marry, also do not break right away from their existing relatives. They bring their families of origin into their new lives and they thus have to make

> a profound double adjustment: to each other as individuals, and to the relatives who surround them. The wife has to reconcile her new obligations to her

[3]Fletcher, R., *The Family and Marriage in Britain,* Penguin Books, Baltimore, 1966.

[4]Zelditch, M., Role Differentiation in the Nuclear Family, in *Family, Socialization and Interaction Process.* T. Parsons and R. F. Bales, Eds., Free Press, Glencoe, Ill., 1955.

husband with her old obligations to her parents, and the husband likewise. The wife has to adjust to the husband's family of origin, and he to hers.[5]

Young and Willmott[6] point this out in their study of families in East London and emphasize that marriage has a modifying influence on all family relationships of each of the partners of a modern family as in the extended family of more primitive societies.

One further milieu factor must be emphasized, since its effect is somewhat of a paradox. The extraordinary acceleration of technological progress has not only outdated parental knowledge and competence, thus depreciating them in the eyes of their children, but has also generated intense counterfeelings in the young against the indescribable horrors associated with the impersonal "red desert" of industrialization. The new generation is turning back to the simplicities of preindustrial times and the values of single-minded parents.

Historical Note

A further indication of how things change and yet manage to remain basically the same is provided by the earliest dynamic study of family life that we have, made in the middle of the fifteenth century by Battista Alberti in four volumes entitled *Della Famiglia.* The first volume of this monumental work deals with the father-child relationship, the second with the husband-wife relationship, the third discusses the formula for a happy marriage, and the fourth inquires into extrafamilial relationships. Curiously enough, and because of the patriarchal structure of the Florentine family of this period, the mother-child relationship is given only minimal consideration. All the main ideas in *Della Famiglia* derive from the classical thought of the time and are dependent on a bourgeois ethic although the author is extraordinarily sensitive to the dynamic reactions that take place. The flavor of a Florentine household of the fifteenth century comes through very clearly and occasionally startles us with its modernity.

The infant, according to Alberti, belongs to the mother and fathers should leave this precious dyad to its own preoccupations.

[5] Fletcher, R., *op. cit.*

[6] Young, M. and P. Willmott, *Family and Kinship in East London,* Free Press, Glencoe, Ill., 1957.

> Alberti writes, I do not like to see babies tossed in the air by their fathers. People are fools not to realize the danger to a baby in his father's hard hands . . . so let the earliest period be spent entirely outside the father's arms. Let the child rest and sleep in his mother's lap.[7]

In the age that follows, the toddler belongs to the family as a whole although he may follow his mother.

> The child begins to make his wants known and to express them in words and the whole family listens and interprets and praises everything he says and does. This is the springtime of development when infinite hopes are founded in the most slender evidence of subtle intelligence and keen memory.

The latency of the boy is when the father comes in.

> It is practical not to keep little boys too long on the lap of the mother but to accustom them to life among men. They should not be left to feminine occupations or to the company of little girls. Their fathers should stimulate them to daring things to counteract the fables of the old women who surround them. The father should provide some sort of consistent model for his child and he should not expect that the child will only copy his good attitudes and behavior. Once the child has incorporated the father's vice, the father, highly tolerant of the vice within himself, may beat it unmercifully in the child.

Alberti remarks:

> One wants to say to them, "you stupid, crazy fathers! How can you expect little ones not to learn the object lesson of your ancient lusts?"

Alberti is also insistent that the father should not punish the children physically without first controlling his own anger. The child may feel that the punishment is deserved but it is the anger, especially in its more sadistic forms, that alienates the child. He suggests that some fathers cannot cope with the disciplinary role and should leave the act of punishment to others more capable of carrying it out judicially. He is also very much against the establishment of a peer relationship with a small child.

> A father must always be a father and act like a father, not pompously but with dignity and not with undue familiarity but with kindness. Every father should remember that love produces more permanent changes than fear and that severity without kindness inculcates hate rather than obedience. A son is a son and should be treated as such, not as a servant.

Alberti considers that the natural unit of the family has a logical structure and function. Families are therefore not artifacts.

[7] Alberti, B., *Della Famiglia,* 1453.

> Since the child comes into the world as a tender and delicate creature, he needs someone to nourish him with diligence and love and protect him from all harm. A woman can do just this, but since she is fully occupied thus, she is in no position to go out and seek provisions. Man, however, being by nature energetic, can go out and bring in things so that he becomes a natural provider. However, he cannot always be sure of returning immediately from the hunt or from the fields, so the woman must learn to save up supplies to cover the period when her husband is away. This involves her in the maintenance of supplies. It seems clear, therefore, that nature has taught mankind the necessity of having two parents both to increase and continue generation and to nourish and preserve those already born. Since more than one family may tax the man's resources too far, it seems natural that he should be the provider for only the one family.

A somewhat jarring note to these otherwise modern tones comes when Alberti discusses the husband-wife relationship. He clearly does not see it as a democratic coalition although he stresses its basis in love. For example, there are many things that one should not discuss with one's wife because it is in the nature of women to be indiscreet.

> One should never, in fact, tell a secret, even a trivial one, to one's wife. Stupid husbands blab to their wives and forget that women themselves can do anything sooner than keep quiet. I make it a rule never to speak with her of anything but household matters or of the children. These I discuss a great deal with her and by so doing she learns the principles of what is required and how to apply them. I do this in part to prevent her from entering into discussions with me concerning more important and private affairs.

However, Alberti insists, as he does with the children, that love makes for a more obedient wife than fear. The woman should not be intimidated but by gentle and devious ways she can be made to come round to the husband's point of view. For example, if she uses make-up, which he abhors, he is not immediately prohibitive.

> I wait until we are alone, and then I smile at her and say, "oh dear, how did you get your face so dirty? Did you by any chance bump into some cooking utensil? For goodness sake go and wash yourself quickly before people see you and make fun of you." She immediately understands what I am getting at and begins to cry but then she goes off and washes off the makeup. Wives will be obedient if their husbands know how to be husbands.

Study Methods

It would seem, from this brief survey, that it takes all sorts of families to make a world and that there are significant variations from one time to another and from one place to another. Throughout this book various methods of approaching the family scientifically or clinically will be found. There are references to questionnaires, living-in experiences, "focal interviewing," "unroofing," clinical investigation, projective techniques, behavioral observations, family group sessions, ecological explorations, and so on. Sometimes the data are anecdotal, sometimes impressionistic, sometimes objective, and sometimes interpretative. The reader can explore these various techniques for himself and sift the information offered from the different sources. It all adds up to very complex evidence and is not easily reduced to cut-and-dried conclusions. At times he may be impressed by the statistical evidence and at others by the personal revelations that seem more true to life, but always, he must bear in mind his own subtle and sophisticated system of prejudices which help to give him a coherent but personal view of the matter.

E. JAMES ANTHONY
CYRILLE KOUPERNIK

February, 1970
St. Louis, Missouri, U.S.A.

February, 1970
Paris, France

Acknowledgments

We acknowledge, with much gratitude, the almost indispensable help that we have received from Mrs. Martha Kniepkamp in the arduous tasks of collating, proofreading, indexing, typing, and retyping manuscripts, deciphering unreadable editorial comments, and coping with a shoal of correspondence with our globally distributed contributors. Without her steady and unflinching responsiveness to urgent editorial pressures, the Yearbook would still be loitering on the hard road to the printers. At peaks of activity she has at times been ably and cheerfully assisted by Mrs. Lorna Drafall. On the French side, Mademoiselle Martine Léage deserves the same gratitude.

The English translation of the papers originally written in French has been skillfully performed by Mrs. Eileen Geist, who combines a perfect knowledge of French with a remarkable mastership of a rather technical terminology.

We also thank our many contributors for making that extra special effort to meet the deadline dictated by the wish of the International Executive to have the book available for the participants of the 7th International Congress of Child Psychiatry and Allied Professions in August of 1970 in Jerusalem.

Lastly, we express our appreciation to our publishers who always made themselves immediately available to deal with knotty problems of production, costs, format, and deadlines when these raised their provocative heads.

E. J. A.
C. K.

Contents

Family Dynamics

Editorial Comment

The three contributions to this section neatly complement one another in presenting different accounts of family functioning which, when put together, offer a fairly complete and theoretically satisfying account of what must be regarded as one of the most complex social organizations in existence. The authors approach their topic from different points of view, sharing a common dynamic basis but varying in the use of transactional concepts. In one, the emphasis is group dynamic, in another, interpersonal, and in the third, environmental. It cannot be said that the three contributions add up to a general theory of the family integrating the intrapsychic and the interactional aspects, but there is an encouraging indication that the psychoanalytic, the transactional, and the ecological might someday be interlaced within a comprehensive and coherent theoretical matrix.

For the psychoanalyst (but not the child analyst), the members of the patient's family are reduced to shadowy projections on the screen of his associations. As Freud developed his theory, the internal representation of the family gradually came to assume major importance, but he himself remained well aware of the relationship of the intrapsychic to the actual. For example, he perceived the meaning and importance of the Oedipus complex in the basic organization of the family from primitive times and related the child's fantasy of the "family romance" to its experience of rejection and the child's tendency to lying to an unconscious communication with lying parents. He also considered that the most devastating effects on personality development occurred when a strong, authoritarian father paired off with a weak, masochistic mother. Today, in Western cultures, we have become more concerned with the reverse combination.

Lebovici asks psychoanalysts to look beyond the Oedipus complex for a better understanding of familial relationships and points to the fact that Freud himself took an additional step in this direction in his study of group phenomena. Lidz, also reared in the psychoanalytic tradition, cannot understand how anyone can promulgate an adequate theory of personality development outside the context of the family and its interpersonal functioning. The family, for him, is a developmental setting, providing the children growing up in it with experience of a miniature social system, the structure of which helps to structure the personality in a lasting fashion. This is a "core experience" without which we would be less than human. Minuchin, expressing his indebtedness to Roger Barker, feels it important to stress the undeniable fact that the outside of the individual has as much significance as the inside in his development, and that the neglected ecosphere is a crucial factor in the understanding and treatment of the disturbed child. The comprehensive study of the child, therefore, entails the investigation of him as an individual, the investigation of the environment in which he lives, and the "linkages" between these two. The child in his family gives place to the broader conception of the child in his environment.

It would seem that the three contributions are concerned in their different ways with the splitting created by traditional theory and perpetuated by traditional practice. The dichotomies of internal and external, intrapsychic and interpersonal, individual and familial are largely in the minds of the observers. In Barker's helpful metaphor, quoted by Minuchin, the freight train brings wheat to Chicago to be sold as food although the business of growing the wheat has nothing to do with the problems of running a train. Unfortunately, the theoretical distinctions may help to create iatrogenically artificial separations within the patient so that he ceases to regard himself as an integrated being in which the whole and its parts are in continuous dynamic relationship with one another. The child is not only a bundle of drives and defenses, nor merely the third component of the Oedipal triad, nor simply a member in good standing of a group association, nor just the product of his environment, all of which sound anonymous, but a unique individual with a personal identity that comes from his being a particular child in a particular family in a particular environment.

The Psychoanalytic Theory of Family

S. LEBOVICI (FRANCE)

Until the psychoanalytic revolution, the theory of family relations was defined by biological, sociological, and moral criteria. The child was first described within the framework of his neurobiological development in which family relationships did not seem to play a role. Weak and innocent, he had to learn everything from his parents who, in turn, had complete authority over him. Thus, the bonds tying the child to his parents were defined by obedience and love. The patriarchal family, which found its prototype in the history of Western civilization, had as its basic point of reference the life of the couple, in which the father, responsible for providing for the needs of the family, had complete authority. The mother, more specifically responsible for nutritional, educational, and household care, was the provider of love.

To be sure, the natural history of family life is considerably more subtle than this simplified schema suggests, because numerous socio-economic and cultural factors are involved which have evolved along with the history of society. For example, in the nineteenth century, with the strides made in urban and technical civilization, the small family took on a specific character which it still possesses to a large extent. But until Freud, the internal conflicts within these small units were only dealt with as tragedy, bourgeois drama, or comic skits.

* Translated by Eileen Geist.

Psychoanalysis has radically changed all this by revealing the conflicting desires and frustrations that are inevitably at work in such groups, and by bringing out the dramatic history of interindividual and intrafamily conflicts. The straightforward and traditional moral framework has given way under pressure from the fantasy life of each of the family members. The closed world of ethics and conflicts of conscience has been superseded by the phantasmagoria of conflicting tensions that express the inner life by way of incessant traumas.

To come to the main point of psychoanalytic theory, family life is definable by the nature and the consequences of a certain prototypical interpersonal fantasy situation, namely the nodal structure of the Oedipus complex.

Freud's Oedipus Complex

It has often been said that it was the young Sigmund Freud's complicated family situation which led him to better discern in his own past the mysteries of Oedipal relations. As the son of an elderly father who had lost status because of his relative inability to surmount economic difficulties, and of a much younger mother, his father's second wife, Freud had grown-up half-brothers and thus was the uncle of nephews who were older than himself. As a child, he was taken care of by an old woman-servant who had a great influence over him and who was fired for stealing, which only served to complicate a family situation already rather difficult to interpret.

We know that in his work with Breuer, Freud discovered the importance of sexual traumas within family life among a certain number of hysterics whose cases have been reported in *Studies in Hysteria* [3]. When his father died, Freud passed through a crisis which was related to the agonizing self-examination which he had been forced to make: he had understood that quite often the sexual traumas of which the hysterics complained had not taken place. In his self-analysis, he came to understand that his memories concerning his dead father were false; his father could not have been a homosexual who had tried to seduce his son; such ideas could only be the product of fantasy life. From then on, he would not only have to track down pathogenic traumas, but also reconstruct the development of unconscious and internalized conflicts that were in the final analysis only the product of instinctual activity (Freud's "Copernican Revolution").

The Oedipus Complex as Basis for the Family

In fact, the Oedipal situation, which constitutes the structural and fantasmic prototype of interpersonal and intrafamilial relationships, can only be understood as the product of the biological dependence of the child and of ambivalent family relationships.

The total dependence of the newborn infant on maternal care can only be satisfied by fusional union. The need for this union is constantly pressing, but it is never fulfilled, and it is at work in the dialectic of desire which provides the structure of the inner life. The father intervenes as mediator and as the image of reality in this union which is the outcome largely of hallucinatory activity.

The universal law that prohibits incest institutionalizes the necessity for this relationship and in so doing creates and maintains family ties. But the desire to transgress this law is reestablished by the psychoanalytic experience which, "anticipating the past," leads us to become aware that man will always want to fulfill this desire for union with his mother and that the nonfulfillment of this wish creates fantasies which characterize for each individual the family world with its internal conflicts.

The purpose of this presentation is not to describe the Oedipus complex and its implications, but rather to show how this fundamental structure, which shapes the destiny of the child and of the man inside the family, originates and how it is organized. This will involve some discussion of the current controversy regarding the relative importance of diachrony and synchrony and the role of history and structure in delineating the beginnings of the family.

Along with every other psychoanalyst, it seems to us that the myth so admirably represented by the tragedy of *Oedipus Rex* defines man's place within the drama of family conflicts. We will discuss certain applications of the study of interpersonal conflicts as set forth in Freudian doctrine, but we cannot extend them too readily or with any certainty to a study of the family group.

The Structure of the Oedipus Complex

To speak of the Oedipal triangle is equivalent, paradoxically, to evoking a dual system of relationships with the inevitable mixed feelings and complexes that bind the child to both his father and mother. The Oedipus complex is rooted in ambivalence: the child loves and desires his mother who must normally frustrate him and thereby provoke his aggressive demands; he wants to eliminate his father but, guilty of wishing this, he also wants to seduce him. Thus, as we have said, the Oedipus complex has both a positive and a negative aspect: the positive aspect in the case of the little boy lies in the totality of his desires which impel him to want his mother for himself alone and to eliminate his father; but this aspect of Oedipal feeling also has a reverse side, since the child's hostility to his father is compensated for by admiration. At the height of Oedipal development, in identifying himself with his father, the boy submits to the father's authority, which is symbolized by what will become the superego — a judicial authority whose severity derives from all the aggressive projections of the child onto the father image. The difficulty of interpreting the Oedipus complex resides in the fact that the child hates his father as a castrator while at the same time he projects all the love that he has heretofore concentrated on himself onto the idealized image of the father. This latter image is called the ego ideal.

The little girl pursues a much more complicated path, since she must turn away from her mother and make a love object of her father. Freud declared that this transformation comes about by way of disillusionment: the little girl discovers her mother's lack of a penis as well as her own lack of one. The trauma inflicted by the discovery of this castration leads her to try and please her father, and turns her away from her mother. In other words, whereas the boy fears castration as the final act of the Oedipal drama, the idea of castration becomes for the girl a fateful point of departure.

There are multiple facets to this long, slow development within the fantasy life and it is the lot of each individual to be forced to face up to this situation.

After the prophecy of the Delphic oracle, the child Oedipus left his foster parents whom he believed to be his real parents, so as not to kill his father. But he could not escape the prophecy that had been made, and thus he murdered Laius. After having vanquished the Sphinx who barred his entry into Thebes, Oedipus became king and married Jocasta, his mother. When the plague came to Thebes, he was presumptuous enough to search for the guilty person who was infuriating the gods and who was none other than himself. Heedless of the warnings of the blind soothsayer, Tiresias, who knew the truth, he, who had solved the enigmas of the Sphinx, conducted the sacrilegious inquiry that led him to the terrible truth that he had murdered his father and was the husband of his mother. His only recourse was exile, into which he went after having blinded himself so as to no longer be able to see the truth that he had to live with from that day on.

Happily, in the course of psychoanalytic treatment, patients generally limit themselves to bringing into the open the truth of the unconscious that has hitherto been only inarticulate desire, without acting on it. Our blind repression about actually knowing the truth of the unconscious does not prevent us from being compelled to bear responsibility for it and suffer from the guilt which underlies it. The truth of the unconscious is such that it makes us reproduce in the totality of our adult behavior the dramas we have lived out imaginatively and symbolically during childhood within our families.

Psychoanalysts believe this to be a universal truth about man. Unquestionably, certain sociological studies have shown family situations in which the Oedipal structure is not clearly identifiable.[1] But the biological development of the child makes it perfectly clear that the Oedipal structure is indeed one of the nuclei on which our destiny is based.

The Mother-Child Union

In fact, the newborn infant, because of his immaturity, lives at first in a state of total dependence. As a result, in the course of his primary infantile experiences, his mother and the nursing care she gives form a unity, the individual components of which can only be differentiated at moments of animal need. During this period his mother is little more than a function and tends only to become personalized

[1] Actually, recent works on this subject do not support Malinowski's questioning of the universality of the Oedipus complex [12, 13].

when she is feeding him. The unity between the child and his mother who feeds him, cares for him, holds him, and supports him has been vividly described by Winnicott [16] and is obviously a powerful figment of the infantile imagination. Everything conspires to make the child feel all-powerful, and this is reinforced by hallucinatory wish fulfillments activated by the pleasure principle that governs his life at this time. During phases of need, the child invests his mother with feelings even though he is not yet aware of her as a person. When she gratifies his needs to the full, she becomes a good mother and when she frustrates him, which is inevitable, the resulting tensions that accumulate transform her into a bad mother. This oscillation between need satisfaction and need frustration helps to create a distinction in the nursing infant between a good and bad maternal image.

When his degree of development allows him to perceive and to recognize the face of his mother and her existence as a separate unit, the child in turn becomes a separate unit in relation to this external object, and it is the recognition of this that forms the basis of his ego. In order to preserve the object investments and the stable functioning of the ego, the child must forego the direct release of his instinctual tensions, and he helps himself to do this by widening his fantasy life. In submitting passively to the introjected wishes of his mother, he introduces a certain order into the fantasies which constitute the first steps in thinking and in the establishment of psychic reality. From then on, the infant is no longer dominated by the desire for hallucinatory fulfillment. When abandoned by the object, he is now capable of reconstructing it in fantasy, which is the way in which introjected fantasies of the good mother come about. Until this crucial development his needs have been satisfied by hallucinatory or real means, but at this point he achieves the capacity for desire. Wishful fantasies are understandably ambivalent, since they are linked to earlier states of need generated from the first experiences of the infant with his mother.

We have also to take into account interruptions of contact between mother and child that tend to develop certain temporal and spatial rhythms related to the fluctuating needs of the child. These interruptions of contact compromise the feelings of omnipotence associated with the hallucinatory fulfillment of desire, and give rise to the sense of powerlessness which challenges the child's original narcissistic cathexis. He learns that he cannot have what he wants (the frustration of desire leading to the fantasy formation of the bad mother), and he must also learn that he is not identical with what he wants to be (the narcissistic trauma resulting from this powerlessness undermines the fantasy of omnipotence derived from the internalized idealized parents on whom the narcissistic energy was invested).

Thus, the infant, faced with this slowly developing history, each successive phase of which – within the limits of the period that we call oral – leaves its mark on him, produces a complex phantasmagoria based on the desire to introject a good mother, and the guilt for doing so aggressively and for robbing his mother of what is best in her. When he comes to recognize her as an independent being, he will feel the need to put her back together again.

This description, given by Melanie Klein, is based on her observation of young children during psychoanalytic treatment. It becomes understandable in the light of our knowledge of the immaturity of the newborn infant and the hazards of a slow development. In fact, the neonatal phase of the human child throws into sharp relief the contrast between the richness of his fantasy life and his relative powerlessness to express himself on the sensory-motor level. As Winnicott [16] has stated, the mother must for a long time adapt herself perfectly to his needs, sometimes, moreover, by neglecting the needs of the rest of the family. She allows the child to experience simultaneously hallucinatory fulfillment of his desires along with the possibility of introjecting a certain external reality. She thereby gives him the sense of living in a continuity, which is what Winnicott calls the *self*. Later, she satisfies his needs to a lesser extent and subjects him to increasing frustrations; in this way, the child lives through the experience of a good mother, even when he devours her, until his contradictory feelings become unified and he widens the domain of the first intermediary possessions between his mother and himself.

The description that we have just given of the infant's fantasy life in his first relationships with his mother leads him from never-attained and always-sought-after fusion to a certain differentiation in which the mother is at the same time and successively good and bad, intact provider and mutiliated prey, creature torn apart and put together again. The experiences which are worked out in fantasies come from her body, and the instinctual drives which are directed toward the maternal object organize themselves around fixation points that the drives of the developing child and the maternal interest and preoccupation tend to establish around the autoerotic zones.

The Dynamic Role of the Father

Until now the father belonged in some cases with the strangers who provoke phobic behavior on the part of the child in the absence of recourse to the mother. In other cases, the relationship of the child with his father may have a typically maternal character. But with the acquisition of the first rudiments of language and with the first differentiation between "yours" and "mine," the father comes into his own. The child distinguishes him from the mother and constructs fantasies of reciprocal possession. His relationship with the mother is in the second person singular: "I" and "thou." He has now to learn, at his own expense, that a third person, the father, has a claim on the mother whom he had thought exclusively his own. In this genetic perspective, it becomes apparent that it is the recognition of the difference between the father and mother that introduces the triangular problem into the family relationship. To put it schematically, it would seem that the little boy's interest lies in projecting onto his father the inevitable frustrations arising out of the relationship with his mother, since his father is both like him and different from him because he is masculine but is stronger and has possession of the mother.

This frustration of maternal origin was inevitable because of the initial dependence on her of the newborn infant. The existence of the parental couple brings the father subsequently into the dialectic of desire and makes him the fantasied agent of frustration and prohibition.

It can therefore be said that mental life, in its inception, is based upon the dual recognition of the mother as an object of desire as well as a medium for satisfying needs and upon the recognition of the difference between father and mother and of the bonds between them that stimulate the emergence of the Oedipal fantasies.

The basic structure of the Oedipal relationship is clearly biological, but what gives this Oedipal material its specific form are the vicissitudes that accompany maturation, starting with the time when needs

the real trauma and this can be expressed through symptoms and such imaginative or symbolic outgrowths as the dream.

With this in mind, it follows that in order to understand familial interrelationships, psychoanalysts must look beyond the Oedipal model and its direct consequences. Freud himself studied group phenomena in one of his essays in which he described the group bond which constitutes the ego ideal [5]. We have already noted that the postulate of a forbidding and punitive superego includes this particular concept which is derived from the ideal image projected onto the father during the earliest narcissistic investments. This identification bond explains why, apart from conflicts and the way in which they are resolved, the family can be considered as a type of social group. Identifying values are brought into play and roles distributed not only on the basis of historically experienced relationships but also in accordance with those ideal values which go to make up a new reality.

On their side, the Kleinian psychoanalysts, such as Bion [1], give even greater importance to what this author calls the "basic assumption" in the organization of the family group; this assumption is concerned with the common bonds which unite, in an ambivalent fashion, all the members of the group to a mother who is felt in fantasy to be the universal provider.

These various hypotheses can certainly be widely applied, but on the practical level they must be adapted to include the two following considerations:

1. Dynamic studies of small groups have widely taken up Freudian ideas about the identification of the members of the group with the ego ideal [5]. However, we cannot reduce the phenomena which are developed within groups to these basic considerations without taking certain methodological precautions; terminological assimilations especially run the risk of leading to erroneous conclusions. For example, it is common practice to speak of identification with the leader of the group, but the psychodynamic studies which have defined the importance of the latter are only indirectly connected with the psychoanalytic theory of the ego ideal.

2. In the same way, the study of roles within the family and of modes of communication observed between members

> can be made in the parlance of psychoanalysis, whereas there would be some hesitation in using concepts whose significance is restricted to the frame of reference of psychoanalytic metapsychology. Thus, the study of the family group can be carried out by psychoanalysts capable of applying their knowledge of small group theory, with the proviso that the interpersonal relationships observed be theorized according to a double model – the structural model of the Oedipus complex and the psychodynamic model of group theory [8].

As psychoanalysts, we can understand the evolution of interpersonal relationships within the family only by taking into account the particular modes of mental functioning of each of the protagonists therein. Moreover, psychoanalysis teaches us that the play of relationships depends much more on the internal organization of conflicts than on the protagonists in the real relationship. That is, the mental makeup, crystallized by the reaction formations which countermand the instincts, constitutes a characterological framework whose rigidity simply does not permit reciprocal adjustment of interpersonal relationships within the family. Those with experience in child psychiatry know that it is extremely difficult to make a prognosis on any disorder without first evaluating the chances of enlisting help from the parents. Unhappily these chances are limited for at least two reasons: (1) the child's difficulties are an integral part of the family's difficulties, his symptom being a product of them; and (2) the pathogenic influence of the family not only gives rise to the childhood disorder but also determines its development and may even, due to the play of inborn fantasies, be responsible for the cultural transmission of family neuroses through several generations.

The Psychoanalyst and Family Psychiatry

For the psychoanalyst, everything would seem to indicate that the family is the best place to look in order to understand and treat children's disorders. For the best results, he would be advised to adopt the concepts, language, and therapeutic approach of those who have specialized in the treatment of neurotic and psychotic families and who generally think in terms of psychoanalytic theory, supplementing the concepts of intrapsychic functioning with concepts of intrafamilial functioning.

In a recent work [9] the author, along with some collaborators, attempted to describe what might be called a neurotic family, that is, one in which the individual neuroses of each of its members act upon one another and are combined. The neuroses do not necessarily have an unfavorable influence on the child's development. In a still unpublished study of a subgroup of a standard population of Paris, we showed that the spread of morbid symptoms among the children of this group was no different from that found in a group of children under observation by consultants at a child psychiatric center. But in the standard group we were able to note how much the masochistic satisfactions that the devoted mothers inflicted on themselves constituted a precious support for the children and often saved them from entering the field of pathology.

Nevertheless, we do not believe that it is justifiable to broaden the psychoanalytic theory of the individual to cover the group. There would seem to us to be no possible overlapping between the organization of the Oedipal relationship and the identifications which model it on the one hand, and the dynamic phenomena of the group on the other, even if there are repercussions between them.

Psychoanalysts, such as Slavson [14] or Foulkes and Anthony [2], who have used the operational concepts of psychoanalysis for the study of groups, have done so cautiously and in a logical fashion. The same prudence should be exercised by those psychoanalysts who use the family approach for diagnostic and therapeutic purposes to define their activity in this new domain by way of a terminology which is specific to it, without necessarily abandoning their own way of looking at things.

Conclusion

This brief presentation cannot hope to summarize all the theoretical and clinical perspectives opened up by psychoanalysis for the understanding of family relationships. We have limited ourselves to showing that the structural model of the Oedipus complex is what the psychoanalyst uses to define the family relationship.

We have also tried to show that this is a natural model with a biological basis and with considerable explanatory strength. It has enabled us to see why the dependence of the human infant determines the entire natural history of its family relationships as they are experienced in fantasy life. The behavior of children and their parents in reciprocal relationships is based on this organization, which tends to repeat itself continuously and constantly in everyday life and activity.

The theory that we have presented is far from being accepted by all psychoanalysts. Some of them, in following the thesis of Ferenczi, recently taken up again by Bowlby, consider that the fundamental relationship of the baby with its mother is that of a primary attachment, centered on and organized around the mother. To support this hypothesis, Bowlby relies on ethological confirmation, particularly on the findings in which successive phenomena follow the release of instinctual behavior after exposure to some specific releasing mechanism [15]. Recent work on aggression [10] seems to strengthen this thesis that, within species, attachment is closely related to aggression. It is the ritualized form of its expression, in modes of behavior which can be innate as well as acquired.

For our part, we believe that psychoanalytic experience does not enable us to leap directly from the study of fantasy life to the study of instinctual behavior patterns. Our experience only enables us to know the outward representations of drives, when their by-products crop up in the form of desire.

The objection could be made that we have not hesitated to use neurobiological references in order to understand the development of the child within the dialectic of his maturation and his relationships. However, it is this basic biological reference that seems to us to constitute a solid foundation for the understanding of the organization and universality of the Oedipal structure.

For this reason, we would dissociate outselves from the Freudian hypothesis, first put forward in *Totem and Taboo* [4] and later in *Moses and Monotheism* [7], in which Freud speculates that the individual history of each one of us reproduces the fate of primitive man who, in the primal horde, gangs up with his brothers to kill his father who then becomes the totem animal. To avoid the recurrence of ritual murder, the incest prohibition establishes itself as the basis for all other prohibitions and taboos.

Nevertheless, when we carefully read Freud's reflections on the exogamic laws of marriage, we can see that the prohibition of incest reflected in them has simply been secondarily institutionalized.

It is a fact, however, that Freud postulated more than once the idea that our mental organization was the outcome of inherited memory traces, and that our individual history was the product of ancestral dramas that we can find again, more or less laid bare, in rites, myths, and dramatic tragedies. Thus, the Oedipal interpretation of these cultural products enables us, according to him, to reconstitute our own history as well as that of our ancestors.

We do not believe that this hypothesis is indispensable to an understanding of the organization of the Oedipal relationship; but our experience as analysts is constantly informing us that the structural nucleus of the Oedipus complex gives a specific shape to the human family.

From this point of view, we have been extremely interested in the thesis recently developed by Mendel in *La révolte contre le père* [11]. He, too, does not believe in the murder of the father, as it has been described by Freud. He thinks that the infant, confronted with his desire for the mother and with the contradiction which characterizes this desire, because of the richness of the fantasies which make it explicit and because of his powerlessness to satisfy them, needs to invent a rival for himself that he projects quite naturally onto the father whom he learns to recognize and whom his mother is at once ready to offer to him as this rival and interdictor. Thus, his aggressiveness and his powerlessness can invest this fantasied rival in more and more complex forms deriving from the Oedipus complex. The same emergence can be observed in the history of mankind when prehistoric man passed from a sacred fusion with nature to its domestication by the use of tools.

Because we have agreed with the set of hypotheses that could cover both the development of the child as well as the evolution of mankind and because we have seen in both the appearance of a father whose power and prohibitions were felt to be a fantasied necessity, does not imply that we are in agreement with the entire theory currently fashionable in certain French psychoanalytic circles. To those engaged in the study of linguistic structures, the Oedipal organization is formed according to the modes of exogamic exchanges which also constitute a basic model, reflecting these same structures. It would be *the father's name* that would lie at the basis of the fantasy regarding paternal prohibition, because the mother calls upon him to compensate for the fact that she cannot gratify the child she has produced without having recourse to the phallic power to which she gains access through intercourse with her partner. In contrast, our entire thesis has attempted to show that the name of the father only appears because the child has need of it in order to escape from the danger of his desires that he cannot dominate. It is undeniable that the mother also uses her husband in her fantasies, but this fact only constitutes an additional proof of the fundamental thesis that maturation cannot, by itself, explain the child's developmental course because this is also determined by his relationship with his parents and by their relationship to each other.

Bibliography

1. Bion, W. R., *Experiences in Groups,* Tavistock Publications, London, 1961.
2. Foulkes, S. H., and E. J. Anthony, *Group Psychotherapy* (The Psychoanalytic Approach), Penguin Books, London, 1957.
3. Freud, S., *Etudes sur l'Hystérie,* 2nd ed., Stand, Paris, 1893
4. Freud, S., *Totem et Tabou,* 13th ed., Stand, Paris, 1913.
5. Freud, S., *Group Psychology,* 18th ed., Stand, Paris, 1920.
6. Freud, S., *Inhibition, Symptôme et Angoisse,* 20th ed., Stand, Paris, 1926.
7. Freud, S., *Moise et le Monothéisme,* 23rd ed., Stand, Paris, 1937.
8. Lebovici, S. and R. Diatkine, La dynamique de groupe, *Psychiatr. Enfant,* V, 1 (1962), 339.
9. Lebovici, S., G. Diatkine, and A. Arfouilloux, A propos de la Psychiatrie familiale, *Psychiatr. Enfant,* XI, 1 (1969).
10. Lorenz, K., *L'agression* (une histoire naturelle du mal) (Trad. V. Fritsch), Flammarion, Paris, 1969.
11. Mendel, G., *La révolte contre le père,* Payot, Paris, 1969.
12. Ortigues, M. C. and E., *Oedipe Africain,* Plon, Paris, 1966.
13. Parin, P., F. Morganthaler, and G. Parin-Matthey, *Les Blancs pensent trop,* Payot, Paris, 1966.
14. Slavson, S. R., *A Textbook in Analytic Group Psychotherapy,* Int. Univ. Press, New York, 1964.
15. Tinbergen, N., *L'étude de l'instinct* (Trad. B. de Zélicourt et F. Bourlière), Payot, Paris, 1953.
16. Winnicott, D. W., *De la pediatrie a la psychanalyse* (Trad. J. Kalmanovitch), Payot, Paris, 1969.

The Family as the Developmental Setting

THEODORE LIDZ (U. S. A.)

The family has everywhere been society's primary agency in providing for the child's biological needs and simultaneously directing his development into an integrated person capable of living in society and transmitting its culture. Any attempt to study the child's personality development or maldevelopment as an autonomous process, independent of the family matrix, distorts as much as it simplifies; it is bound to error, for such abstractions can be made only by eliminating the essential factors in the process. Because the family is ubiquitous, it has often been taken for granted and many of its essential functions overlooked. It is a universal phenomenon because it is an essential correlate of man's biological makeup, the basic institution that permits his survival by augmenting his inborn adaptive capacities. Everywhere the family must meet two determinants: the biological nature and needs of man, and the requirements of the particular society in which it exists, and which it subserves by preparing its offspring to live in it. Therefore, families everywhere will have certain essential features in common even while handling similar problems in differing ways in accord with the ways and needs of the specific society. In this essay I shall attempt to denote the essential functions of the family and the requisites for carrying them out.

Man is born with two endowments: a genetic inheritance and a cultural heritage. His genes transmit his physical structure and his physiological makeup, which as in all other animals, permits his survival within a relatively narrow range of environments; but his unique adaptive techniques are not born in him, are not an inherent outgrowth of his genetic endowment. He is born with a unique brain that permits the acquisition of language which enables him to acquire from those who raise him the adaptive techniques developed by his society for coping with the environment and for living together, and which enables him to develop a personality suited to the specific society in which he happens to grow up. It is a vastly different mechanism for survival and adaptation than other organisms possess, and we can never understand human development and functioning properly unless we take full cognizance of this dual heritage.

Man's biological makeup requires that he develop in a social system and assimilate a culture. The family is an essential derivative of man's biological makeup for it is the basic social system that mediates between the child's genetic and cultural endowments, provides for his biological needs while instilling societal techniques, stands between the individual and society, and offers a shelter within the society and against the remainder of society. The complete dependency of the infant and very small child and the many years it takes until he can cope for himself, require that he be raised by persons to whom his welfare is as important as their own. His dependency and his prolonged attachment to them provide major motivations and directives for his development into a member of the society. The family forms the earliest and most persistent influence that encompasses the still unformed infant and small child for whom the parents' ways and the family's ways are *the* way of life, the only way the child knows. All subsequent experiences are perceived, understood, and reacted to emotionally according to the foundations established within the family. The family ways and the child's patterns of reacting to them become so thoroughly incorporated in the child that they can be considered determinants of his constitutional makeup, difficult to differentiate from the genetically determined biological factors with which they interrelate; a circumstance that greatly complicates the study of his physical development as well as his personality development. Subsequent influences will modify those of the family, but they can never undo or fully reshape these early core experiences.

Although the family is accepted as an essential institution because of its child-rearing functions, we cannot properly understand why the family is omnipresent or how it rears children, unless we appreciate that it subserves three sets of functions which, even though we shall consider them separately, are intimately interrelated. It is likely that no other institution can simultaneously fill these three sets of functions which cannot be met separately without radical changes in our social structure and without grave consequences; and it is highly probable that these functions essential to human adaptation cannot be met separately at all, except under very special circumstances, but must be fused in the family.[1]

Aside from providing shelter and nurturant care for children and concomitantly directing their personality development, the family also subserves essential needs of the spouses and of the society. The family not only fills a vital need of every society by carrying out the basic enculturation of its new recruits, but also subserves other societal functions. The family constitutes the basic social system in virtually every society, the fundamental unit of the larger social system: it forms a grouping of individuals that the society treats as an entity; it creates a network of kinship systems that helps stabilize even an industrial society; it constitutes an economic unit which in some societies is the major economic unit; it provides roles for its members both within the family and within the larger social system; and it provides status, motivation, and incentives that affect the relationships between individuals and the society. The nuclear family is, however, formed by a marriage and it serves to complete and stabilize the lives of the husband and wife. Although these three sets of functions of the family – for the children, for the society, and for the parents – are intimately interrelated and complement one another in many ways, they can also conflict and, indeed, some conflict between them is inevitable. The demands of society can obviously conflict with the needs of the spouses and children as when the husband must enter military service, or when the prevalent beliefs and mores of the broader society oppose those of the parents. I wish, however, to concentrate primarily upon the intricate relationships between the marital relationship and the fulfillment of the parents' needs and the capabilities of a family to carry out its child-rearing functions properly.

[1]The Israeli kibbutz is one carefully planned means of dividing these several basic functions between the child's parents, the nurturing nurse, and the children's home. The parents, however, continue to fill major functions as objects for identification and basic love objects, etc.

Although there are many reasons why people marry – love, passion, economic security, status, to escape from the parental home, to have children, to legitimize a child – marriage is a basic institution in virtually all societies primarily because of man's biological makeup and how he is brought up to reach maturity. Each person grows up in a family, forming essential bonds to those who nurture him, assimilating from them and internalizing their ways and attributes. Within his family of origin, however, he cannot achieve completion as an adult. Minimally, he must be frustrated because he cannot become a parent with its prerogatives and because sexual gratification cannot be united with affectional relationships. In his natal family he has enjoyed the security of being a member of a mutually protective unit in which, theoretically at least, his welfare has been of paramount importance to his parents. He leaves his family with his emotional attachments to it unresolved and with strong conscious and unconscious motivations to bring closure to these emotional imbalances. He moves toward a new union with a person who seems to fill the image of the desired complementary figure sufficiently to be transformed into it, a transformation achieved more readily when his perception is blurred by sexual impulsions. Even if the spouse is selected for him by others, he hopes through the marriage to again achieve the security afforded by a union in which his welfare and needs are of paramount importance to another person – a situation fostered by marriage in which the spouses' well-being and security are intimately if not irrevocably connected.

Marriage is also motivated by the division of the human species into two genders. A couple are not only drawn together by sexual impulsion but also because the two sexes complement one another in many other ways. From earliest childhood the male and female are subjected to gender-linked role training, and thereby acquire – if not also because of their genetic and hormonal differences – differing skills and ways of viewing the world, relating to people, giving and receiving affection. In a general sense, neither a man nor a woman can be complete alone. It is not that opposites attract, but that the two sexes are raised to divide the tasks of living and to complement, modify, and complete one another, as well as to find common purposes sexually and in raising their children.

A marriage can exist with the husband and wife assuming all sorts of role relationships and with very different ways of achieving reciprocity provided they are satisfactory to both, or simply more satisfactory than separating. The customary roles of husband and wife can be reversed with the wife earning the livelihood and the man doing the cooking and housekeeping; they can each remain in their parental homes; one or both may find sexual outlets only outside of the marriage; one spouse may fill a parental rather than a marital role for the other; it can form a sadomasochistic partnership or a source of masochistic satisfaction to both. The variants are countless. However, when the arrival of children turns a marriage into a nuclear family, the spouses' ways of relating must shift to make room for the children. Limits are then set upon how the couple can interrelate if they are also to provide a proper developmental setting for their children.

Although marital relationships are complex, they can be encompassed and studied in terms of the interaction between two persons, including the influence and impact of others and of other situations upon these two persons. A family, in contrast, cannot be grasped in terms of a dyadic relationship for it forms a true small group with a unity of its own. As in all true groups – in contrast to artificial groups such as are organized for sensitivity training and group psychotherapy – the action of any member affects all and the members must find reciprocally interrelating roles or conflict ensues. The group as a unit exacts loyalty requiring that each member give some precedence to the needs of the group over his own desires; and it requires unity of objectives and leadership toward these objectives. Small groups, even threesomes, tend to divide up into pairs that exclude others from significant relationships and transactions and impair or disrupt the group unity. Such requisites of groups in general are heightened and tightened in the family by the intimate living and the intense and prolonged interdependency of its members. Structure, roles, and leadership are necessary to promote the essential unity and to minimize divisive tendencies.

The family is, moreover, a very special type of group with characteristics imposed upon it by the biological differences of its members as well as by the particular purposes it serves. Recognition of these characteristics leads to an appreciation of some requisites of its structure [10].

1. The nuclear family is composed of two generations each with different needs, prerogatives, and obligations. The parents, having grown up in two different families, seek to merge themselves and their backgrounds into a new unit that satisfies the needs of both and completes their personalities in a relationship that seeks permanence. The new unit differs to a greater or lesser degree from their families of origin and thus requires malleability in both partners. The new relationship requires the intrapsychic reorganization of each spouse to take cognizance of the partner. Stated in very simple terms, the ego functioning of each is modified by the presence of an alterego including the id, ego, and superego requirements of the alterego. Wishes and desires of a spouse that can be set aside must be differentiated from needs that cannot be neglected.

   The parents are properly dependent upon one another, and children must be dependent upon parents, but parents cannot properly be dependent upon immature children. The parents serve as guides, educators, and models for offspring. They provide nurturance and give of themselves so that the children can develop. Though individuals, as parents they function as a coalition, dividing roles and tasks in which they support one another. As basic love objects and objects for identification for their children, who the parents are, how they behave, and how they interrelate with one another and not simply what they do to their child and for their child are of utmost importance to the child's personality development.

   The children, in contrast to their parents, receive their primary training in group living within the family, remaining dependent upon the parents for many years, forming intense emotional bonds to them, and developing by assimilating from their parents and introjecting their characteristics, and yet must so learn to live within the family that they are able to emerge from it to live in the broader society; or, at least, to start families of their own as members of the parental generation.

2. The family is also divided into two genders with differing but complementary functions and role allocations as well as anatomical differences. The primary female role derives from woman's biological structure and is related to the nurture of children and the maintenance of a home needed for that purpose, which leads to an emphasis upon interest in interpersonal relationships and emotional harmony – an expressive-affectional role. The male role, also originally related to man's physique, is concerned with the support and protection of a family and establishing its position in the larger society – an instrumental-adaptive role.
3. The relationships between family members are held firm by erotic and affectional ties. The parents who seek to form a permanent union are permitted and even expected to have sexual relationships. While all direct sexual relationships within the family are prohibited to the children, erogenous gratification from parental figures that accompanies nurturant care is needed and fostered; but it must be progressively frustrated as the need for such primary care diminishes lest the bonds to the family become too firm and prevent the child's investment of interest and energy in the extrafamilial world. The de-erotization of the child's relationships to other family members is a primary task of the family [5].
4. The family forms a shelter for its members within the larger society. Theoretically, at least, members receive affection and status by ascription rather than by achievement, which provides a modicum of emotional security in the face of the demands of the outside world. However, the family must reflect and transmit the societal ways, including child-rearing techniques appropriate to each developmental phase, and the culture's meaning and value system, and so forth, to assure that the children will be able to function when they emerge from the family into the broader society.

These fundamental characteristics of the nuclear family, and correlaries derived from them, set requisites for the parents and their marital relationship if it is to provide a suitable setting for the harmonious development of their offspring and to foster their children's development into reasonably integrated adults capable of independent existence.

Let us now examine how a family carries out its essential functions with respect to its offspring. The child does not grow up to attain a mature workable personality simply through the nurturance of inborn directives and potentialities but requires positive direction and guidance in a suitable interpersonal environment and social system. He does not simply mature into an integrated and adaptable person unless fixations occur because of some innate tendency, some emotional trauma, or some flaw in maternal nurturance during the pre-Oedipal phases of his development. The positive molding forces have been largely overlooked because they are built in to the institutions and mores of all societies and into the ubiquitous family which has everywhere unknowingly carried out the task of directing the child's potential into an integrated structure. The family must foster and direct the child's development by carrying out a number of interrelated functions. I shall consider them under four headings: (1) the parental nurturant functions that must meet the child's needs and supplement his immature capacities in a different manner at each phase of his development; (2) the dynamic organization of the family which forms the framework for the structuring of the child's personality or, perhaps stated more correctly, channels and directs the child into becoming an integrated individual [1]; (3) the family as the primary social system in which the child learns the basic social roles, the value of social institutions, and the basic mores of the society; and (4) the task of the parents to transmit to the child the essential instrumental techniques of the culture, including its language. We must examine the nature of these essential contributions to understand human personality development and maldevelopment.

The Parental Nurturant Function

This is the one requisite of the family that has been specifically recognized by most developmental theories, has been the focus of intensive study and, therefore, does not require careful elaboration here. We are concerned with the nature of the nurturance provided from the total care given to the helpless neonate to how the parents foster an adolescent's movement toward independence from them. It concerns more than filling the child's physical needs, it involves his emotional needs for love, affection, and a sense of security; it includes providing opportunity for the utilization of new capacities as the child matures. Proper nurture requires parents to have the capacities, knowledge, and empathy to alter their ways of relating and their attitudes to the child in accord with his changing needs. The degree of constraint provided a 9-month-old is unsuited for a toddler and the limits set for a 15-month-old would restrain the development of a 3-year-old child. The capacity to nurture, or for a mother to be maternal, is not an entity. Some mothers can nurture a child properly so long as he is almost completely dependent, but become apprehensive and have difficulties as soon as he becomes a toddler and can no longer be fully guarded from dangers inherent in his surroundings. Some have difficulties in allowing the child to form the erotized libidinal ties essential to the development of the pre-Oedipal child, whereas others have difficulties in frustrating the child's erotized attachment during the Oedipal phase. Some mothers cannot feel secure about the child's ability to manage without them when he must start school, and others will have particular difficulty when genital sexuality appears during the child's adolescence. However, unstable parents are often disturbing influences throughout the course of the child's development and such panphasic influences are often more significant in establishing personality traits or personality disturbances in offspring than are fixations at a specific developmental period. Although the mother is the primary nurturant figure to the child, particularly to the small child, and usually the family expert in child rearing, her interrelationship with the child does not transpire in isolation but is influenced by the total family setting. It is obvious, even though often overlooked, that a mother's capacity to nurture properly is influenced profoundly by her marital interaction with her husband, by the demands of another child, and by the relations between her children, and that the father's relationships with the children can profoundly influence her maternal behavior. Her capacities to give of herself to a child are affected by the emotional input that she receives from others.

The quality and nature of the parental nurturance that a child receives will profoundly influence his emotional development – his vulnerability to frustration, and the anger, aggressivity, anxiety, hopelessness, or helplessness he experiences under various conditions. As Erikson [4] has pointed out, it influences the quality of the basic trust he develops – the trust he has in others and in himself. It influences his sense of autonomy and the clarity of the boundaries that are established between himself and the parental persons. It contributes to the child's self-esteem as a member of his own sex. It lays the foundations for trust in the reliability of collaboration and the utility of verbal communication as a means of solving problems. The child's physiological functioning can be permanently influenced by the manner in which the parental figures respond to his physiological needs. It is apparent even from these brief comments why so much attention has properly been directed to the parental nurturant functions and how profoundly they influence personality development; but, they are only one aspect of what a child requires from his parents and family.

The Family Structure and Personality Integration

Let us now turn to consider the relationship between the dynamic organization of the family and the integration of the personality of the offspring. Although the family organization differs from society to society and with social class and ethnic group within a society, it seems likely that the family everywhere follows certain organizational principles because of its biological makeup. The family members must find reciprocally interrelating roles or distortions in the personalities of one or more members will occur. The division of the family into two generations and two genders minimizes role conflict, tends to provide a conflict-free area into which the immature child can develop, and directs him or her to grow into the proper gender identity which forms the cornerstone of a stable ego identity. All groups need unity of leadership but the family contains two leaders – a father and a mother. Unity of direction and organization requires a coalition between the parents that is possible because of the different but interrelated functions of the father and the mother. *For the family to be conducive to the integrated development of its offspring, the spouses must form a coalition as parents, maintain boundaries between the generations, and adhere to their respective gender-linked roles.* These essentials may sound all too simple until we explore the consequences.

THE PARENTAL COALITION

As I have just noted, any small group requires unity of leadership but the family has two leaders. The mother, no matter how subjugated, is the expressive-affectional leader concerned with the stability and harmony of the home and with satisfying the nurturant and emotional needs of the children. The father as the instrumental leader supports and protects the family and usually establishes its position in the society. A coalition between the parents is necessary not only to give unity of direction but also to provide each parent with the support essential for carrying out his or her cardinal functions. The wife, for example, can better delimit her erotic investment to maternal feelings when her wifely sexual needs are being satisfied by her husband. The tendency of small groups to divide up into dyads that create rivalries and jealousies is diminished markedly if the parents form a unity in relating to their children. The child's tendency to possess one or the other parent for himself alone – the essence of the Oedipal situation – is overcome if the parental coalition is firm, frustrating the child's fantasies and redirecting him to the reality that requires repression of such wishes. If the parents form a coalition not only as parents but also as a married couple, the child is provided with adult models who treat one another as alteregos, each striving for the partner's satisfaction as well as for his own. The child then grows up valuing marriage as an institution that provides emotional gratification and security and, thus, gains a long-range goal to pursue.

The child properly requires two parents: a parent of the same sex with whom he can identify and who serves as a role model to follow into adulthood; and a parent of the opposite sex who becomes a basic love object, and whose love and approval is sought by identifying with the parent of the same sex. However, a parent can fill neither role effectively for a child if denigrated, despised, or treated as a nonentity or, even as an enemy, by the spouse. If the parents are irreconcilable in reality, they are apt to become irreconcilable introjects in the child causing confused and contradictory internal directives. Parents can, of course, form a reasonably satisfactory coalition in respect to their children despite marital discord, and to some extent, despite separation. They not only can agree about how the children should be raised, but support their spouses to the children as worthwhile persons and good parents even if their ways and ideas differ.

When serious failures of the parental coalition occur, the growing child may invest his energy and attention in the support of one or the other parent; or in seeking to bridge the gap between them rather than investing his energy in his own development. The child sometimes becomes a scapegoat with his problems magnified into the major source of dissent between the parents and he comes to feel responsible for their friction. A child may willingly oblige and assume the role of villain in order to mask the parental discord to retain the two parents he needs. The child may also be caught in the impossible situation in which behavior intended to please either parent elicits rebuff from the other. When the parents fail to achieve a coalition, there are many ways in which the child becomes subject to conflicting motivations, directives, and standards that interfere with the development of a well-integrated personality.

THE GENERATION BOUNDARIES

The failure to achieve a parental coalition will often also lead to infractions of the generation boundaries within the family. The division into two generations provides a major structuring influence upon the family. The parents are the nurturing and educating generation and provide adult models for the child to emulate. The child requires the security of dependency for many years to be able to utilize his energies in his own development; and a child's personality becomes stunted if he must emotionally support the parents he needs for security. The division into generations lessens the dangers of role conflict and furnishes the space free from competition with a parent into which the child can develop. A different type of affectional relationship exists between parents than between a parent and child. Yet the situation is complicated because of the intense dyadic relationship heightened by erogenous feelings that properly exists between a mother and each pre-Oedipal child, and by the slow differentiation of the child from his original symbiotic union with the mother. The generation division serves to aid both mother and child overcome the bond – a development that is essential to enable the child to first find a proper place as a boy or girl member of the childhood generation within the family and then to invest his energies in peer groups and schooling, and in gaining his own identity. Parents can inappropriately breach the generation boundaries in a number of ways such as: utilizing a child to fill needs unsatisfied by the spouse; by the parent acting as a rival to a child; by a mother failing to establish boundaries between herself and a son; by a father behaving more like a child than a spouse and offering his wife little except satisfaction of her needs to mother. The most obvious disruption of generation lines occurs in incestuous and near-incestuous relationships in which a parent overtly or covertly gains erotic gratification from a child. When a parent uses a child to fill needs unsatisfied by the spouse, the child can seek to widen the gap between the parents and insert himself into it. He finds an essential place in completing the life of a parent and need not – and perhaps cannot – turn to the extrafamilial world for self-completion. The Oedipal situation thus remains unresolved, for its proper completion depends upon having a family in which the parents are primarily reliant upon one another, or upon other adults. Further, if one parent feels excluded by the child, the child's fears of retribution and retailiation are not simply projections of his own wishes to be rid of a parent, but are based upon the reality of having a jealous and hostile parent.

When the generation boudaries within the family are confused, the ensuing role conflicts distort the child's development in many ways, some of which I have indicated. The child's proper place within the family is invaded; rivalries with parents absorb energies and foster internalized conflict; a parent's dependency upon a child occupies the child prematurely with completing the life of another rather than with developing his own ego structure defined by clear boundaries. Aggressive and libidinal impulses directed toward parents become heightened rather than undergoing repression and gradual resolution, and are controlled only through strongly invested defensive mechanisms.

THE MAINTENANCE OF GENDER-LINKED ROLES

The formation of a workable parental coalition usually depends upon the abilities of both parents to assume their respective gender-linked roles in general accord with the cultural pattern and to permit the other to fill his or her role. Although, as already noted, some couples can achieve a reasonable reciprocity when filling deviant roles, their children's development will be affected deleteriously.

The maintenance of the appropriate gender-linked roles by parents in their coalition plays a major role in guiding the child's development as a boy or girl. Security of gender identity is a cardinal factor in the achievement of a stable ego identity. Of all factors entering into the formation of personality characteristics, the sex of the child is the most decisive. Confusions and dissatisfactions concerning sexual identity can contribute to the etiology of many neuroses and character defects as well as perversions; and probably all schizophrenic patients are seriously confused concerning their sexual identity. The attainment of proper sex-linked attributes does not occur simply because a child is born a boy or girl, but is acquired by role allocations that start in infancy, and through role assumptions and identifications as the child grows older. Clear-cut role reversals in parents can obviously distort the child's development, both when they are in the sexual sphere as when a parent is overtly homosexual, or when they concern the task divisions in maintaining the family. A child whose father performs the mothering functions, both tangibly and emotionally, while the mother is occupied with supporting the family can easily gain a distorted image of masculinity and femininity. The common problem, however, is more subtle: the inability of the mother to fill an affectional-expressive role or of the father to provide instrumental leadership for the family. A cold and unyielding mother is more deleterious than a cold and unyielding father while a weak and ineffectual father is more damaging than a weak and ineffectual mother. More explicitly a cold and aloof mother may be more detrimental to a daughter who requires experience in childhood with a nurturant mother to attain feminine and maternal characteristics and an ineffectual father may be more deleterious to a son who must overcome his initial identification with his mother, as well as his early dependency upon her to gain security in his ability to provide for a wife and family. Whereas the sharing of role tasks has become necessary in most contemporary families, leading to some blurring of gender-linked roles, there is still need for the parents to maintain and support one another in their primary gender-linked roles.

A child's difficulties in identifying with a parent of the same sex because this parent is unacceptable to the other whose love the child seeks, can be heightened by the homosexual tendencies of a parent. The mother may be basically unacceptable to a father with homosexual proclivities simply because she is a woman. The daughter responds by seeking to be boyish, or to gain the father's approval by being intellectual, or through some other means that does not threaten him by feminine appeal. Similarly, if the mother is consciously or unconsciously rivalrous with all men, a son can easily learn that masculinity will evoke rebuff from her, and the fears of engulfment or castration by the mother become greater and more realistic sources of anxiety than fears of retaliatory castration by the father.

Although other factors can foster difficulties in the achievement of a secure gender role and identity – such as parents conveying the wish for the child to be of the other sex, or a need to avoid incestuous entanglements – a general assurance of a proper outcome is provided when the parents adequately fill their own gender roles and each is accepted and supported if not cherished in living out these roles within the family.

In considering the relationships between the family structure and the integration of the offspring's ego development, we have been indicating a set of factors in personality development that has scarcely been explored. Still, a little consideration leads us to recognize that the provision of proper models for identification, motivations toward the proper identification, security of sexual identity, the transition through the Oedipal phase, the repression of incestuous tendencies by abolescence, and many other such factors are affected profoundly by the family organization. Unless the parents can form an adequate coalition, maintain boundaries between the generations, and provide the appropriate gender-linked role models by their behavior, conflicts and role distortions will interfere with the proper channeling of the child's drives, energies, and role learning.

The Family as a Social System

The form and functions of the family evolve with the culture and subserve the needs of the society of which it is a subsystem. It is the first social system that the child knows and into which he grows, and from it he must gain familiarity with the basic roles as they are carried out in the society in which he lives: the roles of parents and child, of boy and girl, or man and woman, of husband and wife, and how these roles impinge upon the broader society and how the roles of others impinge upon the family and its members. Although roles can be considered as units of a social system, they also become part of the personality through directing behavior to fit into roles and by giving cohesion to personality functioning. Individuals do not learn patterns of living entirely from scratch but in many situations they learn roles and then modify them to specific individual needs [12].

Within the family the child also learns about basic institutions and their values, such as the institutions of the family, marriage, extended family systems, institutions of economic exchange, and so on; and values are inculcated by identification, superego formation, teaching, and interaction. The wish to participate in or avoid participation in such institutions is a major motivating force and directive in personality development. It is the function of the family to transmit to the offspring the prescribed, permitted, and proscribed values of the society and the acceptable and unacceptable means of achieving goals [3].

Within the family's social system a child is involved in a multiplicity of social phenomena that leave a permanent imprint upon him, such as the value of belonging to a mutually protective unit; the rewards of renouncing one's own wishes for the welfare of a collectivity; the hierarchies of authority and the relationship between authority and responsibility. The family value systems, role definitions, and patterns of interrelating with one another enter into the child through the family behavior far more than through what he is taught or even what is consciously appreciated by the parents.

The Family and Enculturation

The major techniques of adaptation that man requires are not inherited genetically as part of his physical makeup but are transmitted through the cultural heritage that is a filtrate of the collective experiences of his forebears. I am considering the process of enculturation separately from the process of socialization. It concerns that which is transmitted symbolically from generation to generation rather than through societal organizations, but there is obviously considerable overlap. Enculturation of the young cannot be considered discretely from socialization, for social roles and social institutions are also part of the cultural heritage. It is a topic that has received increasing attention in anti-poverty programs where it becomes increasingly apparent that the cultural deprivation of the children is no less important than their social and economic deprivations. They cannot learn readily because they have not been provided with the symbolic wherewithal for abstract thinking and breadth of experience to reason adequately to guide their lives into the future. In a complex industrial and scientific society such as ours the family obviously can transmit only the basic adaptive techniques to its offspring and many of the instrumentalities of the culture must be conveyed by schools and other specialized institutions.

The cultural heritage includes such tangible matters as agricultural techniques and food preferences, styles of dress and housing, and arts and games, as well as less tangible conceptualizations such as status hierarchies, ideologies, religious beliefs, and the values and behavior that are accepted as axiomatic, as divine commands, or simply as the only proper standards and that are defended by strong taboos. The topic cannot be encompassed even in meager outline here, and I shall consider only a single aspect – the transmission of language, not simply as an illustration, but because the totality of the enculturation process depends so very greatly upon it.

Because the capacity to acquire language is innate in humans and because virtually all intact children learn to speak, we are apt to overlook the complexities of the process of learning language and the central importance of language to ego functioning. We required the linquistic anthropological studies of Sapir [11] and Whorf [13] to appreciate that the specific language that a person utilizes profoundly influences how he perceives, thinks, and experiences. We also needed the studies of schizophrenic patients and their parents to understand how greatly faulty and distorted language usage can affect personality development and functioning.

Among the most crucial tasks performed by the family is the inculcation of a solid foundation in the language of the society. Language is the tool of tools, the means by which man internalizes his experience, can think about it, try out alternatives, conceptualize a future, and strive toward future goals rather than simply seek immediate gratifications. After the first year of life the acquisition of almost all other instrumental techniques – that is to say, almost all other learning – depends upon language; and cooperative interaction with others, which is so critical to human adaptation, depends upon the use of a shared system of meanings. Indeed, the capacity to direct the self, to have any ego functioning at all, depends upon having verbal symbols with which one constructs an internalized symbolic version of the world which one can manipulate in imaginative trial and error before committing oneself to irrevocable actions.

To understand the importance of language to ego functioning, we must appreciate that in order for anyone to understand, communicate, and think about the ceaseless flow of his experiences, he must be able to divide his experiences into categories. Each culture is distinctive in the way in which its members categorize their experiences, and each child must learn his culture's system of categorizing not only to be able to communicate with others in the society but also to be able to think coherently. No one can start from the beginning and build up his own system of categorization. Each language is the resultant of thc cumulative experiences of that ethnic branch of mankind.

Categories are formed by abstracting common attributes from experiences or objects that are never precisely identical to bestow some sort of equivalence upon them; thus providing the world with some coherence and regularity that enables prediction. The vocabulary of the language is, in essence, the catalogue of the categories into which the culture divides its world and its experiences. Thus, the words of the language have a predictive capacity upon which we base much of our action, and without the predictive capacity derived from the meaning of words our world would remain far more aleatory. We expect a "summer" to recur annually; that a "streptococcal infection" but not a "viral infection" will respond to penicillin. The proper learning of words and their meanings and of the syntax of the language is essential to human adaptation, but there is no assurance that it will be taught or learned correctly. The correctness and the stability of the child's learning rests upon his teachers, primarily upon the members of his family.

In general, the child uses words to attempt to solve problems. Stated simply, meanings are established rapidly or slowly, with certainty or uncertainty according to how effectively and consistently proper usage attains objectives for the child. The process depends upon reciprocal interaction between the child and his tutors; the consistency between the teachers; the cues they provide; the sounds to which they respond or remain oblivious; the meanings which they reward consistently or sporadically, or indicate are useless, ineffectual, undesirable, repugnant, or punishable. Obviously many other factors are also involved in the attainment of language, and I wish only to note the importance of the family in the process. The categorizing of experience through the abstraction of common attributes, the labeling of categories by words, and the attainment of meanings of words by defining the critical attributes designated by the word are essential both to ego development and to ego functioning. The infant is not born adapted to survive in an average expectable environment as Hartmann [6] has stated. Rather each society, in order to survive, has developed a set of instrumental techniques and institutions that take infants' essential needs into account as a vital factor. Very largely through the use of linguistic tools, the child learns the culture's techniques of adaptation more or less adequately, and he gains an ability to delay the gratification of basic drives, to internalize parental attributes, directives, and teachings, to consider group needs as well as his own, and to be motivated by future security as well as by drive impulsion. Through the categories provided by the language he learns, the world in which he lives, his own needs, and the behavior of others gain some degree of order and predictability.

It seems quite likely that the parental styles of behaving, thinking, and communicating, and their uses of specific patterns of defenses are critical factors in the development of various personality types and character traits in their children through direct example and through the reactions that such styles produce in the child. When Wynne and Singer [14] documented that parents with amorphous and fragmented styles of communicating are apt to produce schizophrenic children; when Bateson and Jackson [2] formulated their "double-bind" hypothesis of schizophrenia; and when my colleagues and I noted how schizophrenic patients had been taught to misperceive, deny the obvious, be suspicious of "outsiders," and so forth [7], a new dimension was added to the study of personality development as well as of psychopathology. We might surmise, for example, that the parents of obsessional patients are often obsessional themselves, unable to tolerate expressions of anger in themselves or in their children, and actually teach the use of isolation, undoing, and reaction formation as a means of handling hostility and anxiety both by their own behavior and by what they approve and disapprove in their children. These obsessional parents would be apt to use rigid bowel training and seek to limit the young child's autonomy and thus foster ambivalence, stubbornness, shame, and undoing defenses in many ways other than through bowel training. These are conjectures, but we have noted that the parents of upper-middle-class delinquents inculcate patterns that certainly contribute to their offspring's delinquency. They teach, "do as I say, not what I do." Indeed, they ofter seem to be saying, "it doesn't very much matter what you do, it's the way things look that counts." Language is often used to gloss over transgressions and make things look satisfactory.

Personality development cannot be studied or understood abstracted from the family matrix in which it takes place. The child-rearing techniques and the emotional quality of the nurturant care provided the child which have been the major foci of attention in the past, important as they are, do not encompass the topic. The child must grow into and internalize the institutions and roles of the structured social system as well as identify with persons who themselves have assimilated the culture. He acquires characteristics through identification but also by reactions to parental objects and through finding reciprocal roles with them. His development into an integrated person is guided by the dynamic organization of the family in which he grows up which channels his drives and directs him into proper gender and generation roles. His appreciation of the worth and meanings of both social roles and institutions is affected by the manner in which his parents fill their roles, relate maritally, and behave in other institutional contexts. Superego development derives from the internalization of directives and superegos of two parents and will be inconsistent if the parental directives are contradictory or if the parents cannot form a workable coalition. The capacities to have the verbal tools necessary for the collaborative interaction with others, to think, and to direct the self depend greatly upon the tutelage within the family and upon the parents' styles of communicating. It becomes clear that numerous sources of deviant personality development open before us when we consider the implications of this approach [9].

In the study of personality development and in the search for guidelines to assure stable emotional development, the emphasis upon what parents should or should not do to the child, for the child, and with the child at each phase of his development has often led to neglect of larger and more significant influences. Who the parents are; how they behave and communicate; how they relate to one another as well as to the child; what sort of family they create, including that intangible, the atmosphere of the home, are of paramount importance.

Bibliography

1. Ackerman, N. W., *The Psychodynamics of Family Life*, Basic Books, New York, 1958.
2. Bateson, G., D. D. Jackson, et al., Towards a theory of schizophrenia, *Behav. Sci.*, 1 (1956), 251–264.
3. Bell, N. and E. Vogel, eds., *A Modern Introduction to the Family*, Free Press, Glencoe, Ill., 1960.
4. Erikson, E., Growth and crises of the "healthy personality," in *Symposium on the Healthy Personality, Vol. 2: Problems of Infancy and Childhood*, M. J. E. Senn, ed., Josiah Macy, Jr. Foundation, New York, 1950.
5. Flugel, J. C., *The Psycho-Analytic Study of the Family*, Hogarth Press, London, 1921.
6. Hartmann, H., *Ego Psychology and the Problem of Adaptation*, Int. Univ. Press, New York, 1958.
7. Lidz, T., A. Cornelison, et al., The transmission of irrationality, in *Schizophrenia and the Family*, by T. Lidz, S. Fleck, and A. Cornelison, Int. Univ. Press, New York, 1965.
8. Lidz, T., *The Family and Human Adaptation*, Int. Univ. Press, New York, 1963.
9. Lidz, T., *The Person*, Basic Books, New York, 1969.
10. Parsons, T. and R. Bales, *Family, Socialization and Interaction Process*, Free Press, Glencoe, Ill., 1955.
11. Sapir, E., *Selected Writings of Edward Sapir in Language, Culture and Personality*, Univ. California Press, Berkeley, Calif., 1949.
12. Spiegel, J., The resolution of role conflict within the family, *Psychiat.*, 20 (1957), 1–16.
13. Whorf, B., *Language, Thought, and Reality. Selected Writings of Benjamin Lee Whorf*, J. Carroll, ed., M.I.T. and John Wiley & Sons, New York, 1956.
14. Wynne, L. C. and M. T. Singer, Thought disorder and family relations of schizophrenics: II. A classification of forms of thinking. *Arch. Gen. Psychiat.*, 9 (1963), 199–206.

The Use of an Ecological Framework in the Treatment of a Child

SALVADOR MINUCHIN (U. S. A.)

A child's behavior is caused by many factors. Some are "inside" the child, like neurons, brains, and glands, as well as memories, motivations, introjects, and drives. "Outside" the child are factors like his parents, his siblings, his family's socioeconomic status, his house, his school (teacher, peers, and curriculum), his neighborhood, his neighborhood peer group, the hue of his skin, television, and many others.

The major theoretical systems in child psychiatry have always been concerned with the influence of both internal and external factors on the development of the child. Particular emphasis has been put, in theory, on the importance of the family and the way the child, an organism with biological and psychological needs, negotiates those needs within the nurturing and socializing unit called the family.

But the techniques of intervention which have been developed by child psychiatry have been aimed almost entirely at the child as a separate organism. Though the *theories* subscribed to have taken account of the importance of external factors in the child's development, the techniques used to change the child have not. Therefore, the context of interventions has been psychiatrist plus child.

This approach to therapy requires an awareness of only two people. The context of the intervention is not recognized as important;

*The author would like to acknowledge the assistance of Frances Hitchcock in preparing the manuscript for this chapter.

the behavior of the child in the therapy session is assumed to be typical, somehow unaffected by his surroundings. The therapist and the child are involved in transactions in which the therapist perceives himself as an observer-participant.

Family therapy, with its wider focus, has not been accepted by child psychiatry in the United States. Perhaps this is because family intervention requires a theory that can encompass at least three people, constantly involved in transactions with one another. The theory also must take into account the processes which constantly occur "across the boundaries" between family members, family subunits, and between the family and significant extrafamilial influences.

Family therapy's focus is necessarily wider than that of traditional child psychiatry, but even family therapy has tended to limit its interventions to the family, without extending its fields of intervention to the school, the neighborhood, or in some cases, even the extended family [22].

Now these traditional concepts of the explanation of behavioral phenomena and techniques for intervention are being challenged by a combination of new theoretical systems such as general systems theory [29], communications [31], group dynamics [7, 30], ecology [4-6], and new techniques of intervention which stem from family therapy [1, 10, 13, 14, 18, 20, 22, 26, 32, 33, 34], encounter groups [3, 23, 27], and community psychiatry [2, 16, 23, 25].

The work of Roger G. Barker [4-6], who has studied child behavior as affected by the different contexts of various natural settings, is an example of approaches which can be used as steps towards a more inclusive theory of behavior and change-producing intervention. Baker, a psychologist, writes:

> The psychological person who writes essays, scores points, and crosses streets stands as an identifiable entity between unstable interior parts and exterior contexts, with both of which he is linked, yet from both of which he is profoundly separated. The separation comes from the fact that the inside parts and the outside contexts of a person involve phenomena that function according to laws that are different from those that govern his behavior [4, page 6].

In other words, to study the child, three elements must be studied independently. One is the child as an individual, the second is the environment in which his behavior is observed. Third, the linkage between these two elements must be studied. What processes are occurring across the boundaries which separate the individual child from his environment, and what is the nature of the mutual impingement of child and environment which is occurring?

Here is a key to one of the problems that have handicapped the development of a more inclusive interventive system in psychiatry. Psychiatry has been concerned with the development of a unified science. It has approached extra-individual units with the assumption that somehow the laws of group dynamics ought to be similar to the laws governing individual dynamics. The concept of the "undifferentiated family ego mass" [9] and the concepts of multiple transference used by some group therapists and family therapists [15] are examples of attempts to stretch individual concepts and adapt them to use with nonindividual theories and techniques [20]. This attempt to extend concepts developed for one theoretical context to use with another may well be inappropriate.

Barker's metaphor is helpful here [4]. He pictures a freight train crossing the plains of the Midwest, carrying wheat to Chicago. The laws which govern the growth of wheat are quite separate from those which govern the motion of the train. The laws which govern the motion of the train are quite different from those which will regulate the price of the wheat, and so on. Each of these are separate areas, which can be studied separately according to separate conceptualizations. But the market analyst who wants to predict the cost of flour may well have to take all of them into account.

The child psychiatrist operating within an ecological framework is in the position of that market analyst. He can study his patient in different contexts, determing those contexts' significance and their relationship to each other. Then he can determine where and how intervention will be maximally effective.

For the ecological psychiatrist working with children, the child's family will usually be the most significant area for intervention, although the school, peers, neighborhood, and others may sometimes be as significant.

In his terms, the family is a behavioral setting which comprises the child.[1] From this point of view, the family is an extra-individual unit with regulatory power over the behavior of its members. At the same time, each member of the family has a separate identity; he is an

[1] I am indebted to Barker [4] for his discussion of behavioral settings, which I have adapted here for the discussion of the family.

individual as well as an interacting member of the family unit. The members of a family will exhibit the characteristic pattern of behavior which pertains to that family. At the same time, all the family members will encompass the family rules in their own individual, differentiated ways.

The B family (which will be discussed later in this paper) is a good example of the regulatory power of a family unit. The B's are very much upper-class, respectable, proper Quakers. They pride themselves on the absence of disagreement in their family life, treasuring a seemly consensus in their family functioning. They have also firmly incorporated the philosophy of reverence for life. When the older son reached adolescence and began to disagree with his father, the family rules made it impossible for him to disagree openly. So he remained a respectful, obedient child while developing a syndrome of *anorexia nervosa*, not eating because he maintained that eating destroys life.

The child and the family, then, are systems with properties of their own, each closely interrelated with the other. The same is true for subunits of the family, such as the spouses or the sibling group. The separate subunits have their own structure and dynamics, and at the same time they are interdependent with the family and larger surrounding systems. Though all these systems may be operating independently at their own levels, they still have strong linkages across their system boundaries. And the boundaries of every system are more or less permeable, depending upon the system and the surrounding circumstances.

The family as a system has standing patterns, programs, and goals. It also has ways of communicating and interacting which maintain these programs and goals. Whenever the family's accustomed methods of interaction are threatened by extra-familial forces or the deviation of a family member, the family network is activated to preserve the usual equilibrium.

At the same time, the family system is responding to pressures from the individual members. For example, when a child enters adolescence and has to adapt both to his family and to an increasingly important peer group, he exerts pressure for more autonomy. If the family is to continue as a healthy, growth-encouraging unit, it must evolve from the family of a young child to the family of an adolescent. It was the inability of the B family to make this kind of adjustment that resulted in the appearance of pathology in its older son.

But ordinarily, there will be extensive adjustments in areas of regulation and control, and the family's regulatory system will consequently change.

The concept of ecological psychiatry can take the many different factors influencing a child's development into account. And as in Barker's metaphor of the train, the different areas of significance can be analyzed without any demand that the laws governing them be conceptualized as somehow interrelated. Studies of the child's level of free fatty acid when subjected to specific stresses, studies of memory, perception, motivations, introjects, and so on, are potentially useful to the broad systems approach. And other studies, such as studies of the family system, will clearly be relevant. Families with engaged and disengaged characteristics may be studied in terms of the regulation of family members and the network for the development of controls. Large families and families with only children can be studied along this variable. The different social nets of families in small towns, slums, and kibbutzim can be studied from the point of view of the linkage between context and family (which hitherto has been the concern of sociology) and the relationship of the family members via intrapsychic linkages (which has hitherto been the field of psychologists and psychiatrists). Studies of this sort will add greatly to our understanding of individual and family dynamics, and within the concept of ecological psychiatry, there is no demand that the *studies* necessarily be related to one another.

In terms of therapeutic *intervention*, however, connections must be made. This will necessitate the study of the links which connect the child and his family, the family and the school, the family and the neighborhood, and so on.

It is in terms of change-producing interventions that the ecological framework indicates changes in the field of child psychiatry. Traditional child psychiatry has operated with the assumption that successful therapeutic intervention within the behavioral setting which comprises psychiatrist and child will produce changes in the intrapsychic life of the child. These changes will, in turn, ensure changes in his relationships with his ecology. The ecological framework challenges this assumption, and a number of corollaries which have accompanied it are also brought under review.

One corollary is a lack of understanding or concern about the influences of the contexts of behavior. The assumption has been that if the psychiatrist observes the child at play in a dyadic interaction with the psychiatrist himself, he is observing a sample of the child's typical behavior. The psychiatrist usually assumes that he is functioning only as a recorder of the child's behavior.

But from an ecological point of view, the therapist is seen as a manipulator as well as an observer and recorder. In other words, he must be influencing the child's behavior even if he is only recording it. In fact, usually he actually dominates the system of transactions between himself and the child because he provides and regulates input.

Another corollary which is challenged is the notion that one can intervene with the child alone. Because the child is a member of ecological settings other than therapist-child, the therapist's interventions with the child will resound in these other settings, whether the therapist intends this or not. And the results of his interventions with the child may produce counterreactions that will have profound effect on the therapeutic task.

These challenges to traditional child psychiatry operate at the same time to the advantage of the child psychiatrist because a realization of the importance of the child's ecology opens new avenues of intervention. Because he recognizes that interventions with the child will have effects on his significant surrounding systems, and vice versa, the therapist is no longer limited to intervening with the child alone. He can intervene with the family, the neighborhood peer group, the school, and many other parts of the child's ecosystem, and thus reach the child from many different points of approach.

I would like to illustrate the advantages of an ecological approach to a child by presenting the B case. This family came to our attention because the oldest son, Stephen, aged 15, had developed eating fads so restrictive that in the last three months he had lost 30 pounds, or about 25 percent of his body weight. He had become a vegetarian a year before on the grounds of reverence for life, and had gradually cut out more and more foods. Now he was eating only those fruits from which he could remove the seeds and plant them. He would eat apples but not strawberries, for instance. He refused to eat dairy products because his using milk might deprive a calf.

Stephen's pediatrician had told his parents that this was a case of *anorexia nervosa*, that Stephen's symptoms suggested schizophrenia, and that his recommendation was hospitalization and force feeding with concomitant psychiatric treatment. The pediatrician based his recommendation on the medical literature concerning *anorexia nervosa*, in which it is considered that *anorexia nervosa* cannot be treated successfully in the home. The first report of a fatal case, in 1895, suggests that the presence of the mother caused the downhill course [12]. And in two cases described in depth by Falstein, Feinstein, and Judas [12], both patients regressed when they were returned home from the hospital, planning to continue therapy on an out-patient basis.

Because of the threat to life involved, the descriptions available have been drawn largely from the study of children who have been hospitalized – that is, they have been separated from their natural ecology and placed in a new behavioral setting, one in which they are labeled seriously ill. Although some authors maintain that there is a consistent history of early struggles between children and parents over feeding and being fed as the battleground on which issues of autonomy and control have been fought [17], there is no study of the *anorexia nervosa* patient within his family. As a result, the available literature presents the problem only from a strictly intrapsychic point of view.

This intrapsychic approach, which "zooms in" on the individual in isolation, recognizes that *anorexia nervosa* can occur as a symptomatic phase in divergent psychiatric disorders.

> Eating may be equated with gratification, impregnation, intercourse, performance . . . growing . . . castrating, destroying, engulfing, killing, canibalism. Food may symbolize the breast, the genitals, feces, poison, a parent, or a sibling [12, page 765].

The same authors emphasize the importance of the position of the adolescent in the family and internalized family conflict, but even here the field of observation is narrowed so that family conflicts are seen as somehow having moved inside the child. Where the starvation is considered an expression of hate and defiance against a mother who puts a great deal of emphasis on eating, this is considered to be the expression of an Oedipal conflict.

In the available literature, the boundaries of pathology are the child's skin. Concomitantly, the interventive techniques traditionally used with *anorexia nervosa* are directed only to the child. The interveners have no strategy other than separating the child from his natural contexts through hospitalization. Treatment in the hospital may be successful, but there is strong possibility of regression outside the hospital [12].

If Stephen's pediatrician's recommendation had been followed, he would probably have been hospitalized after an individual interview. Prolonged treatment in the hospital would have followed. It would probably have included physiological measures such as the use of insulin and chlorpromazine [11], individual psychotherapy, and perhaps behavior therapy [8]. Some therapy with the parents might have been included. This would mostly have concentrated on the mother, since the intrapsychic theory of *anorexia nervosa* postulates a symbiotic mother-child relationship [12].

But Stephen's family refused to accept the pediatrician's recommendation. They felt that Stephen's problem must be a family problem, and they carefully reviewed city agencies until they found one which would take them into treatment as a family.

Since ecological psychiatry is concerned with the context of both diagnosis and treatment, we usually begin by exploring the child's most significant context, his family. Therefore, the first interview in Stephen's case was a family interview, not an individual interview.[2]

The observation of a child in his family presents different explanations of his behavior, depending on the observer's point of observation and the focus of his observation. The therapist in this situation is like a movie camera. He can zoom in and focus on an individual, as the intrapsychically oriented approach does. But he can also widen his focus to include dyads, triads, the whole field, or any particular part of the field. (And he must realize that his presence changes the field he is observing, just as the fact that their picture is being taken causes people's behavior to change. Reciprocally, his behavior is in part regulated by the subjects of his observation.)

For the ecologically oriented therapist it makes no sense to look at the child in isolation. Even when we zoom in on an individual, he is still seen as a member of a mutually regulatory group. Thus we could not see Stephen simply as a sick child. We saw him as an interacting unit of various relationships.

The relationship of Stephen and his father was the most salient interaction in the first interview. The father was the family member who was responding most to the presenting problem, Stephen's ill-

[2] The therapists on this case are Salvador Minuchin, M.D. and Harry J. Aponte, A.C.S.W.

ness. Stephen's reaction to his father's very demanding control was a passive lack of response which clearly triggered increased effort on the father's part.

When we changed our focus to include the husband-wife dyad, we noticed a rather similar interaction between the spouses. The mother was very passive. She allowed her husband to dominate the family. Reciprocally, it was her very passivity that continually forced him to assume almost all of the executive power in the family.

When we broadened our focus to include Stephen, father, and mother, we noticed the similarity of the two dyads and also recognized that the family's overwhelming concern for Stephen was covering up a problem in the spouse submit. We could also hypothesize that Mrs. B's resentment of her husband was expressed in a covert encouragement of Stephen's rebellion against his father.

Broadening our focus to include the fourth member of the family, Matthew, 13, we realized that this was a family in which three members declared themselves healthy and the fourth, Stephen, accepted and furthered the label, sick and weak. At the same time, there was another hidden three to one alliance. The mother and children were united in a passive coalition which triggered the father to control excessively because the three saw the father as actually a very frail person who would collapse if any stand were taken against him. Therefore, they protected him by maintaining an extraordinary passivity which promulgated the family myth that he was a very strong executive.

As a family group, the B's were very low key. They spoke softly and politely, with long pauses between interchanges. They did not evidence strong conflicts, and they were very obedient to the therapists. At points of stress, they took refuge in bantering and smiles.

Any description of a family system is necessarily static, given the nature of our descriptive language. Language is designed for sequences, so it is difficult to describe the continuous reciprocity of a systems intervention. The therapist reacting to, for instance, the mother's passivity must always keep in mind the way in which her passivity organizes the father to take control, which keeps her passive, and so on.

In spite of this sort of complication, the ecological point of view is very advantageous because it means that several levels of intervention are open. In this case, it was necessary to intervene promptly because of the threat to life represented by Stephen's refusal to eat.

After the first half of this first interview, which lasted 2 hours, we intervened at the total-family level by assigning a family task. This was Friday, and the family had already been scheduled for another clinic appointment on Monday. Over the weekend, the whole family was to eat only what Stephen would eat. The mother and father had to agree to this task, which they obediently did. Matthew was not given a vote; he had to go along if his parents did.

The selection of this particular task forced the family members to organize around problems of regulation and control. A task is one way of creating a specific context within which the family members must interact. In this case we selected this particular task centering on control partly to test our hypothesis that Stephen's not eating was a reaction to a serious imbalance of power in the family, and partly to change the family's perception of the problem. We wanted to mobilize them around an issue that had some possibility of solution via family interaction – that is, control – instead of around a problem they could not solve, Stephen's *anorexia nervosa*.

At the same time, this task changed the family labels. For months they had been deadlocked in a focus on Stephen and his illness. Stephen was seen as weak, sick, and in need of protection. Stephen himself accepted and furthered the label of himself as somehow weak and victimized (a structure that hospitalization would have strengthened).

This task changed that label. The parents were redefined as powerless. Stephen was redefined as the family member in control. Matthew's not being given a vote defined him as a helpless victim of the family's inability to resolve the conflict.

This task also functioned as a diagnostic device. By assigning a task which makes the family perform in ways it is not accustomed to, the therapist can test the family's flexibility of response. Making the family interact in a situation which cannot be met by their automatic responses tests the limits. Sometimes a task will do this by requiring that the family act in completely different ways. Other tasks, such as this one, intensify the tempo or impact of the natural family transactions.

The task performed a further function. We hoped to create crisis in the family by increasing the affective intensity of the situation. This technique of producing change by inducing crisis is based on our experience that a certain type of family, with rigid patterns of interacting, cannot change unless they are jolted out of their usual methods of interacting. The B family found it impossible to negotiate conflicts. Conflicts were always detoured or de-fused. We hoped that by creating a sharp conflict which could not be detoured or de-fused, we would force them to deal with the situation.[3]

When the mother and father agreed to follow Stephen's diet for the weekend, the therapists gave them their home phone numbers, with instructions to call them at any time during the weekend.[4]

The family had a miserable time, with hunger and resentment against Stephen building up. On Monday, during the session, we learned that on Sunday afternoon the father had shut himself in the garage, with Matthew watching, and turned on the car motor. As he later said, he did not want to commit suicide, but he did want Stephen to come and save him so Stephen would be taught a lesson. Matthew ran to get his mother, however, and the mother got the father out of the garage. In the session, Stephen said he had known his father was in the garage and what his father wanted of him. He had determined not to go to him, even if it meant his father's death.

With this task, then, several things were made clear. The father's method of control through guilt and Stephen's negative involvement with his father became unmistakably evident. The father's drastic reaction illustrated the extent to which a problem that had been conceptualized as Stephen's was built into the structure of the family.

In the session, the senior therapist attacked Stephen, his now obvious control of the family, and his value system of himself as the suffering protector of all living things. The therapist labeled Stephen as a despot who cared about all life except his own family, instead of as a victim of that family.

This relabeling shifted Stephen from the down position to the position of active controller of the family. Now, in the context of this

[3] This is an example of the use of iatrogenic crisis [19, 21].

[4] When a therapist organizes a crisis situation in a family, he must insist that he is available at any time and will respond to any call. Mr. B's reaction points to the danger of this type of intervention. Whenever it is used, the family must be cautioned as to the possibility of ensuing crisis, and they must know the therapist is available.

structural change, the therapists again elected to intensify and explore the nature of the father-Stephen interaction. This time, both the mother and Matthew were labeled as powerless by the task assigned.

The father and Stephen were instructed to debate and decide, in the session, whether or not the family should continue to follow Stephen's diet. After a prolonged, no-decision struggle, the therapist intervened. He stated that a decision had been reached and that Stephen and his father had agreed that the whole family should return to a normal diet.

The therapists then indicated that they would be making a home visit and asked if they might come in two days. The therapists would eat with the family, and Stephen would plan the menu with his mother.

That evening the father phoned the senior therapist, saying that Stephen was refusing to eat dinner. Stephen maintained that he had only agreed that the rest of the family should stop following his diet; he intended to continue.

The therapist instructed the father to demand that Stephen honor the agreement but finally agreed to let Stephen go on a full vegetarian diet, starting that moment. He explained to the father that in this way Stephen would experience himself as successful in negotiating with his father, and that the father would also experience a successful negotiation. About an hour later, the father called back to say that he had followed this strategy and Stephen had eaten a full vegetarian meal.

The initial crisis was solved. Stephen was now back on a full vegetarian diet, soon including dairy products; and in a month he attained a normal, if low, weight. The parents were instructed to disengage completely around the problem of eating, and soon no difficulty existed in this area.

This ended the case of *anorexia nervosa*. Among the many interventions available with an ecological approach, the therapists had elected to focus on the father-Stephen dyad and had organized a crisis in a context of heightened struggle for regulation and control. This manipulation had highlighted a specific, narrow problem in the family's interactional field. Because of the seriousness of the presenting problem, priority had been given to the biological concern for survival.

Once the clinical picture moved from the acute illness of one family member to the chronic imbalance of the family, the therapists were free to broaden and change their foci. They made other home visits, sometimes driving out in response to a summons from the father to help negotiate another confrontation. Different family units were explored. There were separate interviews with the parents, Stephen was seen in individual interviews, there were sibling unit interviews, and we intervened at the level of peer group interaction by including Stephen in an adolescent group *via* an adolescent who joined the therapeutic team over the summer. In short, we used a variety of strategies, always keeping in mind the importance of specific contexts and the influence of transactions across systems.

For instance, two days after the second session we changed both the context of the interviews and the function of the therapists by making our first home visit, as arranged.

In the clinic sessions, the therapists had functioned as active manipulators of the field, introducing new situations and new rules, pushing the family, and observing the ways they responded to being pushed. In the family's home setting, the therapists functioned quite differently. They now were gathering data in the family's natural context, observing and becoming part of the family household as guests, affecting their data as little as they could in a visit lasting over 5 hours. They discovered many of the strengths of the family. Both boys acted as competent hosts, showing the therapists their rooms and the various articles in their rooms which reflected their many keen interests. The parents were also proud to present the positive aspects of their lives. They gathered a great deal of information about significant members of the extended family which would later be useful in therapy.

Although the family's battles were no longer being waged around Stephen's eating, they were still going on, of course. A new conflict area now arose; Stephen refused to talk. He kept silent for long periods of time, and when asked a question, often refused to answer. In this way the family's communications were now transacted in a way which was remarkably similar to that of the old eating conflict, though now in an area which was not life-threatening.

From an intrapsychic point of view, Stephen's dynamics could be interpreted in the same way, regardless of the change in symptomatology. But from an ecological point of view, a significant change had occurred. The family had moved away from its crippling focus on Stephen and his problems and had begun to understand the problem in their negotiation of conflicts. And the introduction of the therapists as significant members of the ecosystem meant a structural change in the form of negotiators who could help the family transact its area of confrontation.

The therapists also began interventions in the extrafamilial sphere. From an ecological framework, there are many behavioral settings that can be utilized as pathways for the introduction of change [2, 28]. In work with adolescents, an obvious pathway is the adolescent peer group.

In general, the adolescent patient in therapy is expected to become free to move towards extrafamilial contacts by himself in the measure in which he improves in negotiating and developing autonomy in the family. But it seemed to the therapists that Stephen needed practical help in negotiating the complexities of adolescent society. As a member of a very enmeshed family, he had never made friends outside the family. He spent whole days at home, usually closeted in his bedroom, playing with his white rat. Occasionally the therapists were successful in persuading Stephen to go out, usually to the library, but this seemed to be the extent of his sorties outside the home.

In order to further one of their goals – increasing an age-appropriate autonomy in Stephen – the therapists decided to intervene at the interface between the family and the adolescent peer group. We introduced an adolescent therapist to the therapeutic team – a boy who would be Stephen's friend. This was accepted without difficulty by the family.

We looked for an adolescent who would have some of the nonjudgmental acceptance that some groups of "hippies" have. We chose a 15-year-old with hair longer than Stephen's, easy contact with adults, the ability to make friends easily, a capacity for benign, age-appropriate disengagement from his own family, and a thorough knowledge of the geography of teen-aged Philadelphia. He saw Stephen twice a week or so for 4 to 6 hours at times the boys arranged together. He introduced Stephen to a group of his friends, and Stephen became a silent and marginal group follower.

The adolescent therapist also served an interesting function for Stephen's parents. He attended the family sessions once a week, and the B's soon began to question him eagerly about his relationship with his family. They asked about his responsibilities, the extent of his autonomy, and so on. He served as a teacher for the entire family. The parents began to learn about "model family relationships" from an adolescent from a less enmeshed family; and at the same time, Stephen was carefully watching another adolescent dealing with adults, talking with them in respectful but independent fashion, and easily preserving his autonomy without the need for continuous confrontation.

The B family has now been in treatment for about 4 months. There has been no eating problem since the first 4 days of treatment. The focus of intervention has now shifted away from Stephen to the problems between the spouses. Though many problems remain in the family, the prognosis is good.

Of the many interventions at many levels made in this family, the techniques discussed were highlighted because they illustrate some of the alternative methods of intervention which the ecological approach gives therapists.

This ecological approach brings its difficulties. One of them is the loss of therapeutic control consequent upon the broadening of the therapist's field. Because his areas of intervention are spread, his power in each area is diminished. Instead of the easily controllable dyadic setting, he is faced with many variables in many settings. This is an understandable source of the resistance to this model of therapy found in traditional child psychiatry.

If one takes this approach as a problem and a challenge to the field, it means that the child psychiatrist must change. He must build a large and flexible repertory of techniques for differentiated diagnosis and interventions. Then the very difficulties of this approach contain opportunities for the therapist to pick his area and method of intervention. If one pathway is blocked, there are many others.

Bibliography

1. Ackerman, N. W., *Treating the Troubled Family*, Basic Books, Inc., New York, 1966.
2. Auerswald, E. H., Interdisciplinary vs. ecological approach, *Fam. Process*, 1968, 7, 202-215.
3. Bach, G. R. and P. Wyden, *The Intimate Enemy: How to Fight Fair in Love and Marriage*, Morrow, New York, 1969.
4. Barker, R. G., *Ecological Psychology: Concepts and Methods for Studying the Environment of Human Behavior*, Stanford University Press, Stanford, 1968.

5. Barker, R. G. (ed.), *The Stream of Behavior*, Appleton-Century Crofts, New York, 1963.
6. Barker, R. G. and P. V. Gump, *Big School, Small School*, Stanford University Press, Stanford, 1964.
7. Bion, W. R., *Experiences in Groups*, Basic Books, Inc., New York, 1959.
8. Blinder, B. J., A. J. Stunkard, D. Freeman, and A. L. Ringold, Behavior therapy of *anorexia nervosa:* effectiveness of activity as a reinforcer of weight gain, Paper presented at the 124th Annual Meeting of the American Psychiatric Association, Boston, May 1968.
9. Bowen, M., The family as the unit of study and treatment, *Amer. J. Orthopsychiatry*, 1961, *31*, 40-60.
10. Bowen, M., The use of family theory in clinical practice, *Comprehensive Psychiatry*, 1967, 7, 345-374.
11. Crisp, A. H. and F. J. Roberts, A case of anorexia nervosa in a male, *Postgrad. Med. J.*, 1962, *38*, 350-353.
12. Falstein, E. I., S. C. Feinstein and I. Judas, Anorexia nervosa in the male child, *Amer. J. Orthopsychiatry*, 1956, *26*, 751-772.
13. Haley, J. D. *Strategies of Psychotherapy*, Grune & Stratton, New York, 1963.
14. Jackson, D. D. and J. H. Weakland, Conjoint family therapy: some considerations on theory, technique and results, *Psychiatry*, 1961, *24*, 30-45.
15. Kramer, C. H., *Psychoanalytically Oriented Family Therapy: Ten Year Evolution in a Private Child Psychiatry Practice*, Family Institute of Chicago, Chicago, 1968.
16. Leopold, R. L. and L. J. Duhl (eds.), *Mental Health and Urban Social Policy*, Jossey-Bass, San Francisco, 1968.
17. Lesser, L. I. *et al.*, Anorexia nervosa in children. *Amer. J. Orthopsychiatry*, 1960, *30*, 572-580.
18. MacGregor, R. *et al.*, *Multiple Impact Therapy with Families*, McGraw-Hill, Inc., New York, 1964.
19. Minuchin, S. Conflict resolution family therapy, *Psychiatry*, 1965, *28*, 278-286.
20. Minuchin, S., Family therapy: technique or theory? in J. Masserman (ed.), *Science and Psychoanalysis*, Vol. XIV, Grune & Stratton, New York, 1969, pages 179-187.
21. Minuchin, S. and A. Barcai, Therapeutically induced family crisis, in J. Masserman (ed.), *Science and Psychoanalysis*, Vol. XIV, Grune & Stratton, New York, 1969, pages 199-205.
22. Minuchin, S. *et al.*, *Families of the Slums: An Exploration of Their Structure and Treatment*, Basic Books, Inc., New York, 1967.
23. Perls, F. S. *Gestalt Therapy Verbatim*, Real People Press, Lafayette, California, 1969.
24. Rice, K. *The Enterprise and Its Environment*, Tavistock Press, London, 1963.
25. Riessman, F., J. Cohen and A. Pearl (eds.), *Mental Health of the Poor*, The Free Press of Glencoe, New York, 1964.
26. Satir, Virginia M., *Conjoint Family Therapy: A Guide to Theory and Technique*, Science and Behavior Books, Inc., Palo Alto, 1964.
27. Shutz, W. C., *Joy: Expanding Human Awarenesss*, Grove Press, New York, 1967.

28. Speck, R. V., Psychotherapy and the social network of a schizophrenic family. *Fam. Process*, 1967, *6*, 208-214.
29. Von Bertalanffly, L., *General Systems Theory*, George Braziller, New York, 1969.
30. Watson, G. (ed.), *Concepts for Social Change*, NEA, Washington, D.C., 1967.
31. Watzlawick, P., Janet H. Beavan and D. D. Jackson, *Pragmatics of Human Communication: A Study of Interactional Patterns, Pathologies, and Paradoxes*, W. W. Norton & Co., Inc., New York, 1967.
32. Whitaker, C. A., Psychotherapy with couples, *Amer. J. Psychotherapy*, 1958, *12*, 18-23.
33. Wynne, L. C., Some indications and contraindications for exploratory family therapy, in I. Boszormenyi-Nagy and J. L. Framo (eds.), *Intensive Family Therapy*, Harper and Row, New York, 1965.
34. Zuk, G. H. and I. Boszormenyi-Nagy, *Family Therapy and Disturbed Families*, Science and Behavior Books, Palo Alto, 1966.

Family Vulnerability and Family Crisis

Editorial Comment

The human infant is born with many vulnerabilities and is generally conceded to be among the most helpless and immature of nascent organisms. During a prolonged childhood it slowly develops a survival capacity so that its security and well-being become more and more its own concern and less a function of caretakers. The transition from this relatively hazardous phase of life is mostly brought about by the combined forces of maturation and family environment. It is quite true that the infant is born with a certain degree of resilience and resistance, but it is its life in the family that furnishes it, by both conscious and unconscious precept, with a basic repertoire of defenses, coping skills, social aptitudes, cultural accomplishments, and technical abilities that serve it in good stead during the stresses and strains of development. The combination of genetic equipment and learned behavior establishes in time a "likeness" to the family that remains more or less imprinted for the remainder of life. This fundamental reaction type becomes as permanent and as unchanging as the child's name although many modifications and modulations may be superimposed with later experience. The interplay of the two factors—the diathetic and the environmental—punctuates the course of the life cycle and renders it far less predictable than would otherwise be the case.

The first three contributions to this section concern themselves with the factor of disposition or diathesis as it effects vulnerability. Lois Murphy, more than anyone else, has traced the evolution of coping and defensive behavior from birth onwards and no one is better qualified to analyze the differences between the two mechanisms without which our capacity to deal with the daily pressures of existence would be negligible. Greenberg considers the vulnerability of the infant, "free from congenital neural defects," in relation to the natural safeguards provided by the mother, in the absence of which the child becomes prone to atypical development. In spite of his careful research design and the use of controls, the author's results do not quite rule out the possibility that the mother's over-stimulating or understimulating behavior is secondary to the stimulus provided by the infant, an alternative that both Erikson (in his postulate of "sending power") and Escalona have considered. The innate or "constitutional" point of view is lucidly exposed by Chess. She points out that the recognition of vulnerability is one of the most important tasks of the clinician and requires special care on his part to prevent the perpetuation of a self-fulfilling diagnosis. The three diagnostic profiles that she offers have the virtue of simplicity and are clearly within the competence of the average parent to understand. This fact, in conjunction with the constitutional point of view, may certainly help to alleviate some of the iatrogenic guilt foisted on parents, but the more sophisticated may find reasons for dissatisfaction in the "externality" of the system. The four crisis papers deal with separation, death, disease, and unemployment as they effect the child and/or his family. Anthony and Veil focus on the family setting, whereas Bowlby and Parkes and Michael Rutter examine the critical developments in terms of the individual. The two authors dealing with bereavement are contented here to draw attention to its often devastating effects on the individual adult and the individual child, both in the present and in the future. What is less fully described and discussed, and may well be a stimulus for further investigation, is the influence of loss on family life and the ways in which the surviving members look to one another for solace, surrogation, and emotional support. The vicissitudes of detachment, searching, and reattachment behavior within a family group surely need to be explored transactionally. Rutter presents a masterly review of the various factors that might be involved in the differential vulnerability of the two sexes and explores the question more specifically for himself in terms of parental illness. The topic has been explored less rigorously, but more dynamically, by other authors with confusing results. For example, in a paper published a few years ago, the authoress sympathized with the problem of being male and consequently "handicapped," since the mortality and morbidity figures for boys were higher at almost every stage of life and boys were definitely more "retarded" than girls during the whole of childhood development. Psychoanalytic authors, on the other hand, are notoriously prone to view women as defective and to center the female psychology around this point. Here Rutter examines the various alternatives whether boys and girls may respond differently to stress, or perceive stress differently, or model themselves on different parents, or experience different types of child care. What he does not consider are the dynamic implications of difference within the family system of relationships, but then he does not pretend to be a family therapist but remains what he is and what is needed more than anything else in our science today, a fact-finding psychiatrist.

In Anthony's study, the ability of the family to cope with stress is found to depend on its previous history and the extent to which it has achieved integration, solidarity, and organization. To this extent, the "good" families may actually thrive on stress, whereas the more poorly adjusted ones may take a progressive course to final deterioration. Veil finds effects that are not too dissimilar in the case of unemployment. There are the same early stages of shame, rejection, inferiority, and loss of family solidarity culminating in later stages of defeat, dependence, and despondency. Whether the workings of the Oedipus complex are as sensitive to unemployment as Veil suggests remains to be seen, but it is an interesting supposition.

We cannot neglect to comment on the finding by Hinkle and Wolff (quoted by Rutter) that the healthiest group of people in any population were middle-aged spinsters with full-time jobs who had never sought marriage. These "maiden aunts" are a feature of many cultures, particularly British, in which they function as helpful, conscientious, hard-working, and indispensable adjuncts to family life. Without them, many families would be the poorer and the culture itself would undoubtedly suffer. What then is the reason for their relative invulnerability, their mental and physical healthiness? Can it have something to do with their somewhat selfless approach to life? A research project on aunts seems highly indicated if we hope to clarify this complex problem of vulnerability, and we say this without facetiousness.

The Problem of Defense and the Concept of Coping

LOIS BARCLAY MURPHY (U. S. A.)

The concept of coping as a process and an effort has been used and implied at least since the twenties, for instance, in Bernfeld's *Psychology of the Infant* (1929) [1]. Beyond this, psychoanalytic uses of the concept of mastery, and more broadly, the ego, involved or implied processes leading to mastery and expressing ego strength. Recently the term coping has been used by some writers to imply successful management of a dilemma rather than the positive efforts involved. It is then placed in opposition to "defense," which is sometimes erroneously seen as leading to pathology (despite the extensive literature on healthy and universal defense structures shaping character).

Following some years of incidental study of coping methods of young children [12], I began a series of studies in 1953 at the Menninger Foundation which focused on this aspect of child development. In one paper [13], I discussed the contribution of temporary defense mechanisms to coping in early childhood. In the present paper I would like to carry this discussion further, in the context of some of the psychoanalytic discussions of defense and coping, particularly those of Anna Freud and Dorothy Burlingham.

*This paper is based upon studies supported by USPHS Grants M680 and 5 R12 MH9236, by the Gustavus and Louisa Pfeiffer Foundation, and the Menninger Foundation; and also by the USPHS Grant MH10421, Children's Hospital of D.C.

The Problem of Defense

The first edition of Anna Freud's *The Ego and the Mechanisms of Defense* was published in 1936 and since then it has been the basic manual for the study of defense mechanisms. It is of the greatest importance that only a few years after Freud's *Ego and the Id* [8] Anna Freud was approaching this topic not only in terms of its contribution to the understanding of pathological processes but also in terms of its contribution to the understanding of normal personality development. This is hinted in her chapter headings and in the table of contents. Her book is divided into four parts, the first of which is entitled: "Theory of the Mechanisms of Defense," with a first chapter titled, "The Ego as the Seat of Observation," thus placing what H. Hartmann referred to as "autonomous ego functions" in relation to ego mechanisms which were defensive. Following a discussion of method in the "Application of Analytic Technique to the Study of Psychic Institutions," Anna Freud continued to "The Ego's Defensive Operations Considered as an Object of Analysis." The latter dealt with the role of analysis of the defensive measures against the instinct; transformations undergone by the affects, and resistances of the ego and their relation to symptom formation.

Next, she reviewed briefly the history of the concept of defense from its first appearance in 1894 in Freud's study, "The Defense Neuropsychoses" [5], through discussions of the etiology of hysteria, further remarks on the defense neuropsychoses in the appendix to "Inhibition, Symptom, and Anxiety." Following this come the nine methods of defense which had up to the time of her writing been described in the theoretical writings of psychoanalysis: regression, repression, reaction formation, isolation, undoing, projection, introjection, turning against the self, and reversal to which she adds the tenth, sublimation, with the comment that it pertains rather to the study of the normal than to neurosis.

The last chapter in the first section presented an "Orientation to the Processes of Defense According to the Source of Anxiety and Danger." This prepares the reader for the next sections with examples of the *avoidance* of *objective pain* and *objective danger* which Anna Freud considered the preliminary stages of defense; *denial in fantasy, denial in word and act,* and *restriction of the ego* are the three patterns dealt with in this section.

In the next section, dealing with *identification with the aggressor,* and the combination of projection and identification in behavior which appears altruistic, comparisons are made between the defense patterns or strategy first worked out in the study of patients to examples of normal behavior in everyday life. The final section deals with defenses motivated by fear of the strength of the instincts, as is common during adolescence and at menopause.

Throughout, Anna Freud is constantly aware of and carries the reader into applications of the concepts of defense to the understanding of normal behavior. As would be natural in that part of the discussion dealing with analytic technique, her discussion of defenses is constantly oriented toward the process and sequences of response which can be seen during the analytic hour; by following through the mechanisms of defense especially in instances where impulses do not emerge in direct form in the analytic situation, she points out that it is possible to fill in a gap in a patient's memory of his instinctual life, and to acquire information which fills in gaps in the history of his ego development or the history of the transformations through which his instincts have passed [4].

She discussed in some detail the ego's defense against the *affects* associated with instinctual impulses—love, longing, jealousy, mortification, pain, and mourning—and with hatred, anger, and rage—the impulses of aggression. If the instinctual demands with which they are associated are to be warded off, these affects must submit to all the various measures to which the ego resorts in its efforts to master them, that is, they must undergo metamorphosis. She stated that whenever transformation of an affect occurs whether in analysis or outside it, the ego has been at work and we have an opportunity of studying its operations.

In longitudinal records of children studied over an extended period of time, we see clear examples of changes in affect in the rise and decline of fears before and after the Oedipal period parallel with the emergence of intense aggressive and erotic feelings at about the age of four and their subsequent *management* by *channeling,* and *relinquishment* as the ego makes investments in new interests and activities with peers. Among normal children we see the intensity of affect and apparent urgency of the *drive reduced while fantasy themes persist;* affect may even change to humorous exaggeration or superior derogation in successive levels of defensiveness. Here we see normal uses of defense resources to cope with everyday conflicts, frustrations, and pressures in their relations with restrictive adults especially.

Anna Freud noted that one and the same ego can have at its disposal only a limited number of possible means of defense, but that these are used differently at different times: at particular periods in life and according to its own specific structure, the individual ego (and we can add, this includes healthy egos) selects now one defensive method, now another—maybe repression, displacement, or reversal—and these it can employ both in its conflict with the instincts and in its defense against the liberation of affect.

In comparing free association with the process of play as described by the English school for child analysis, she remarks,

> Interruptions and inhibitions in play are equated with the breaks in free association. It follows that if we analyze the interruption to play we discover that it represents a defensive measure on the part of the ego comparable to resistance to free association.

Anna Freud does not completely accept the equation between free association and play, but this observation has value beyond the sphere of analysis—breaks or shifts in topic, tempo, style or role of play, social interaction, conversation, or other activity often involve defense against an impulse which threatens to express itself in action, words, or emotional expression.

Thus, by observation of shifts in the level of cognitive-affective expression in responses to the CAT, we can focus on the points which involved special threat for each child and the effect of the anxiety aroused by this threat on the level and style of his integration.

Anna Freud stated that the term defense is in fact the first expression of the dynamic standpoint in psychoanalytic theory, after its first use in 1894 in Freud's study, "The Defense Neuropsychoses" [5], it was employed in several of his subsequent works [6, 7] to describe *the ego's struggle against painful or unendurable ideas or affects.* This term was abandoned for a time and replaced by that of repression.

The special point of interest for us here is the concept of the struggle of the ego, and for our purposes it is any struggle of the ego, whether against painful or unendurable ideas or affects, or against the situations or stimuli in the external environment which if not controlled would arouse such affects.

The Concept of Coping

Since the term defense mechanism was appropriated for the intrapsychic maneuvers, transformations, and other operations dealing with affects and instincts, another term is needed to refer to the ego's dealing with the actual external or objective situation itself. In 1926 [9] Freud stated that the old concept of defense could be advantageously used again if it were employed "explicitly as a general designation for all techniques which the ego makes use of in conflict which *may* lead to a neurosis"; he suggested that the word "repression" be retained for the special method of defense described in the early studies. Repression is thus one psychic process serving the purpose of *protection* of the ego against instinctual demands. Freud first referred to the processes of turning against the self and reversal as "vicissitudes of instinct," but Anna Freud comments that from the point of view of the ego these mechanisms also come under the heading of methods of defense.

> For every vicissitude to which the instincts are liable has its origin in some ego activity. Were it not for the intervention of the ego or of the external forces which the ego represents, every instinct would know only one fate—that of gratification.

The use of the small word "may" (lead to neurosis) implies that this does not necessarily happen, but there is a risk. Actually, there are risks in any coping efforts as well. Military adventures involve active coping strategies but may end in defeat; so may many ordinary coping efforts in the lives of all of us.

When a child is anxious about possible consequences of dangerous impulses he may repress the impulse and phobically avoid tempting situations. Actually most defense mechanisms involve both intrapsychic changes, transformation of affects and of impulse, and also of interaction with the external world. But suppose the ego merely avoids the situation, conscious of its fear and of the danger in the situation, without any repression or transformation of affect or impulse. In such instances we can say the child is *"coping with the situation" by evasion, turning away, avoidance, and so forth.* If these initial avoidances lead to constellations of activity which are adequate to protect the individual from the threat in the situation and which lead to other gratifications, the avoidance pattern may be adequate in itself without involving the deeper transformation of affect and instinct. This is apt to occur when adequate substitutes are found and a safe form of gratification takes the place of the threatening one. Anna Freud used the term "control" of affective life to describe the normal way of handling or coping with everyday conflicts.

In further discussion of the role of symptoms, she remarked, "If the ego employs repression, the formation of symptoms relieves it of *the task of mastering its conflicts,* while if it employs the other defensive methods, it still *has to deal with the problem."* Here "the task of mastering its conflicts" and of "dealing with the problem" are normal, everyday demands which life places on the individual. These coping efforts or "coping" is simply a shortcut for these concepts.

In other words, coping is a broader concept than that of defense mechanism as the defense concept has been classically used. We find Anna Freud repeatedly referring to the problem of *mastery of impulse,* not with any assumption that defense mechanisms are the only resources the ego brings to mastery but that these resources are involved where other methods fail. From time to time she also *comments explicitly that defenses are not necessarily of a pathological character, particularly such defenses as displacement.*

In stating that the ego is "ready to ward off affects associated with prohibited sexual impulses if these affects happen to be distressing, e.g. pain, longing, mourning," Anna Freud pointed out that this simple defense against primarily painful affects corresponds to the defense against the primarily painful stimuli which impinge upon the ego from the outside world. In other words, she almost suggests that the intrapsychic defense pattern is modeled on the overt behavior in relation to objective external stimuli.

Later Anna Freud pointed out a relationship between defense and what we are calling coping as follows:

> When the ego has taken its defensive measures against an affect for the purpose of avoiding 'pain,' something more besides analysis is required to annul them if the result is to be permanent. The child must learn to tolerate larger and larger quantities of pain without immediately having recourse to his defense mechanisms.

She added it must be admitted that "theoretically it is the business of education rather than of analysis to teach him this lesson." Here she made it clear that the analysis of defense as such is not sufficient when the defense itself has arisen for the purpose of avoiding pain, that the analysis of defenses cannot be successful unless the coping methods of the child become increasingly successful and take over the job of helping the child to cope with painful experience.

While Anna Freud's clarification of the functioning of defense mechanisms is basic to all psychoanalytic thinking, her use of the term coping is much less well known. For this reason, it is important to give examples of the direct and indirect ways in which she uses the concept.

In *Infants without Families* [3, p. 61] we find an illustration of her direct use of the word "coping":

> The first family setting is the framework within which the instincts and emotions of the child grope towards their first objects. A child can never completely possess these objects but in this first display of its feeling it learns 'to love,' to cope with its instinctual forces and thus lay the foundations for its character formation, a process which entails a great deal of discomfort. It is this first parent relationship which a child repeats, sometimes in a lessened, sometimes in an intensive degree on the parent substitutes, if they are offered, in a residential institution.

In other words, the coping patterns developed in one setting are drawn upon in new situations.

Moreover, her records of the behavior of individual children include examples of *coping* efforts like the following: [3, p. 97]

Pauline, 4½ years old, who usually adopts a motherly attitude toward a younger little boy who was very anxious, advised him to "cover himself right over" as she always did during the time of an evening air raid. Here she appeared to make a positive use of the comforting value of covers, possibly due to the sheer gratification of the contact experienced, perhaps due to its association with tucking in activities by the mother or to its connection with tactual experiences of bodily closeness; perhaps also an ostrich-like element of hiding may be present.

Anna Freud also said that the ego does not defend itself only against the pain arising from within. In the same early period in which it becomes acquainted with dangerous internal instinctual stimuli, it experiences "pain" which has its source in the outside world. The ego is in close contact with that world. The outside world is a source of both pleasure and pain. "A little child's ego lives as yet in accordance with the pleasure principle; it's a long time before it's trained to bear pain." She saw the little child as too weak to oppose the outside world actively, to defend himself against it by means of physical force, or to modify it in accordance with his own will.

> . . . as a rule the child is too helpless physically to take to flight and his understanding is as yet too limited to see the inevitable in the light of reason and submit to it. In this period of immaturity and dependence the ego, besides making efforts to master instinctual stimuli, endeavors in all kinds of ways to defend itself against the objective 'pain' and dangers which menace it. . .

So she observed that while analytic observation has been focused primarily "on the inner struggle between the instincts and the ego, of which neurotic symptoms are the sequel, *the efforts of the infantile ego to avoid pain by directly resisting external impressions belong to the sphere of normal psychology.*" Their consequences may be momentous for the formation of the ego and of character but, she felt, they are not pathogenic.

This is a direct invitation to the study of those efforts of the child to avoid pain by its own direct activity in its dealings with the environment. Oddly enough this invitation of 1936 was not accepted by those working in normal psychology. It remained for the analysts themselves, including Anna Freud and others dealing with the behavior of children subjected to bombing, evacuation, and so forth during the war to give case records of children's ways of handling the threats and stresses of this period. Studies of hospitalization, Bowlby's work on separation from mother, and other comparable studies began to fill in this major gap.

This is despite the fact that the experience of fear itself and the child's expression of fear, had been studied to a considerable extent by Gesell [10], Jersild and his associates [11] and others in the discipline of child psychology. Lacking a dynamic orientation, none of these observers of children focused on the child's way of dealing with the stimuli for fear, or his ways of managing himself, or his environment so as to avoid pain, threat, and the experience of being frightened.

A few clinically trained psychologists such as Saul Rosenzweig and Eugene Lerner [12], together with Lewin and his associates, did focus briefly on the child's reaction to frustration. These tended to be concerned with the actions following frustration; in Lewin's records and in Lerner's records there were notations on the direct efforts of the child to attack the frustrating object, or to escape from it by leaving the field. However, these coping methods were only noted incidentally and were never brought into the spotlight of research in child development.

In another discussion the children's ways of handling losses of maternal care are described.

> Motherless children in orphanages care for their bodies in an unexpected manner. Sometimes it is hard to get the children to take off their rubbers. They say they might catch cold. All the bogeys concerning the child's health which had troubled their mothers in the past are taken over by the young children themselves after separation or bereavement. They substitute themselves for their mothers by perpetuating the bodily care received from her [3].

In *Young Children in Wartime* [2] we find illustrations of more complex expressions of protest, complaint, and finally denial in coping with a prolonged threat. In May 1941, the gardener reported that a bomb had fallen in the garden without exploding. The area was roped off and children were not allowed to go into the garden. This is a place where they had been accustomed to play. The weather was warm and sunny and the children obviously did not like this arrangement at all. A bomb at a great distance may be an object of horror. A bomb, on the other hand, which settles down so near to one's own household is somehow included in it and soon becomes an object of familiarity. It is true that on the first day an unexploded bomb is contemplated with respect and suspicions. When it delays exploding, the reaction in the people around is not, as one should expect—one of thankfulness and relief. The reaction is rather one of annoyance with it which develops into contempt for the bomb as the days go by. The bomb is treated more like an imposter who has formed us into an attitude of submission under false pretenses. In the end, when no one believes in its explosiveness any more, it sinks down to the position of being a bore. At this stage a nine-year-old girl, Constance, was heard to say in an angry tone: "I wish the bomb would explode so that we can use the garden again." Finally a group of children dashed for the garden entrance and when caught and brought back, one insisted, "There is no bomb," at which all the children screamed in chorus, "There is no bomb! We are going out in the garden!" Pamela then came in again and said firmly, "It has exploded."

In her broad survey of psychological reactions in *Young Children in Wartime* [2] Anna Freud also reviews the experience to which the children were exposed and her observations of the children's responses:

> All our bigger children have had their fair share of war experiences. All of them have witnessed the air raids either in London or in the provinces. A large percentage of them has seen their houses destroyed or damaged. All of them have seen their family dissolved, whether by separation from or by death of the father. All of them are separated from their mothers and have entered community life at an age which is not usually considered ripe for it. The questions arise which part these experiences play in the psychological life of the individual child, how far the child *acquires understanding* of what is going on around it, how it *reacts emotionally,* how far its anxiety is aroused, and *what normal or abnormal outlets it will find to deal with these experiences* which are thrust on it.

Thus she outlined the problems of coping with stress, the cognitive and affective factors in and the need for examination of behavior channels used by the child in his effort to deal with it. She continued:

> It can be safely said that all the children who were over two years at the time of the London "blitz" have *acquired knowledge* of the significance of air raids. They all *recognize* the noise of flying aeroplanes; they *distinguish* vaguely between the sounds of falling bombs and anti-aircraft guns. They *realize* that the house will fall down when bombed and that people are often killed or get hurt in falling houses. . . . They fully *understand the significance* of taking shelter. Some children who have lived in deep shelters will even *judge the safety of a shelter* according to its depth under the earth. . . . The children seem to have no difficulty in understanding what it means when their fathers join the Forces. We even overhear talk among the children where they compare their fathers' military ranks and duties. . . .

She went on to say that the children were similarly ready to take in knowledge about the various occupations of their mothers, though the constant changes of occupations made this slightly more difficult. Mothers of 3-year-olds would play out, changing backwards and forwards between the occupations of railway porter, factory worker, bus conductor, milk cart driver, and so on. The mothers visited their children in their varying uniforms and proudly told them about their new war work until the children were completely confused. Though the children seemed proud of their fathers' uniforms, they often seemed to resent it and felt *estranged when their mothers appeared in unexpected guises.*

Anna Freud remarked that it was especially hard for *children to get any understanding of the reason why they were being evacuated* despite the fact that they actually did live in London with their mothers during the worst dangers. Being sent to the country afterwards when London seemed quite peaceful made no sense to them. They felt that if "home" was as much in danger as all that, their mothers should not be there either. Their feeling about home was intense: "home" was the place to which all children were determined to return, irrespective of the fact that in most cases they were aware that it had been destroyed.

"The *understanding of catastrophes* to their homes like the death of father, had little to do with reasoning," Anna Freud comments. The children met the usual psychological difficulties of grasping the significance of death at such an early age. Their attitude to the happening was completely a matter of emotion.

But she observed that children who had the support of their parents were able to endure the most severe experiences of bombing without traumatic shock while children separated from their parents suffered profoundly. Another classic observation was that the experience of *aggression in the external world was tolerated by the child because of the importance of the experience of aggressive impulses* from within: instead of turning away from the destructions of war in instinctive horror "the child may turn towards them with primitive excitement." She commented on the enormous difficulty of educating children toward control of aggression while they were living in a world where destruction was an everyday matter—a difficulty endlessly repeated in the decade of the sixties.

Beyond the fact that children in London who had the support of stable parents were not traumatized by experiences of being bombed, she commented on the ease with which children became accustomed to the very real and severe threats, giving illustrations of children who initially paid attention to the dropping of bombs during an air raid, then lost interest and turned their attention to a storybook. We are not told whether just *getting used to* the noise was the dominant pattern or whether the child came to the conclusion that since there was nothing he could do about it he might as well turn away from it to concern himself with more satisfying things, or the third possibility that a strong desire to *shut out* the anxiety-provoking noise and escape into the satisfactions of his book was involved.

Anna Freud proceeded from these observations on children's ways of coping with *"objective anxiety"* to the ways in which a second kind of anxiety is handled. She observed that after the first years of life the individual learns to criticize and overcome in himself certain instinctive wishes, or rather he learns to refuse them conscious expression. He learns that it is bad to kill, to hurt, and to destroy, and would like to believe that he has no further wish to do any of these things. He needs the support of control in the external world to sustain this attitude and when he sees killing and destruction going on outside, it arouses his fear that the impulses which he put away will be aroused again. She noted that the small child in whom inhibitions against aggression have not yet been established is free of the abhorrence of air raids, but the slightly older child who has just been through this fight with himself will be particularly sensitive to their menace, and will have real outbreaks of anxiety when bombs come down and cause damage.

The *fear of his own conscience,* developed out of fear of parental authority, also influences the child's reaction to external threats. Fear of ghosts and bogeymen develops as reinforcements of the real parental authorities and of the inner voice conscience, and various figures of the external world serve as symbols for them. Policemen who may arrest them, gypsies who might steal or kidnap, lions or tigers who could come and eat them, earthquakes which might shake their houses, thunderstorms which might threaten them, or religious teachings may dominate the entire picture so that everything else is left aside and the child is primarily afraid of the devil and of hell or afraid that God can see everything and punish him for his sins. Such children are as afraid of sirens and of bombs as they are afraid of thunder and lightening; Hitler and German planes may take the place of the devil.

In order to cope with such fears, the children made repeated demands for extra protection, for the supporting presence of the mother, for someone to stay near their bed or hold their hands until they fell asleep. When air raids and bombs stop, these children return to their old fears of ghosts and bogeymen.

Children who lost their fathers as a result of bombing turned away from their memories in quiet times as much as possible and were "gay and unconcerned" in their play with the other children. But this effort to forget could not be sustained during the recurrence of an air raid which brought back their memories, and their tendency to repeat their former experience.

> For these children every bomb which falls is like the one which killed the father, and is feared as such. One of our war orphans, in contrast to all other children, is immensely excited when he sights any bomb damage, new or old. Another, a little girl of six, transfers this fear and excitation from bombs to accidents of all kinds, to the sight of ambulances, talk of hospitals, of illnesses, of operations, in short to every occurrence which brings the fact of death (of her father) back to her mind.

Adults did not anticipate the children's ways of coping with being placed in the homes economically superior to their own.

> Children who are billeted on householders who are either above or below the social and financial status of their parents will be very conscious of the difference. If urged to adapt themselves to a higher level of cleanliness, speech, manners, social behavior or moral ideals, they will *resent* these demands as criticism directed against their own parents and may *oppose* them.

Some children refused new clothes, and hung on to torn and dirty things from home. With young children this might have been just an expression of a desire to cling to the familiar; with older children it is a refusal to be unfaithful to the standard of their homes.

Here we see the variety of patterns of emotional response aroused by the experience and the ways in which the child handled his anxiety about it, whether in terms of overt direct effort to get support, or with various defense mechanisms including a tendency to deny the objective reality or to deal with it through fantasy displacements and the like. The ways in which these children kept themselves "normal" through experiences which adults ordinarily would have expected to be devastating and disintegrating to the child included a variety of combinations of direct coping methods and defense mechanisms which appear to have been relinquished when the stress diminished, among the normal children.

In contrast to the healthy use of support and also of denial, escape into storybooks, fantasy, and projection—all used in egosyntonic ways which contributed to the maintenance of the integrity of the child—we are told of children who were not able to get adjusted to foster homes or to the nurseries which were set up to provide conditions as adequate as possible to take care of children separated from their mothers.

> ... Not many children present as frightening a picture as Patrick, three and a half years old, who found himself reduced to a state in which compulsive formula and symptomatic actions played the largest part; or Beryl, four years old, who sat for several days on the exact spot where her mother had left her, would not speak, eat or play, and had to be moved around like an automaton.

Even apart from these unusual cases we have seen long, drawn-out states of homesickness, upset, and despair which are certainly more than the average inexperienced foster mother can be expected to cope with.

Anna Freud noted that no similar states of distress were seen in children in the London shelters which housed mothers and children. Thus she documented the capacity of children to cope with severe stress when the supporting mother is at hand.

Precursors of Coping and Defense

Records of infants observed at the age of 1 month, 2 months, and 3 months, provide evidence for activities of a variety of sorts which might be regarded as precursors of later defense mechanisms or, more comprehensively, coping styles. In common with very simple organisms such as a worm or an ant, a very tiny baby will turn its face or body away from a threatening stimulus, shut its eyes to shut out such a threat, curl into itself, and so forth. Some babies will also push away, bat at, or in some other way crudely attack a stimulus which is a source of discomfort, such as an uncomfortable blanket pushing at its face. A baby's cry, at first doubtless a primitive discharge mechanism of the organism, soon becomes incorporated into a technique for obtaining help. It is used as communication, expression, demand as well as an outlet for anger, fear, discomfort, anxiety. As soon as the development of motor skills and the beginnings of locomotion make it possible for the baby to turn over, creep, pull, or push himself away from the stimulus, his primitive turning away or shutting his eyes is extended to the possibility of removing his body, and as fast as fine motor control develops his initial amorphous batting and pushing away yields to more refined methods of hitting at or throwing away in protest.

These are all active ways of defending one's self against discomfort or external stress—that is, ways of directly coping with it. However, as memory, imagery, and fantasy develop, the baby's resources are extended so that it is no longer necessary for him to depend solely on these active dealings with the external environment. Thus we can see a continuum between the earliest methods of active coping and later methods of defense, some of which become patterned into defense mechanisms.

A simple model would be like this: the baby turns away from a threatening stimulus. This makes it possible for him to *forget*. Or independently, or parallel with forgetting, to *deny* the existence of the threat. When forgetting is sustained and maintained consistently, we refer to repression.

It is hardly reasonable to assume that all forgetting is repression under emotional conflict since when the infant is very young, such a multitude of stimuli are pressing upon him in succession that memory must be regarded as an achievement in itself and forgetting as a normal consequence of the shifting of attention from a previous stimulus to a new and more absorbing one. Enduring memory may very likely depend upon the development of constellations of organized traces which can capture new impressions and integrate them into an already established configuration in the very early months, while it is possible for massive, pervasive, deeply disturbing experiences to leave an enduring impression, or for crucially significant events occurring at a time when thresholds are low, to be imprinted in an enduring way. However, thousands of relatively irrelevant impressions from the point of view of the baby's early economy are only momentarily registered. Probably only those impressions which are received repeatedly, or in a context of deeply significant affect can be expected to endure. We can only speak of repression then when we are talking about traces which would otherwise be retained or remembered. Repression takes more energy than forgetting. It is easy to forget things of no consequence. It is hard to repress those which cause us deep conflict or anxiety.

When the baby reaches an age where the threat comes from the reaction of the environment to something he has done, whether it is a matter of biting his mother's nipple while nursing or throwing something out of his playpen or high chair which is frustrating or annoying to him, we find the beginning of anger at the external person who punishes or reproves for the painful or socially destructive action.

It is not uncommon when one observes forceful, spirited babies to see a quick, angry, defiant, accusing look against the grown-up who has slapped the baby's hand or protested against an action of the baby's. It is as if the baby said, "It is you who are bad, not I." This quick exchange referring blame, accusations, protest, and danger to the outside, to the adult seems to serve the purpose of forestalling recognition of her acceptance of guilty feelings by the baby, in those cases where the baby maintains a proud autonomy after such accusing looks at the grown-up. In some instances a baby may follow such an angry accusation with a shy, withdrawing, retreating appeal as if for forgiveness or for reinstatement of love, a look expressive of reparation. This is a distinct next step, however.

What I am first of all concerned with here is the origins of projection in an atmosphere of exchange of anger set off by some unintentional damage by the infant. By the age of 3 or 4 years such processes have gone far enough so that babies (for example, Martin Saunders in our group) have developed a pattern of anticipating blame, protest, accusation, or punishment from the adult and forestalling it by projecting threat to the adult in a way which takes into account the possibility of their threatening behavior, and retreating to an over-controlled or safe area where dangerous activity will be avoided, thus taking no risk. In other words, an early experience of exchange of hostilities leading to a pattern of projection of threat and guilt to the grown-up can become a mechanism which operates automatically and autonomously, thus becoming a defense mechanism.

In the early stages of turning away, denial, repression, and projection, we can see the steps in the baby's actual behavior. After an end product such as projection has been repeated to the point where it becomes crystallized into a mechanism, the child does not go through these steps and the pattern can no longer be broken down—*in exactly the same way that other higher units are established* which then become autonomous and capable of incorporation into still more complicated configurations of response, the *defense mechanism has become an autonomous response pattern.*

By the age of 3 or 4 years most children have already developed a repertoire of such autonomous mechanisms, defense mechanisms which played their part in the total resources of coping used by each child. This was true of all the children in the Coping Project regardless of the overall level of happiness or adjustment or prognosis of future comfortable development as seen by the psychiatrist. In fact, when we look at the repertoire of defense mechanisms as such utilized by the most comfortable and happy children as compared with those about whom we are worried, we find no evidence that a statistically different range of defense mechanisms could be found. We have to look in another direction for differences between these two groups of children.

We can say further that the most normal and happy of our children drew upon defense mechanisms as part of their total strategy for coping, with considerable flexibility and with changing emphases over the period during which we observed them.

We often see that denial is used in the service of mastery and is supported by the cognitive processes which might in turn be regarded as contributing to the maintenance of the defense; or perhaps we can simply say the two go hand in hand. Certainly the cognitive mastery and the denial are both important in the total process of coping with fear of thunder.

As we go through sequences of defense it seems very clear that one defense mechanism yields to another; projection of fear onto a little brother is essentially another form of denial; or perhaps we could say, used in the service of denial as part of the total process of outgrowing a fear.

As we follow the development of efforts to master fears and other stresses on the part of our children, we are struck then by the flexibility with which they use defense mechanisms as part of the total coping strategy. This flexibility includes the capacity to use one mechanism at one time and another later as well as the capacity to use different ones together, when they are needed. An important point here is the fact that we see this not just in an inhibited, withdrawn child who is unable to deal directly with the environment and thus develops defense mechanisms as substitutes for active efforts with the environment which he might otherwise be able to make. The same child who uses defense mechanisms flexibly is very direct in his ability to seek comfort from his sister, to go to his parents' room, to actively snuggle into bed himself when frightened by thunder, and so on. The defense mechanisms appear not as substitutes for active efforts, or as a result of failure to make active efforts, but rather go hand in hand with his active efforts as part of the total coping program, as it were.

Up to this point we have dealt with the development of defense mechanisms as we ordinarily talk about them and with their place at different points in the child's total coping effort at any given time in the child's development. We used the phrase "the place of the defense continuum in the total coping process" because we saw a continuity between the baby's first efforts to turn away even through such a limited act as shutting its eyes or turning its head, to later efforts to turn away bodily, efforts to deny and repress, then subsequent patterns of projection and the like. We speak then of a developmental continuum in the emergence of defense mechanisms as autonomous response patterns which have developed by a series of steps from more primitive defense measures, but which, once reaching a state of effective operation at a more complex level, function at that level automatically without going through the preliminary steps.

We cannot see the whole process adequately, however, unless we also look at the defensive use of normal ego functions which are part of the child's total cognitive, motor, and affective development. All normal babies respond with varying degrees of vivid interest in visual, auditory, and tactual stimuli as fast as their neurological development provides the equipment for responsiveness to the stimuli of the outside world. Babies differ widely in their use of such stimuli. The analysis of records of infants shows wide differences between the tendencies of certain babies to pay more attention to faces and people than to things, or to pay more attention to colorful , shiny, and in other ways interesting objects, in contrast to faces. Our knowledge is not at a point where it is possible to stand on firm ground in any theory regarding the basis for such differences between eager excitement about and response to *things* as compared with faces. (Controlled studies of differences between babies whose first oral gratifications come through being nursed or being fed while held, cuddled, and smiled at by the mother as compared with babies who are played with very little and fed by bottles held on mechanical bottle holders might contribute something to this distinction.) At present we can only observe that wide differences can be seen in very young babies.

Illustrations from Normal Development

One of the babies with a strong interest in objects was Trudy who was born at a time when her family actually fostered such an interest. With father busy completing an advanced professional degree, mother helping to support the home and caring for an older child, neither parent had the time for play with and spontaneous exchanges with the baby, Trudy, which subsequent children in the family received. Trudy had a cradle gym and was very much interested in it, playing with the toys which dangled above her chest with great enthusiasm. This interest persisted, and by the time she was in nursery school, she was a child who enjoyed puzzles and other types of play with the objects and toys of nursery school very much. She did not make contact with other children readily. Her nursery school teacher felt this as a lack and may have communicated some of her restlessness and dissatisfaction with Trudy's limited use of the social opportunities of the nursery school. At any rate, it is striking that by the time Trudy was 7 or 8 years old in elementary school, where her teacher expressed great appreciation of the intellectual skills she had developed, Trudy now began to expand into very much more active spontaneous social relationships with children, and was, at the age of 8, possibly the most popular child in her group. This social ease utilized, in fact, the intellectual ease which had developed from early infancy and which was now accepted as important and praiseworthy in the school situation.

This is a brief summary of many hundreds of pages of data on Trudy; what we are interested in here is the fact that what began as an autonomous ego function mainly observing, analyzing, making relationships between her perceptions and concepts of objects was utilized by her beyond the time it might otherwise have occupied in her early months in lieu of the attention from parents which she would have been getting if they had not been so busy. Accepted by them as a source of strength, since she was in a family of intellectual interests, it contributed to her identification with her parents and thus received constant reinforcement at home.

It seems fair to say in this instance that interest in such things as manipulating and thinking about objects, putting them together, and solving puzzles, developed in a conflict-free fashion through her initial years in the family because these activities were satisfying to her in themselves, were accepted and appreciated by the family, and fitted in with her identification with her parents' intellectual activities which were so predominant at that time. In nursery school it is quite possible that an exaggeration of her interest in puzzles was used defensively and with more conflict primarily because of the lack of enthusiasm or suspiciousness of the nursey school teacher. Being in an intellectual family, however, the supports at this age were strong enough so that whatever conflicts and unhappiness arose in nursery school around her intellectual interests and activities with puzzles were not deep enough to outweigh the positive gratifications which were intrinsic in the first place and reinforced by the family interest in the second place. By the time she got to elementary school, where intellectual performance was expected, she was able to retrieve and build on the foundations of autonomous ego functioning and her enthusiasm for the intellectual activities.

It is particularly dramatic in this connection that her I.Q. increased 24 points between the age when she was tested at the time she was in nursery school and the test when she was 8 years old. At the latter stage, she was more spontaneous and outgoing, generally free from inhibition, as well as functioning more enthusiastically in cognitive terms. During the period of conflict and defensiveness in the use of cognitive functioning, she was constricted, we may assume. Later, despite the fact that cognitive functions had been utilized defensively for a period, she was able to recapture her enthusiastic immediacy of satisfaction and she blossomed into richer cognitive functioning; because of it and parallel with its acceptance and appreciation in a social group, she blossomed likewise into much more creative social activity. It is interesting to note that along with her popularity and leadership in the group, traces of the unhappiness and insecurity she had had earlier in nursery school were hinted in her concern about insecure children in the school group, children who were different, as she might have felt different in nursery school. This sensitivity to difference included unusual social awareness and creativity in relation to Negro children or other minority group children in the school group, even at this age when many children handle sensitivity to difference by activities aimed toward protecting their own status.

At the period of her flowering, Trudy's I.Q. was 146, suggesting that this was a perceptive and sensitive little girl whose perceptiveness might have contributed to a more than average sensitive reaction to her nursery school disapproval of intellectuality.

With many another child, knowledge, the desire to know, to have questions answered, to solve problems, is utilized defensively in certain situations parallel with their use as spontaneous expression of childish response to the world about them when they were free from threat. At the same time, in some children, the defensive use of the drive for knowledge interferes with spontaneous autonomous delight in intellectual functioning. In Martin's case the intellectual interest appeared to be pushed so hard because of a need to outstrip an older brother. In his case the intellectual functioning rarely seemed to go on in the atmosphere of delight, enthusiasm, mastery, and ease characteristic of others. Typically, Martin produced his answers and his thoughts in an atmosphere of anxiety and tension and a need to prove something [14].

Conclusions

In general, the children in this normal group use defense mechanisms and autonomous ego functions in a mutually supportive way; cognitive functions per se are able to be enjoyed in many instances quite spontaneously, at the same time that they might be used in other situations as part of a coping process which included defense mechanisms. Further, we could see that the balance of spontaneity and enthusiasm attending cognitive functioning shifts from one period to another, cognitive functions being utilized as part of a defensive process during a period of stress as in the case of Trudy. Also, we saw that while cognitive functions might serve a temporarily defensive function, they could be retrieved for more spontaneous experiencing when the situation changed and a defensive role was no longer needed. Finally, in the case of one or two children under a chronic, persistent, competitive pressure, cognitive functions were used for defense so consistently as to become embedded in a defensive character structure, and thus were much less accessible to the flexible and happy use typical of most children [15].

The patterning of defense mechanisms as part of total coping varies with different children, and outcomes vary. Neither defense mechanisms nor specific coping devices inevitably lead to pathology, or guarantee normal development. The latter is a complex outcome of interactions between the balance of vulnerabilities and strengths and their interaction with the sequential patterns of stress and support from the environment [13, 16].

Bibliography

1. Bernfeld, S., *Psychology of the Infant* (Translated by R. Hurwitz) Routledge & Sons, London, 1929.
2. Burlingham, D. and A. Freud, *Young Children in Wartime: a Year's Work in a Residential War Nursery,* Allen & Unwin, London, 1942.
3. Burlingham, D. and A. Freud, *Infants Without Families; the Case for and against Residential Nurseries,* International Universities Press, New York, 1944.
4. Freud, A., *The Ego and the Mechanisms of Defense,* International Universities Press, New York, 1946,
5. Freud, S., The Neuro-Psychoses of Defence, *Standard Edition,* 3 (1894), 45-61.*
6. Freud, S., Further Remarks on the Neuro-Psychoses of Defence, *Standard Edition,* 3 (1896), 162-185.
7. Freud, S., The Aetiology of Hysteria, *Standard Edition,* 3 (1896), 191-221.
8. Freud, S., The Ego and the Id, *Standard Edition,* 19 (1923), 3-66.
9. Freud, S., Inhibitions, Symptoms and Anxiety, *Standard Edition,* 20 (1926), 77-175.
10. Gesell, A., *Developmental Diagnosis: Normal and Abnormal Child Development. Clinical Methods and Pediatric Applications,* 2nd ed., Hoeber, New York, 1947.
11. Jersild, A. T. and F. B. Holmes, Children's fears. *Child Develpm. Monogr.,* 20 (1935), 356.
12. Lerner, E. and L. Murphy *Methods for the Study of Personality in Young Children,* Society for Research in Child Development, National Research Council, Washington, D.C., 1941.
13. Murphy, L., *Personality in Young Children,* Basic Books, New York, 1956.
14. Murphy, L. B., A longitudinal study of children's coping methods and styles, *Proceedings of XVth International Congress of Psychology,* Brussels, 1957, 436.
15. Murphy, L. B., Coping devices and defense mechanism in relation to autonomous ego functions, *Bulletin of the Menninger Clinic,* 24, 1960.
16. Murphy, L. B., et al.,*The Widening World of Childhood: Paths toward Mastery,* Basic Books, New York, 1962.

**The Standard Edition of the Complete Psychological Works of Sigmund Freud,* 24 Volumes, translated and edited by James Strachey. London: Hogarth Press and the Institute of Psycho-Analysis, 1953–

Atypical Behavior during Infancy: Infant Development in Relation to the Behavior and Personality of the Mother

NAHMAN H. GREENBERG (U. S. A.)

INTRODUCTION

A basic premise of this chapter is that the appearance of unusual behavior in infants indicates faulty development, a vulnerability to stress, and a greater probability for later development of abnormalities in cognitive, sensorimotor, social, and emotional functions. It is also assumed that the development of atypical behavior among infants free of congenital neural defects, or of other major birth abnormalities, is a consequence of inadequate, insufficient, inappropriate, faulty, or abusive infant care and stimulation. The actual infant care and stimulation patterns constitute the maternal behavior observed as infant-mother interactions and are thought to be derivatives of maternal personality although such connections are difficult to delineate and document.

*Supported in part by the Department of Mental Health, State of Illinois, in part by the City of Chicago Board of Health, and by the Childrens Bureau, Department of Health, Education and Welfare.

†Supported in part by a Research Scientist Development Award MH 13, 984 from the N.I.M.H.

The purpose of this paper is to report findings from studies designed to discover early forms of atypical behavior and to trace their development in infants, to describe and measure the interactions between these infants and their mothers, and to learn about the personality of these mothers.

Research on the development of atypical behavior during infancy, especially the study of family-reared babies, has received scant attention. With some notable exceptions, such as Spitz [71, 75], A. Freud [28], a few descriptions [10, 14, 25, 30, 43, 54, 67, 79], and clinical reports [63, 64] by pediatric and psychiatric physicians, human research in this area has been more or less confined to studies of consequences of nursery environments on the development of infants reared in institutions [29, 62, 69, 74, 76] and to effects of experimental interventions designed to alter atypical behavior observed among institutionalized retardates [80]. Studies of atypical behavior and of developmental abnormalities among family-reared infants have been few in number [2, 37, 57, 78], although recent public and professional interest in seriously abused and neglected children has led to an increasing number of clinical reports [3, 13, 18, 49].

There are compelling needs and strong arguments for raising the priority of research in these areas and to learn much more about the development of atypical behavior during infancy. There is an impressive body of evidence to support the idea that the first few years of life have an inordinate influence on the development of intellectual, learning, and psychosocial functions. Although it is not necessary to detail here the evidence supporting this theory, it is relevant to indicate that the evidence comes from a variety of research, and especially from animal experimentation. There is a wide array of findings which demonstrate that learning and problem-solving abilities can be increased when experimental animals are reared in particularly designed perceptual and stimulation environments [5, 27, 42, 45]. It is relatively easy to design environments in which to rear experimental animals who will develop a susceptibility to extreme and unusual behavior [5, 66] or who will fail to differentiate the specialized behavior necessary for the subsequent development of cognitive and social functions [5, 42, 44, 45]. There is evidence from both human and animal behavior which reveals that the "traditional" timetable of behavioral maturations can be hastened, slowed down, or even aborted by environmental events [36, 62, 70, 81]. Indeed, even neural, neurophysiological, and neurochemical structures and functions are vulnerable to the stresses created by altering the natural stimulus environment in which experimental animals are reared. Such changes in the neural makeup

Table 1a Atypical Behavior of Infancy

DISORDERS OF FEEDING AND OF THE GASTROINTESTINAL TRACT

1. DISTRUBANCES OF SUCKING (E.G., WEAK SUCKING RESPONSE, UNCOORDINATED SUCKING)
2. BODY HYPERTONICITY, OVERSTIMULATED BY SUCKING
3. REGURGITATION AND VOMITING
4. AVOIDANCE OF OR REFUSAL TO FEED FROM A BOTTLE AND/OR BREAST
5. REFUSAL OF SPECIFIC FOODS
6. REFUSAL TO CHEW
7. NONACCEPTANCE OF NEW DIETS OR CHANGES IN DIETS
8. ANOREXIA
9. "BOTTLE-FIXATION" ACCOMPANIED BY AN EXCLUSION OF OTHER FOODS (NUTRITIONAL ANEMIA)
10. FOOD FADS (OTHER THAN BOTTLE FIXATION)
11. EXCESSIVE EATING (OVEREATING; BULIMIA, HYPERPHAGIA)
12. RUMINATION
13. PICA, INCLUDING COPROPHAGIA AND TRICHOPHAGIA
14. CELIAC DISEASE
15. MALNUTRITION (UNDERFEEDING)

DISORDERS OF ELIMINATION

1. DIARRHEA
2. CONSTIPATION
3. PSYCHOGENIC MEGACOLON
4. ENCOPRESIS
5. WITHHOLDING STOOLS

RHYTHMIC (STEREOTYPICAL) PATTERNS OF BODY MOTILITY

1. HEAD-ROLLING AND HEAD-NODDING ACCOMPANIED NYSTAGMUS (SPASMUS NUTANS)
2. BODY-SWAYING (BODY-ROCKING)
   i. NORMATIVE
   ii. REPETITIOUS
   iii. EXCITATORY
3. HEAD-BANGING
   i. REPETITIOUS
   ii. AGITATED

of organisms may be concomitant with and fundamental to the limitations, constrictions, and deviations in intellectual and emotional functions observed when the rearing of organisms occurs under conditions of insufficient and inappropriate care or extreme stimulation [59, 66].

Table 1b Atypical Behavior of Infancy

DISORDERS OF HABIT FORMATION (HABIT PATTERNS, FOCAL ATYPICAL BEHAVIOR)

1. DISTURBANCES OF SLEEP
   i. RESISTANCES TO SLEEP
   ii. DROWSINESS
   iii. FITFUL SLEEP
   iv. HYPERSOMNIA
   v. HYPOSOMNIA AND INSOMNIA
2. BREATH HOLDING
3. AEROPHAGIA
4. BITING AND CHEWING OF SELF (e.g., OF LIPS, TONGUE, NAILS AND OTHER BODY PARTS)
5. BITING AND CHEWING OF OTHERS
6. GRINDING OF TEETH (BRUXISM)
7. SUCKING HABITS (e.g., OF THUMB, FINGER, LIPS, AND INANIMATE OBJECTS)
8. SPITTING
9. PULLING AND PICKING OF SELF (e.g., OF LIPS, NOSE, AND OTHER BODY PARTS)
10. TRICHOTILLOMANIA (PULLING OUT OF HAIR, e.g., SCALP AND EYEBROWS)
11. RUBBING OR STROKING OF SELF
    i. MASTURBATION
    ii. OF BODY PARTS OTHER THAN GENITALIA
    iii. STROKING OF SELF WITH INANIMATE OBJECTS

EXAGGERATIONS OF BEHAVIOR STATE OR AROUSAL

1. OVERACTIVITY
2. EXCESSIVE CRYING OF EARLY INFANCY (SO-CALLED "COLIC")
3. HYPERSENSITIVITY ASSOCIATED WITH A HYPERALERTNESS
4. HYPERTONICITY
5. FUSSINESS AND RESTLESSNESS
6. LETHARGY, WEAKNESS, HYPOACTIVITY (ENERGY IMPOVRISHMENT)
7. EXCESSIVE DROWSINESS
8. HYPOTONICITY

There are other timely reasons for increasing research on early atypical development in humans. There are increasing interests in the study of early environments, interests originating in an escalating concern for the disadvantaged families. The high rate of mental illness, delinquency, and unemployment together with a tradition of poor educational performance and family instability among the children of poor families has generated strong interests in their environment and in their development. Earlier studies [22, 47, 55, 58, 80] and more numerous recent observations on child-rearing practices in poor families [4, 11, 19, 48, 61] suggest a consensus view that children reared in poor families are exposed to limited social and emotional resources and live in a climate of intellectual impoverishment, which severely disadvantage the children who are inadequately prepared for productive futures. Parental and child-rearing behavior in the very poor families has been characterized as harsh and disciplinarian with limited interpersonal warmth [78, 83]. Children are squelched – they are taught compliance [20, 22, 50]; curiosity and inquiry are discouraged if not punished [11, 47, 50, 61]. The amount of talk between parent and child is limited in amount, in variety, and in purpose [20, 61, 78]. When these patterns are considered in the context of large families, marital instability, and disorganizing economic and familial crises, the child-rearing environment in the very poor families takes on a description of disproportionate quantities of inappropriateness, few if any enriching events and stimulations, neglect in long-range planning, and the use of harsh if not abusive stimulations. These conditions begin to assume a striking resemblance with those experimentally contrived environments in which major behavioral and morphological abnormalities can be developed.

These inferences and deductions are difficult to support or refute since the information needed to test them is not yet available. The data which are required include direct observations of maternal behavior and of the specific care techniques and stimulations of these infants by their parents, particularly their mother. It is well known that more than a few of the children from the very poor families develop quite well even by middle-class socioeconomic standards. The fact of being reared in a very poor family is not a sufficient explanation for the "maladaptations" in later life. The outcome to which children from the very poor are, at least in theory, destined can also be the fate of children from middle-income and affluent families. The child-rearing practices – the techniques of care and characteristics of stimulation of infants by their mothers – stem from various sources, including culture and subculture factors, but may well be more closely related to overall personality attributes. In our studies on atypical development during infancy, subculture and personality factors are separately examined.

CONCEPTS AND PHENOMENOLOGY OF ATYPICAL BEHAVIOR OF INFANCY

The course of healthy development during infancy is revealed in the infants who are acquiring more varied, discrete, and complex behavior patterns which subserve the emergence of an increasing array of organized motoric, perceptual, cognitive, and other mental functions. These acquisitions increase the infants' capacities to benignly tolerate and assimilate increasingly complex and intense internal (visceral) and external (somatic) stimulation and for a growing range of varied experiences. These are features of developmental progress which are described as follows:

1. Behavioral plasticity: that is, the capacity for more varied options or greater selectivity in behavioral responses. This results from the buildup of discrete behaviors which provide increasing numbers of complex structures that subserve attentional, cognitive, social, and related psychological functions.
2. Behavioral regulation: that is, the increasing capacity for more ordered and regulated behavior. This results from the buildup of varied patterns and their organization which unites various behaviors into functional sets and systems.
3. Stimulation tolerance: an increasing capacity to benignly tolerate and assimilate more complex and intense somatic and visceral stimulations (e.g., novel tasks, "stresses") without behavioral and inner disruption.

The development of these characteristics is also conceptualized as gains in levels of adaptation, and is assumed to stem from continuing sequential differentiation of neural, neurophysiological, and neuroendocrine apparatus and functions. Stimulations significantly influence the extent and character of the differentiations, the functional ordering of neural matrices, and the sensory thresholds established during early development. How the infants "experience" and react to any stimulation will depend in part on various quantitative, qualitative, and temporal properties of stimulation. Neural and neurophysiological differentiations and subsequent development will be influenced by the various characteristics of early stimulations, the consequences of which may be observed in the attributes of adaptation.

Table 1c Atypical Behavior of Infancy

DISORDERS OF MANIFEST AFFECT

1. CHRONIC, EXCESSIVE OR UNCONTROLLABLE CRYING WITH SCREAMING
2. MARASMUS
3. DEPRESSION
4. PROLONGED AND UNDUE INFANTILE STRANGER REACTION
5. PROLONGED AND UNDUE INFANTILE SEPARATION REACTION

ATYPICAL DEVELOPMENTAL PATTERNS
GENERAL OR IN SPECIFIC AREAS, e.g., MOTOR, SOCIAL, LANGUAGE, ADAPTIVE

1. PHYSICAL
   i. ACCELERATED
   ii. RETARDED (FAILURE TO GROW, FAILURE TO THRIVE)
   iii. UNEVEN
2. MATURATIONAL PATTERNS (SPECIFY AREA AND TYPE)
   i. ACCELERATED
   ii. REGRESSION (e.g., LOSS OF WALKING, TALKING)
   iii. LAG IN CEREBRAL INTEGRATION
   iv. RETARDED (ENVIRONMENTAL, HOSPITALISM, DELAYED LATERALITY)
   v. UNEVEN (INCLUDES PSEUDOMATURE PATTERNS)

DISORDERS OF EARLY OBJECT RELATIONS

1. AVOIDANCE RESPONSES (e.g., HEAD-TURNING, CRAWLING AWAY)
2. FETISHISM OF INFANCY---ATTACHMENT TO INANIMATE OBJECTS
3. ABSENCE OF MATERNAL SEPARATION RESPONSE (ATYPICAL IF NOT OBSERVED BY THE 9th OR 10th MONTHS)
4. PROLONGED AND UNDUE INFANTILE STRANGER REACTION
5. PROLONGED AND UNDUE INFANTILE SEPARATION REACTION ACCOMPANIED OR REPLACED BY ATYPICAL BEHAVIOR (e.g., SILENT BODY-ROCKING AND TOTAL WITHDRAWAL)

OTHER BODILY (VISCERAL) DISTURBANCES

1. SKIN COMPLAINTS
2. RESPIRATORY COMPLAINTS

Thus, through use and stimulation, functional neural matrices or networks are organized and sensory thresholds are increased [40]. These functional combinations of differentiated elements subserve the organization and regulation of behavior, and their steady development provides for the gains in levels of adaptation, that is, an increase in behavioral plasticity, behavioral regulation, and gains in tolerance for stimulation.

The assumption is made that developmental progress and steady gains in adaptation are being achieved when the following are satisfied by empirical criteria:

1. Decreasing amounts and episodes of undue or prolonged inner strain.

2. Fewer major or persistent behavioral upheavals, breakdowns of behavioral patterns or the loss of their integrity, such as might occur when extreme stimulation overwhelms an infant and leads to a frenzied state.
3. Fewer signs of an habitual use of generalized random hyperactivity, of unusual forms of behavior, or of a reliance on avoidance responses.
4. Fewer and more transient losses of existing functions during stress such as frustration, unless the disuse of a function is associated with the emergence of higher order functions.
5. No indications of developmental arrestations which will deprive the infant of functions yet to emerge.

The appearance of atypical behavior is taken as evidence of a departure from these properties of development. This is observed when normal, useful, and socially desirable patterns of behavior are misused, disrupted, fail to appear, or stop their activity. Thus, when feeding evokes distress, when the sight of a bottle or face leads to avoidance (e.g., facial turning-away and the expression of pain), when in later months an infant displays no relief in reuniting with his mother after a short separation, we can observe the consequences of disrupting forces and discover misuse and loss of functions. Atypical behavior is also observed in the diversion of newly acquired motor skills into depleting and socially useless stereotypical hypermotility patterns. When an infant acquires the motor skills enabling the hand-knee position and crawling but spends inordinate amounts of time body-rocking and only a fleeting moment in crawling, it becomes reasonable to conclude that a new motor pattern needed for exploratory behavior and the expansion of experience has become subverted.

Empirical evidence of atypical behavior is found in disturbed feeding and elimination, in rhythmic hypermotility patterns, in a variety of focal habits, exaggerations of behavior state, and in the faulty development of major sectors or areas of behavior. A list of these phenomena, based on our own observations and the observations reported by other investigators [2, 10, 15, 30, 35, 57, 67, 75, 79], is included in Tables 1a, 1b, and 1c.

MATERNAL BEHAVIOR AND PERSONALITY IN RELATION TO THE ATYPICAL BEHAVIOR OF INFANCY

The responsibility for atypical behavioral development among infants has in part been attributed to inadequate, insufficient, inappropriate, faulty, or abusive infant care and stimulation. It is assumed that such undesirable experiences are due to attributes of the mothers' behavior in their choices of stimulations and infant care techniques used to regulate state, gratify needs, and to comfort. Healthy development is nurtured by the mothers' interactions with the infants' sensorimotor modalities which bring into play sucking, looking, hearing, touching, and awareness of position and movement. By regulating the infants' behavior states, the mothers also protect them from being overwhelmed by extreme inner excitation. In such ways, the stimulation characteristics of infant-mother interactions are thought to effect the characteristics of differentiation, the buildup of sensory thresholds and, consequently, the early development of adaptation.

In summary, maternal behavior is thought to play a major, but not exclusive, part in the stimulation variance through the following processes:

1. The selection of stimulations that the infant receives, thus helping to shape up the sensory environment.
2. The activation of differentiation and maintenance of the functional integrity of neurosensory and neuromotor apparatus through stimulation.
3. The increase and decrease of sensory thresholds with stimulations.
4. The change of behavior states or arousal through stimulation which facilitates, impairs, regulates arousal or dissipates excessive inner tension; such stimulation occurs during pacification or soothing, during attention and alerting behavior. These shifts in arousal constitute an inner source of stimulation.
5. The specific infant care techniques, such as feeding, on visceral and somatic stimulation.

If atypical development can indeed be induced and maintained by insufficient, inappropriate, or extreme stimulation, it seems reasonable that the more favorable environment for the progress of normal differentiation and adaptation is one that provides "rich" stimulation; that is, repeated sensory stimulation of mild or moderate intensity, varied in type with perhaps some balance between constancy and novelty and presented appropriate to the infant's state and needs. The levels of stimulation need to vary but clearly not to include excesses on the high or low side of overstimulation and stimulus deprivation.

It is important to separate out negligence and abuse ascribed to cultural conditions from that due directly to the person responsible for infant care. If neglect is thought of in terms of deficiencies, restrictions, or the absence of specific environmental stimulations and care needed for an infant to thrive, then a number of general and specific circumstances qualify for such conditions. For example, ignorance, famine, and poverty may be irreversible, in any immediate sense, and infant neglect may occur as a consequence. Faulty information combined with insufficient resources for educating an uninformed mother engaged in undesirable infant care practices may also contribute to infant negligence. A mother suffering from a serious mental disorder that includes aparthy, isolation, and disinterest in her environment may create conditions of negligence.[1] In terms of actual experiences, the babies in each of the three conditions may go through very similar, perhaps almost identical, experiences in their care and sensations. This is not to suggest that maternal attitudes and emotions do not influence the characteristics of infant care and stimulation. Rather, the background and personality of a mother might be the roots of negligence or of the failure to respond with warmth and nurturance. Each must be carefully assessed especially if an understanding of the relative importance of their contribution is to be utilized in prevention and treatment. The utilization of a comparative design should aid the discovery of significant differences between mothers and subcultures whose infants thrive and mothers and subcultures whose infants do not thrive.

[1] See the chapter on "The Mutative Impact of Serious Mental and Physical Illness in a Parent on Family Life" by E.J. Anthony, in this book.

It is assumed that a favorable mother-child relationship involves mutual satisfaction and pleasure and that the mother's capacity to recognize and evaluate the needs of her own child, and her ability to achieve gratification within her own unique personality pattern, influence the development of adequate maternal behavior. The importance of childhood events and experiences, such as the mother's own mother-child relationship and the woman's identification with her own mother on subsequent mothering is emphasized by Benedek [8]. The reciprocal element of the mother-child relationship and the importance of the mother's experience is indicated by Benedek's statement that:

> the capacity of the mother to receive from the child, her ability to be consciously gratified by the exchange and to use this gratification unconsciously in her emotional maturation is the specific quality and function of motherliness.

Benedek [8], more so than others, emphasizes the idea that for both infant and mother, developmental processes are intensively interactive and begin at conception. Therefore, an assessment of the mother's adjustment during pregnancy may help anticipate future maternal behavior.

The mother who gains gratification from interaction with her infant is thought to acquire confidence in her mothering abilities; this may greatly influence not only further mother-child interaction, but also aid in the fulfillment of her role as a woman.

A number of reports [21, 26, 77] suggest that the emotional status of mothers during pregnancy significantly affects the infant. Emotional stress and anxiety during pregnancy were associated with less favorable infant adjustment. Gravid infrahuman subjects have been experimentally subjected to extreme stimulations resulting in morphologically damaged offsprings. It is difficult to extrapolate such findings for application to humans. But it is reasonable to seriously entertain the general idea that rather alien emotional and environmental conditions impinging on gravid women, especially during the critical first trimester of pregnancy, may sufficiently alter inner physiological and biochemical conditions and the processes of embryogenesis as to cause untoward events for a developing fetus. The nature of such alterations and the emotional conditions necessary and sufficient to bring them about are not well known or understood in the human.

Some Types of Atypical Behavior in Infancy

The three groups of aberrant behavior most commonly seen are:

Rhythmic hypermotility patterns
A significant lag in the rate of weight gain
Feeding problems, including pica

These are not the only atypical forms of behavior, but they are the predominant ones. In general, the findings reported in the literature are not the result of systematic study and are not correlated with observed infant-mother interactions, which is why our own study was undertaken.

RHYTHMIC (STEREOTYPICAL) HYPERMOTILITY PATTERNS: BODY-ROCKING, HEAD-ROLLING, AND HEAD-BANGING

Most reports of rhythmic hypermotility in infants are of body-rocking and consist of case reports with rather elaborate theoretical statements or of reports on the development of body-rocking in nursery-reared and institutionalized infants [29, 62, 74]. A few of the reports include information on the infant's developmental background and on antecedent behavior and events.

One of the earliest stereotypical motor patterns is *Spasmus nutans* or head-rolling (nodding) usually accompanied by nystagmus. Originating in the earlier months of infancy, the onset of *Spasmus nutans* has been ascribed to inadequate visual stimulation [66], although a clinical study by the author [35] suggests other prior stimulation conditions.

The lack of empirical data on body-rocking and head-banging is in contrast to a rather sizable body of theory [15, 51, 52]. Body-rocking is considered a form of "autoerotic" phenomena, while head-banging is considered a form of "autoaggression." Greenacre [52] and Brody [14] classify body-swaying using subjective designations of affectomotor behavior.

A *normative form,* a bouncing body-rocking, is considered common when the infant is in transition between one state of neuromuscular maturation and another [14, 52]. A *repetitious form* of monotonous rocking is thought to be soothing and "autoerotic." There is an *agitated form* involving rapid, energetic, and excitatory rocking. Thought to be autoaggressive, this body-rocking is accompanied by head-banging. It is thought of as an "autoerotic" behavior pattern (others include thumb-sucking, coprophilia, coprophagia, and genital play) and a consequence of institutional upbringing, since it has been a frequent finding among nursery-reared infants and institutionalized children. Body-rocking is thought to be rare in family-reared infants. Head-banging is occasionally reported, usually for illustrative purposes and as clinical evidence in formulations on the genesis and vicissitude of aggression.

BODY-ROCKING AND INSTITUTIONAL REARING

In his studies on hospitalism [74], Spitz compared the incidence of body-rocking, coprophilia, and genital play ("autoerotic phenomena") among three groups of infants. One hundred and seventy infants were observed in a nursery environment where the mothers remained responsible for their own infant's care within the institution; 61 infants were observed in a second environment, termed "Foundling Home," where infant care was in the hands of nursery personnel and the care was poor; the third group consisted of 17 infants reared within their own families, described as involving "excellent mother-child relations." Of the 170 "nursery" infants, 140 were observed to manifest autoerotic behavior; this included 87 infants who engaged in body-rocking. Spitz concluded that body-rocking and genital play were mutually exclusive, since of the 87 infants displaying rocking, only 7 were observed to engage in genital play. The "Foundling Home" infants exhibited practically no autoerotic behavior, as only 4 infants engaged in body-rocking. Among the family infants, only one of 17 evidenced body-rocking, the remaining 16 were all observed to engage in genital play.

Spitz's data are among the most extensive reported in this area, and the nursery population (institutional, with the mother responsible for care) is particularly pertinent for our studies, since body-rocking was a frequent finding and some data regarding the "nursery" infant mothers are reported. About one-fourth of the mothers of the "nursery" infants with body-rocking were evaluated with psychological tests and were described as generally "infantile, extroverted with alloplastic tendencies, lacking the faculty to control their aggression. . . presenting outbursts of negative emotion, of violent hostility." Spitz observed that the babies were alternately exposed to intense outbursts of love and equally intense outbursts of hostility and rage. The mothers of the "nursery" infants were characteristically inconsistent, impulsive, and subject to swift changes in mood.

From his observations and from developmental tests of the infants, Spitz concluded that the babies were retarded in social adaptation, that is, in their relation to a libidinal object and in their manipulative ability. Spitz [74] interpreted these findings as reflective of faulty object relations and stated that:

> the disturbance with which we were confronted in the case of the children whose main autoerotic activity consists in rocking is one of complete incapacity to form object relations. . .the whole body of the infant is subjected to autoerotic stimulation. The activity is an objectless one. . .

A. Freud reports body-rocking among infants who received excellent care in an institutional nursery. She also refers to autoerotic gratification in the young child, and designates thumb-sucking, body-rocking, and head-knocking. Of the latter two she states that these are "...rare under family conditions. . .what is responsible is evidently the fact of institutional life itself."

PSYCHOANALYTIC CONCEPTUALIZATIONS

Approaching the subject of body-rocking and self-attacking behavior on strictly theoretical grounds, Kris [51, 52] was of the opinion that body-rocking is associated with inadequate maternal stimulation and that autoerotic behavior is linked to an absence of satisfactory ties to the mother. Spitz [72] remarked that aggression must be neutralized and this requires a relationship with the love object. However, a loss of the object, according to Spitz, results in the infant having himself as the only available object and thus self-attacking behavior develops from self-directed aggression. These processes are thought to lead to hyperactivity, autoagressive and externally directed aggressive behavior.

Suggestions have been made that the origins of severe body-rocking can be ascribed to environments which are understimulating and/or overstimulating. The high incidence of body-rocking among infants reared in situations of deprivation and neglect gives support to the idea that insufficient somatic stimulation is an important precondition for severe body-rocking. It has also been suggested that body-rocking can develop in infants exposed to excesses of kinesthetic stimulation while relatively lacking stimulation in other sensory modalities. These are also the conditions in which faulty or insufficient affectional ties with a maternal person emerge. This type of development is viewed as a basis for infants to prefer a heightening of self-stimulation and body-rocking. These are essentially the same as conditions of high arousal and excitation and it is of interest that insufficient stimulation and excesses of stimulation will both increase the levels of arousal. Conditions of high arousal and excitation may lead to diffuse, agitated, rhythmic movements of the whole body. A more moderate type of body-rocking will modulate such behavior in its soothing and lulling effects.

Bringing together ideas from psychoanalytic theory and observations from neurophysiology and infant behavior may provide a way of unifying contributions to enhance our understanding of atypical development. The establishment of credibility, however, rests with appropriate empirical data that describes and defines the sensory environment impinging on the infant and the response characteristics of babies.

FAILURE-TO-THRIVE

The infant who is nonthriving suffers from generalized retarded growth and malnutrition despite the availability of adequate food. The usual criterion is height or weight below the three percentile value for the infant's age and sex [49, 82]. It is characteristic for such infants to gain weight rapidly if, when admitted to a hospital, they receive good care. Failure-to-thrive has been related to low birth weight, birth complications, developmental retardation, and adverse environmental conditions [1, 49, 82]. Congenital heart malformation, cystic fibrosis, hypothyroidism, mental deficiency, and renal disorders have also been found, but it is where we observe no probable physical cause of the growth retardation that psychological variables are of particular importance. Many cases are a complex interaction of physical, nutritional, and psychological factors such as in failure-to-thrive associated with pica and nutritional anemia.

Most reports do not clearly delineate failure-to-thrive from maternal deprivation. Although most studies deal with the occurrence of the syndrome in institutional infants, this syndrome occurs in infants reared at home by their own mothers. Several published cases described the occurrence of failure-to-thrive in infants and children living in families [49] and in these instances, failure-to-thrive has been related to parental neglect and rejection, and to poor infant-mother relations. Disturbances in the mother-child relationship are considered the primary problem, and the failure-to-thrive is thought to reflect resulting "emotional" disturbances on body functioning. Although the circumstances of the families varied, most were of low socioeconomic status. This may well be a sampling bias since most cases are drawn from clinic populations. The marital status of mothers varied; the absence of the father was observed in a number of cases and there are reports of family violence. There is little mention about prenatal events. The mothers are often described as depressed, lacking emotional warmth toward the infant, and unable to provide protective care for the infant. Some of the mothers are also described as anxious, indifferent, rejecting, inadequate, or unable to experience gratification in their maternal role.

From the present literature it appears that "idiopathic" failure-to-thrive is associated with parental neglect, rejection, and depression, but so far the studies have not included controls and have been largely descriptive.

PICA[2]

Pica, or perverted appetite, exists as early as 6 months of age and is a habit of ingesting large quantities of nonnutritious substances. In various instances, pica may be secondary to an organic problem, for example, parasitic disease or malnutrition. In others, however, no organic disturbance can be found, and it is reasonable to assume that, in general, pica has psychological or mental origins. A distinction is made between pica and malacia, the latter being a craving for bizarre foods – but food nonetheless.

Pica is a problem because of the danger of lead poisoning which, when not fatal, may cause severe and permanent brain damage. It is difficult to know how much has been caused by the lead poisoning and how much may have existed prior to the pica. It may well be that brain-damaged children are more susceptible to pica. Such qualifications, however, do not detract from the dangerous pica-lead poisoning relationship. Exact statistics on the true incidence of lead poisoning are hard to find, although one estimate has 112,000 to 225,000 young children contracting lead poisoning each year in the United States. If infections are excluded, lead poisoning is the most common childhood disease in urban communities.

[2]See the chapter "The Child with Pica and His Family" by F. Millican and R. Lourie in this volume.

However, such data remain scanty and very general although pica is considered most prevalent among the poor. The necessary information, including the assessment of pica prevalence in middle and upper socioeconomic groups, remains to be done. The overall incidence of pica in one clinic population was 46 percent in the Black people and 25.5 percent in the White people. Pica was highest in low-income families, and apparently more accepted in families of Black people. Poor economic conditions and faulty housing were associated with the greater availability of paint and plaster chips. In addition, due to their living circumstances, the mothers of children with pica were thought to be unable to watch their children. Another study [41] found low hemoglobin and ascorbic acid in children with pica – but which came first, the pica or anemia, could not be determined. This same study found the following social factors to be significant: unmarried mothers, residential mobility, major familial emotional problems, and poor play facilities. Most cases of paint poisioning in children occur in areas characterized by overcrowded living quarters, by poor economic conditions, by inadequate maintenance of housing, and by nonparental supervision of young children [33].

A Study of Mothers of Atypical Infants

SUBJECTS AND THEIR SELECTION

Mothers and infants were referrals from the out-patient and in-patient service of the Department of Pediatrics. The referrals were made by pediatricians using the following criteria:

1. *Age of infant:* less than 30 months.
2. *Atypical behavior:* one or more of the atypical forms of behavior listed in the tables of atypical behavior (Tables 1a, 1b, and 1c).
3. *Physical health:* no major medical disease, including congenital neural defects and other serious birth abnormalities.
4. *Previous hospitalizations:* no prior hospitalization or institutionalization of longer than two weeks duration.
5. *Maternal separation:* no maternal separations longer than two weeks.

The experimental group consisted of 42 mothers and their infants with atypical behavior. Although they were successive referrals from the Pediatric Services, wo do not know if the sample was random and we do not know how many infants satisfied the above criteria and were not referred. Twenty of them were referred from the pediatric in-patient service.

As controls, we selected 16 male infants who showed no evidence of atypical behavior but who were being seen in the Pediatric Clinic for inguinal hernias prior to surgical repair. Individual mothers of these 16 infants were matched for socioeconomic and marital factors with 16 of the 20 mothers in the experimental group, and their infants were matched for ordinal position.

DATA COLLECTION PROCEDURES

Data on each mother and her infant were collected systematically according to the following protocol:

1. *For each infant*
   a. *Medical data.* Efforts were made to collect all available prenatal, paranatal, and pediatric data including information on physical growth and observations pertinent to accessing overall development.
   b. *Infant Behavior Inventory* (IBI). This is a two-part questionnaire designed to discover and record specific forms of atypical behavior, to trace their chronology, and to determine patterns or combinations of behavior. Part I of the IBI contains 39 items for use with infants up to 6 months of age. Part II contains an additional 28 items and with Part I is administered to infants between the ages of 10 and 24 months.
2. *For assessing maternal attitudes and personality*
   a. *Clinical interviews.* Tape-recorded, semi-structured interviews were designed to learn about the mother's history and family background and to obtain data to permit objectified evaluations of some broad dimensions of personality and maternal attitudes.

b. *Projective psychological tests.* Rorschach, Thematic Apperception, and Draw-A-Person tests were administered to each mother. The data were used to make independent assessments of the mother's motivations and personality structure. Detailed case reports and a predictive interpretation regarding the infant-mother interaction were made for each case.

c. *Personal history questionnaire.* Each mother completed a self-administered questionnaire of more than 100 items which covered several different areas including self, family, medical data, education, interests, and occupational history.

d. *Parent-Child Relations (PCR) Questionnaire.* This questionnaire, developed by Roe and Siegelman [68] was selected to assess the mother's attitudes and feelings toward her own mother. The form contains 130 statements about parental behavior which the mother marks according to its truth concerning her own mother.

3. *For assessing maternal behavior*

a. *Maternal behavior anecdotal descriptions.* Descriptions of interaction between the infant and mother as reported by the mother during interviews.

b. *Motion film-recorded infant-mother interaction in set situations.* Each infant and mother are filmed together following a standard protocol during which a sequence of settings and events occur including:

i. an undirected spontaneous interaction;

ii. a feeding of the infant by the mother;

iii. the presence of a "stranger" with both mother and infant;

iv. the mother leaves the room and the "stranger" is alone with the infant;

v. the "stranger" leaves the room and the infant is left alone; and finally

vi. the mother returns to the room for a reunion scene.

FINDINGS

Four patterns of atypical behavior emerged. One pattern centered about a retarded rate of weight gain and is referred to as the failure-to-thrive syndrome. The second pattern involved pica which was accompanied by lead poisoning. The third pattern consisted of body-rocking and head-banging and is referred to as a patterned hypermotility syndrome. The fourth pattern, with ten atypical forms of behavior, is termed the syndrome of generalized atypicality.

THE FAILURE-TO-THRIVE SYNDROME (N = 26)

The most common characteristic of the experimental infant was a retarded rate of weight gain (see Figure 1). Twenty-six of the 42 infants were classified as failure-to-thrive. Eight of these had persistent and frequent vomiting and regurgitation which may have been significant in the etiology of the insufficient weight gain. Rumination was observed or reported in 4 infants, all of whom suffered from chronic regurgitation. Of 7 infants with anorexia, but without vomiting or regurgitation, 5 cases were in infants with failure-to-thrive.

The failure-to-thrive group also included 4 infants with nutritional anemia, 4 with generalized retardation, and 3 with *Spasmus nutans.* Five of the group were also the victims of parental violence and were diagnosed as battered babies. One of these babies subsequently died of a skull fracture after an assault by its mother. One infant engaged in pica but did not ingest lead-impregnated material.

PICA WITH LEAD POISONING (N = 8)

There were 8 infants with pica and lead poisoning. It is of interest that none were failure-to-thrive by weight and none engaged in body-rocking or head-banging. Three of the 8 pica-lead poisoning infants also had a nutritional anemia. Although there were recent episodes of vomiting in 4 of the group, these were clearly related to the lead poisoning.

PATTERNED HYPERMOTILITY SYNDROME (N = 6)

Of the 6 infants with chronic body-rocking, 5 were also head-bangers and only one qualified as a failure-to-thrive. There was no evidence of concurrent gastrointestinal symptoms or feeding disturbances and there were no pica histories associated with lead poisoning. The one infant with body-rocking and head-banging who was a failure-to-thrive also engaged in coprophagia and trichophagia. *Spasmus nutans* was found as a solitary atypical phenomenon in three infants.

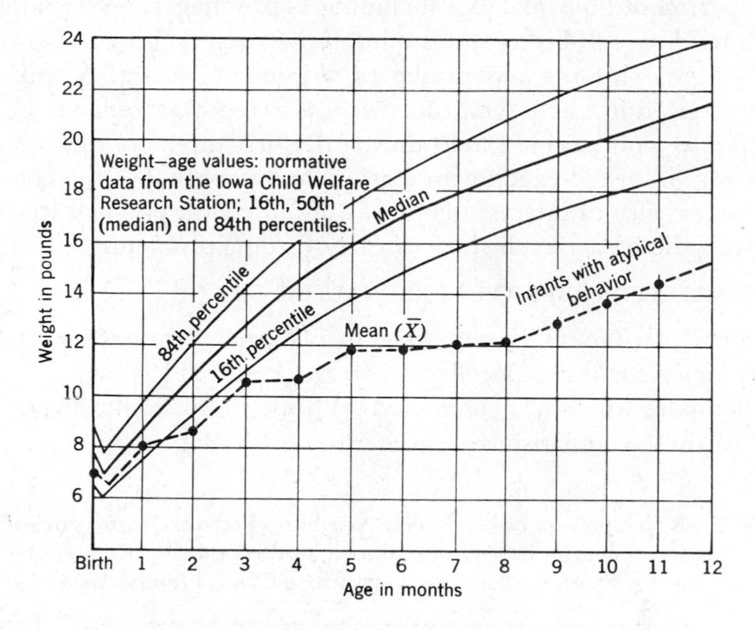

Figure 1 Weight-age relationships from birth to 12 months of age in infants with atypical behavior. The average weights at each month for the M-AI infant Ss are compared with standard weight-age values for controls.

SYNDROME OF GENERALIZED ATYPICALITY

Two infants displayed an array of phenomena which included vomiting and regurgitation, aerophagia, head-banging and body-rocking, trichotillomania, pica including coprophagia and trichophagia, breath-holding, self-biting and rumination as well as failure-to-thrive.

Although 14 infants were presented with complaints of vomiting and regurgitation, these symptoms were also reported to have occurred to a noticeable extent during the first three months of infancy in 33 of the experimental group and in only 2 of the control infants. It is also of interest that 7 of 8 infants with pica and lead poisoning did not give a history of early feeding problems.

MATERNAL ATTITUDES AND PERSONALITY

Maternal Attitudes. A comparison of maternal attitudes was carried out by analyzing the data collected by the Personal History Questionnaire which was completed by both groups of mothers. Some of these comparisons are presented in Table 2.

Table 2 A Comparison of Personality Attributes between Mothers of Infants with Atypical Behavior (M-AI) and Control Mothers (M-CI). Ratings of Personality Variables Are Based on Transcribed Clinical Interviews

PREGNANCY ADJUSTMENT AND MATERNAL ATTITUDE VARIABLES	DIFFERENCES OF STATISTICAL SIGNIFICANCE BETWEEN MOTHER GROUPS (p VALUE)	
	M-AI > M-CI	M-CI > M-AI
1. Number of severe physical symptoms during pregnancy	.05	-
2. "Unhappy-sad" pregnancy	.05	-
3. Similarity between self and own mother	-	.01
4. More similarities like mother than father	-	.05
5. Closeness in characterization of mother	-	.03
6. Perception of mother role	-	.02
7. Child care of affection	-	.01
8. Being needed and activities as source of satisfaction in mother role	-	.01
9. Changes in feelings relevant to having children	-	.03

AN ASSESSMENT OF MATERNAL PERSONALITY

Interview Behavior. In general, the experimental mothers were an apathetic group. They were overtly less active, showed little curiosity, and asked for very little information. They seemed disinterested in the interview, in learning about their infant, or in participating in efforts to get at their babies' problems. They were quite reticent to communicate and were rather unresponsive when questions were posed. Their answers were sparse and if more information was requested, they became irritable, impatient, and reluctant to elaborate. They were without enthusiasm and rarely asked questions of their own.

An Assessment of Some Broad Dimensions of Maternal Personality Using Clinical Interviews. Each tape-recorded clinical interview was transcribed and each maternal subject was assessed on nine 5-point scales by two of four raters.[3] The scales included the following:

Defense organization was based on an assessment of the predominant modes of defense, the degree of flexibility and stability of defense functions, and on the hierarchy of defense operations.

Reality testing was rated on the basis of evidence of intactness, deficiencies, distortions, or confusions.

Capacity for self-observation was assessed on the evidence of the mother engaging in self-scrutiny and introspection.

Frustration tolerance was rated on the evidence of overall ability to tolerate frustration in general, as well as specific frustrations.

Degree of self-object differentiation was rated on the evidence of achievement of structural development with autonomy, stability, and self-awareness.

Anxiety tolerance was rated on an overall estimate of the capacity for tolerating anxiety.

Self-concept was rated on the evidence of the mother's overall attitude toward herself, her self-esteem, and her feelings of adequacy and worthfulness.

Capacity for emotional involvement with others was rated on the mother's ability to engage in relationships with her children and others.

[3]The clinicians who rated each maternal subject included John G. Loesch, M.D., Pamela J. Haley, M.A., Nahman H. Greenberg, M.D., and Joan Klonowski, M.D.

With the exception of anxiety tolerance, which failed to differentiate the two groups of mothers, the control mothers were rated as stronger on the other broad dimensions of personality. The results are summarized in Table 3.

Table 2 A Comparison of Pregnancy Adjustment and Maternal Attitude Variables between Mothers of Infants with Atypical Behavior (M-AI) and Control Mothers (M-CI). Ratings of Pregnancy Adjustment and Maternal Attitude Variables Are Based on Completed Personal History Questionnaires (Parent Information Form II)

PERSONALITY VARIABLE	DIFFERENCES OF STATISTICAL SIGNIFICANCE BETWEEN MOTHER GROUPS (p VALUE)	
	M-AI > M-CI	M-CI > M-AI
1. Defense organization	-	.02
2. Capacity for self-observation	-	.05
3. Reality testing	-	.05
4. Frustration tolerance	-	.05
5. Degree of self-object differentiation	-	.02
6. Anxiety tolerance	-	-
7. Self-image or concept of self	-	.05
8. Overall adaptation	-	.05
9. Capacity for emotional involvement with others	-	.02

A RORSCHACH STUDY OF MOTHERS OF INFANTS WITH ATYPICAL BEHAVIOR

Maternal personality studies have generally been conducted with mothers of older atypical children using nonprojective instruments such as the Minnesota Multiphasic Personality Inventory [31, 32]. Projective instruments such as the Rorschach do not lend themselves readily to objective quantitative methods of content analysis. Although aware of this major issue, we elected to use the Rorschach with the initial sample of mothers because of the rich source of data on the maternal personality which we expected would be generated.

The experimental group consisted of 29 of the 42 mothers. The control group consisted of a sample of 30 women employed at a mail order house; they were drawn from a larger population of normal women forming the subjects of an earlier study [7] and matched to the experimental group for age, education, and socioeconomic class.

The experimental group was administered the Rorschach under the standardized conditions advocated by Beck [7] and scored according to the system utilized by him; each protocol was independently scored by the two psychologists[4] experienced with the Rorschach and scored a third time to rule out clerical errors and reconcile differences in the application of scoring rules. The protocols of the control group obtained from the earlier study by Beck were checked by the psychologists to insure that they were scored according to the same rules applied to the experimental group.

The Beck scores of the two groups were found to differ significantly, by *t* test, on four of the Rorschach determinants: R, F+%, A%, and P. These data are presented in Table 4.

Table 4 Rorschach Variates Differentiating the Mothers of Infants with Atypical Behavior from Control Mothers

MATERNAL Ss	N	R		F+%		A%		P	
		$\bar{X}$	s^2	$\bar{X}$	s^2	$\bar{X}$	s^2	$\bar{X}$	s^2
OF ATYPICAL INFANTS	29	24.17	90.06	74.79	157.00	52.90	259.21	5.66	1.86
OF CONTROL INFANTS	30	28.53	100.2	82.77	107.33	48.73	298.94	6.57	4.80
t SCORES		1.72		2.66		0.96		1.92	

The lower R of the experimental group reflects reduced expressiveness and less intellectual investment in the environment. The F+% indicates their somewhat less effective intellectualized approach in maintaining reality contact. Their higher A% indicates a lower scope of flexibility of imagination, and their lower P represents less conformity with conventional percepts.

THE PARENT-CHILD RELATIONS (PCR) QUESTIONNAIRE

The 130 items of the PCR are scored on ten scales which include loving, protecting, demanding, rejecting, neglecting, casualness, rewarding (symbolic, love), rewarding (direct, object), punishing (symbolic, love), and punishing (direct, object). Using the PCR scales, the experimental and control mothers were compared on their estimations of the relationships with their own mothers or mother surrogates.

[4]The psychologists were Jesse Hurley, M.S. and Robert Lipgar, Ph.D.

By the t test and the f test (analysis of variance), the categories rejecting, demanding, neglecting, and punishing (direct, object) were judged significantly different at the .05 level between the two groups of mothers. The mothers of infants with atypical behavior described their own mothers or mother surrogates as rejecting and demanding, neglectful, and physically punitive.

SUMMARY OF ATTITUDINAL STUDIES

Our data lead us to the unavoidable conclusion that all of the experimental mothers suffered from serious emotional disturbances and with few exceptions could be classified as borderline, pre-psychotic, severe character disorder, and psychotic. In assessing their personalities, we were impressed by the limited range of defenses, the inflexibility, the severely impaired judgment and the poor reality testing. Clinically, while many appeared depressed, most seemed distant, apathetic, withdrawn, and impoverished. They showed little empathy and closeness, and gratifying relations with other adults were almost nonexistent.

Their fantasy life was usually sparse and most often consisted of rather primitive notions and fears with hostility and violence as the essential features of bizarre oral thoughts. Much of their energy seemed devoted to keeping control of their feelings and overt behavior. The world was often portrayed as crude and cruel, a place where people get stung, neglected, gobbled up, hurt, and taken advantage of as they consciously express a desire for trust, nurturance, and closeness. The surface of well-behaved, compliant, quiet, and meek adults was in contrast to these other forces residing just beneath the surface. These mothers impressed us as being severely hostile, yet they were clearly unable to acknowledge hostile impulses and were amazingly unaware that this was a pervasive feature of their personality and of their mood. This was an unmistakable feature even in the five mothers whose infants were the victims of maternal violence and suffered enough severe physical injury to qualify them as battered babies.

MATERNAL BEHAVIOR AND INFANT-MOTHER INTERACTIONS

Patterns of maternal behavior have been investigated by a variety of methods and from many perspectives [84]. In conceptualizing infant development as stages in differentiation and adaptation, maternal behavior is assumed to contribute a major source of the stimulation variance which influences the development of behavioral plasticity, behavioral regulation, and stimulation tolerance.

This section contains a summary of findings from analyses of motion-filmed samples of infant-mother interactions.

SPONTANEOUS AND UNDIRECTED INTERACTION

Play. Distinct differences in the behavior of the two groups of mothers were readily observed during the initial 10 minutes of filmed interaction recorded in an undirected and unstructured situation. The mothers of both groups tended to rely on various toys and dolls, which were available in the room, to occupy the time. The quality of play interaction differed significantly between the two groups of pairs.

The play interaction of the control pairs consisted of mothers and infants doing it together. Play was organized, the mothers were matter-of-fact and, although the play objects were unfamiliar, play itself was not. There was an abundance of chatter from the mother and some cheerfulness. A few toys and dolls were all that were needed to allow satisfactory play. The mothers had no difficulty in maintaining an interest in the situation or in observing their baby. There was an organized quality to the play behavior and time was spent on specific activities.

The interactions of the experimental pairs were quite different. These mothers were either very busy or very inactive and uninvolved. Some mothers alternated between the two behaviors. Four of them remained completely inactive and unresponsive during the initial 10 minutes of filming. The remainder spent the time in sporadic, inconsistent, and poorly organized play. Toys and dolls were not selected from the toybox. Instead, all the toys and dolls were gone through in rapid succession. Attention shifted quickly from one object to another and each change was greeted by exaggerated expressions of interest and enthusiasm followed promptly by the usual blandness.

Facial and Other Expressive Behavior. The facial expressions of the experimental mothers were stereotypical and fixed. Two of these mothers had masklike expressions with little or no facial movement and no glimmer of a smile at any time. Another extreme were the mothers from the same group who displayed a standardized cheerful smile, even as they talked angrily to their babies.

The voices of all these mothers were usually subdued, sometimes inaudible, and usually flat – except when their anger was directed at the infants. When this occurred, their expressionless masks were temporarily lifted.

Gross body movements were restrained and they frequently became immobile if not rigid. Animated behavior was not observed at all. Occasional intense expressions showed themselves as they addressed their babies with negative words and phrases such as "no-no," "you're bad," and "are you getting mad." Although restricted in gross movements, these mothers engaged in an inordinate number of small motor movements; hands busily manipulated small objects, nails were bitten, and lip smacking was prominent.

Some Attributes of Stimulation. A striking feature of 7 experimental mothers was their undisguised and repetitious physical overstimulations. These included moderate slapping, playing biting, mild hitting, vigorous rubbing, harsh stroking, tight grasping, poking, nibbling and a great deal of grooming; all of which were directed to various parts of the infants' body.

Stranger, Separation and Reunion Sets. There were 6 control and 7 experimental infant-mother pairs where the infants were all 9 months of age or older. All the control infants responded to the appearance of the stranger with apprehension and moved closer to their mother; they all cried when their mothers left the room and continued to cry but with varying intensity. They all looked at the door of the room although not all made an effort to go to the door. Their mother's return was greeted with diminution or cessation of crying.

The responses of the experimental infants were less uniform and included withdrawal, avoidance behavior, body-rocking, ordinary crying, severe crying to the extent of shrieking, and sometimes no change in behavior at all. Reunion with the mothers also produced a variety of responses. The infants who were most distressed demonstrated relief. The infants who appeared to have no reaction to their mothers leaving were equally casual to their return, and the body-rocking baby stopped body-rocking on the return of his mother.

Conclusions

This report contains selected findings from a group of studies on the behavior and development of infants with atypical behavior. The results indicate an interaction between atypical behavior in the infants, serious abnormalities in the personality of the mothers, and patterns of maternal care which ranged from neglect and kinesthetic understimulation to robust and sometimes abusive overstimulation. Although certain characteristics of child-rearing and family relationships may be more prevalent among the poor, the results of these studies indicate that if infant atypical behavior is used as a measure of the consequences of inadequate, faulty, or abusive care and stimulation, the fact of economic hardship or poverty is not sufficient to account for the patterns of atypical development and child care which were observed. This does not rule out the possibility of such conditions being more prevalent among the very poor. Indeed, the recent findings from studies of nutritional inadequacies, malnourishment, and starvation among infants and young children in the United States indicate that this may very well be the case. The need is for careful sampling of subjects so that both major culture and subculture variables can be discriminated and their effects measured.

It is unfortunate but true that developmental problems of infancy are often not recognized or they are ignored or their importance minimized. Too often, the problems are dismissed with the prognostic misrepresentation – "he will grow out of it" – a statement which has little if any empirical support. There is no proof that the remission of atypical behaviors indicates the restoration of healthy development. We are not sufficiently alert to early indicators of developmental difficulties and, in spite of our conviction of the importance of early influences on development and later personality, we do not, in general, utilize principles of early intervention to prevent the continuity and buildup of atypical processes. If atypicality were identified early, intervention could perhaps be shorter and more enduring. The nature of intervention programs should depend on empirical evidence and sound principles of development.

Bibliography

1. Adelson, L., Homicide by starvation: the nutritional variant of the "battered child", *Journal of the American Medical Association,* 186, No. 5 (1963), 104-106.
2. Anthony, E. J., Stress in Childhood, in *The Nature of Stress Disorders,* Thomas, Springfield, 1958.
3. Bain, K., The physically abused child, *Pediatrics,* 31, No. 6, (1963), 895-897.
4. Bayley, N., and E. S. Schaefer, Relationship between socioeconomic variables and the behavior of mothers toward young children, *Journal of Genetic Psychology,* 96 (1960), 61.
5. Beach, F. A. and J. Jaynes, Effects of early experiences upon behavior of animals, *Psychol. Bull.,* 51 (1954), 239.
6. Beck, S. J., *The Rorschach Experiment,* Grune and Stratton, New York, 1960.
7. Beck, S. J., *Rorschach's test, Vol. I., Basic Processes,* 2nd ed., rev., Grune and Stratton, New York, 1949.
8. Benedek, T., Toward the biology of the depressive constellation, *Journal of the American Psychoanalytic Association,* 4 (1956), 389.
9. Bennett, E. L., M. C. Diamond, D. Krech, and M. R. Rosenzweig, Chemical and anatomical plasticity of brain, *Science,* 146 (1964), 610-619.
10. Bergman, P. and S. K. Escalona, Unusual sensitivities in very young children, *The Psychoanalytic Study of the Child,* 3/4 (1949).
11. Berlin, I. N., The emotional and learning problems of the socially and culturally deprived child, *Mental Hygiene,* 50 (1966), 340.
12. Bloom, B. S., *Stability and Change in Human Characteristics,* John Wiley and Sons, New York, 1964.
13. Blue, M. T., The battered child syndrome from a social work viewpoint, *Canadian Journal of Public Health,* 56 (1965), 197-198.
14. Brody, S., Signs of disturbances in the first year of life, *American Journal of Orthopsychiatry,* 28 (1958), 362.
15. Brody, S., Self-rocking in infancy, *Journal of American Psychoanalytic Association,* 8 (1960), 464.
16. Bronfenbrenner, U., Toward a Theoretical Analysis of Parent-Child Relationships in a Social Context, in *Parental Attitudes and Child Behavior,* John Glidewell, Ed., Thomas Springfield, 1961.
17. Caldwell, B., and J. Richmond, Programmed day care for the very young child: a preliminary report. *Journal of Marriage and the Family,* 26 (1964), 481.
18. Cebak, V. and R. Najdanvic, Effects of undernutrition in early life on physical and mental development, *Archives of Disease of Children,* 40 (1965), 432.
19. Chilman, S., Child-rearing and family relationship patterns of the very poor, *Welfare in Review,* 3 (1965), 9.
20. Chilman, S., *Growing Up Poor:* an overview and analysis of child-rearing and family life patterns associated with poverty, U.S. Department of Health, Education, and Welfare, Welfare Administration, Division of Research, Washington, D.C. 20221, 1966.

21. Davids, A., R. H. Holden, and G. B. Gray, Maternal anxiety during pregnancy and adequacy of mother and child adjustment eight months following birth, *Child Development*, 24 (1963), 993.
22. Davis, W. A. and R. J. Havinghurst, Social class and color difference in child-rearing, *American Sociological Review*, 11 (1946), 698.
23. Downs, Elinor R., Nutritional dwarfing. A syndrome of early protein-calorie malnutrition, *American Journal of Clinical Nutrition*, 15 (1964), 275.
24. Elizur, A., Content analysis of the Rorschach with regard to anxiety and hostility, *Rorschach Res. Exch.*, 13 (1949), 247-284.
25. Escalona, S., Feeding disturbances in very young children, *American Journal of Orthopsychiatry*, 15 (1945), 76.
26. Ferreira, A. J., The pregnant woman's emotional attitude and its reflection the newborn, *American Journal of Orthopsychiatry*, 30 (1960), 553.
27. Forgus. R. H., Early visual and motor experiences as determiners of complex maze learning ability under rich and reduced stimulation, *Journal of Comparative and Physiological Psychology*, 48 (1955a), 215-220.
28. Freud, A., Contribution of psychoanalysis to genetic psychology, *American Journal of Orthopsychiatry*, 21 (1951).
29. Freud, A. and D. Burlingham, *Infants Without Families*, International Universities Press, New York, 1944.
30. Gardner, G. E., Problems of early infancy, *Journal of American Psychoanalytic Association*, 3 (1955), 506.
31. Goodstein, S. and V. N. Rowley, A further study of MMPI differences between parents of disturbed and nondisturbed children, *J. Consult, Psychol.*, 25 (1961), 460.
32. Goodstein, S. and V. N. Rowley, MMPI profiles of the parents of behaviorally disturbed children and parents from the general population, *J. Clin. Psychol.*, 22 (1966), 39.
33. Griggs, R. C., I. Sunshine, V. A. Newill, B. W. Newton, S. Buchanan, and C. A. Rasch, Environmental Factors in childhood lead poisoning, *Journal of the American Medical Association*, 187 (1964), 703.
34. Greenberg, N. H., Studies in psychosomatic differentiation during infancy, *Archives of General Psychiatry*, 7 (1962), 17.
35. Greenberg, N. H., Origins of head-rolling (spasmus nutans) during early infancy, *Psychosomatic Medicine*, 26 (1964), 162.
36. Greenberg, N. H., Developmental effects of stimulation during early infancy: some conceptual and methodological considerations, *Annals of the New York Academy of Sciences*, 118, 21 (1965), 831-59.
37. Greenberg, N. H., Infant-mother interactional studies: I. The use and method of analysis of cinematographic recordings made in a set (standard) situation, in preparation.
38. Greenberg, N. H. Infant-mother interactional studies: III. A Comparison of interactions between atypical infant-mother and normal infant-mother pairs, in preparation.
39. Greenberg, N. H. The construction and application of an infant behavior inventory for the developmental assessment of infants from birth through two years of age, in preparation.
40. Greenberg, N. H. An adaptional model of infant development, in preparation.

41. Haughton, J. G., Nutritional anemia of infancy and childhood, *American Journal of Public Health,* 53 (1963), 1121-26.
42. Hebb, D. O., The effects of early experience on problem-solving at maturity, *American Psychologist,* 2 (1947), 306-7.
43. Heider, G. M., Vulnerability in infants and young children: a pilot study, *Genetic Psychology Monographs,* 73 (1966), 216.
44. Hunt, McV., *Toward the Prevention of Incompetence in Research Contribution from Psychology to Community Mental Health,* J. W. Carter, Jr. Ed., Behavioral Publications, Inc., New York, 1968.
45. Hymovitch, B., The effects of experimental variations in early experience on problem-solving in the rat, *Journal of Comparative and Psychiological Psychology,* 45 (1952), 313-21.
46. Jacobziner, H., H. Rich, N. Bleiberg, and R. Merchant, How well are well children? *American Journal of Public Health and the Nation's Health,* 53 (1963), 1937-1952.
47. Kantor, M., J. C. Glidewell, I. N. Mensh, H. Darnlee, and M. Gildea, Socioeconomic level and maternal attitudes toward parent-child relations, *Human Organization,* 16 (1958), 44.
48. Keller, S., The social world of the urban slum child: some early findings, *American Journal of Orthopsychiatry,* 33 (1963), 823.
49. Kohler, E. E. and T. A. Good, The infant who fails to thrive, *Hospital Practice* (1969) 54-61.
50. Kohn, M. L., Social class and parental values, *American Journal of Sociology,* 64 (1959), 337-51.
51. Kris, E., Some comments and observations of early autoerotic activities, *Psychoanalytic Study of the Child,* 6 (1951), 95-116.
52. Kris, E., Problems of infantile neurosis: panel discussion, *Psychoanalytic Study of the Child,* 9 (1956).
53. Lesser, G. S., Mental abilities of children from different social-class and cultural groups, *Monographs of the Society of Research in Child Development,* Serial No. 102/30 (1965), 1-114.
54. Leitch, M., and S. Escalona, The reaction of infants to stress, *The Psychoanalytic Study of the Child,* 3/4 (1949), 121.
55. Littman, R. A., R. A. Moore, and J. Peerce-Jones, Social class differences in child-rearing, a third community, *American Sociological Review,* 22 (1957), 294-704.
56. Loesch, J. G. and N. H. Greenberg, Patterns of maternal behavior during early infancy, *presented at the Annual Meetings, American Psychiatric Association,* Los Angeles, Calif., 1964.
57. Lourie, R. S., Studies in bed rocking, head banging and related rhythmic patterns, *Clin. Proc. Child. Hosp.,* Washington, D.C. 5 (1949), 295.
58. Maccoby, E. E. and P. K. Gibbs, Methods of Child-Rearing in Two Social Classes, in *Readings in Child Development,* W. E. Martin and C. B. Stendler, Eds., Harcourt Brace, New York, 1954.
59. Murstein, B. I., The projection of hostility on the Rorschach, and as a result of ego-threat, *Journal of Projective Technique,* 20 (1956), 418-28.
60. Orshanky, M. Children of the poor, *Social Security Bulletin,* 26, 7 (1963), 3-12.

61. Pavenstedt, E., A comparison of the child-rearing environment of upper-lower and very low-lower class families, *American Journal of Orthopsychiatry,* 35 (1965), 89-98.
62. Provence, S. and R. C. Lipton, *Infants in Institutions,* International Universities Press, New York, 1962.
63. Putnam, M. C., B. Bank, and S. Kaplan, Notes on John I.: A case of primal depression in an infant, *Psychoanalytic Study of the Child,* 6 (1951), 38-57.
64. Putnam, M. C., Case study of an atypical two-and-a-half year old, *American Journal of Orthopsychiatry,* 18 (1948).
65. Rank, B., M. C. Putnam, and G. Rochlin, The significance of "emotional climate" in early feeding difficulties, *Psychosomatic Medicine,* 10 (1948), 279-283.
66. Riesen, A., Stimulation as a requirement for growth and function in behavioral development, in *Functions of Varied Experiences,* D. Fiske and S. Maddie, Eds., Dorsey Press, Homewood, Ill., 1961.
67. Richmond, J. B., Some direct observations of disordered behavior in infants, presented in panel on "Classical Forms of Neuroses in infancy and Early Childhood," *Journal of American Psychoanalytic Association,* 10 (1962), 571.
68. Roe, A., A parent child relations questionnaire, *Child Development,* 34 (1963), 355.
69. Schaffer, R. R. and W. M. Callender, Psychologic effects of hospitalization in infancy, *Pediatrics,* 24 (1959), 528.
70. Skeels, H. M., Adult status of children with contrasting early life experiences, *Monographs of the Society for Research in Child Development,* 31, No. 3, (1966), Serial No. 105, 1-65.
71. Spitz. R., Anxiety in infancy: a study of its manifestations in the first year of life, *International Journal of Psychoanalysis,* 31 (1950), 138.
72. Spitz, R. and K. M. Wolf, Autoerotism: some empirical findings and hypotheses on three of its manifestation, *Psychoanalytic Study of the Child,* 3/4 (1949).
73. Spitz, R., Anaclitic depression, *Psychoanalytic Study of the Child,* 2 (1946), 313-42.
74. Spitz, R. Hospitalism: an inquiry into the genesis of psychiatric conditions in early childhood, *Psychoanalytic Study of the Child,* 1 (1945), 33-72.
75. Spitz, R., The psychogenic disease in infancy, *Psychoanalytic Study of the Child,* 6 (1951), 255-274.
76. Stone, L. J., A critique of studies of infant isolation, *Child Development,* 25 (1954), 9.
77. Wallin, R. and R. P. Riley, Reactions of mothers to pregnancy and adjustment of offspring in infancy, *American Journal of Orthopsychiatry,* 20 (1950), 616.
78. Walters, J. and R. Cannon, Interaction of mothers and children from lower-class families, *Child Development,* 35 (1964), 433-440.
79. Weil, A. P., Some evidence of deviational development in infancy and early childhood, *Psychoanalytic Study of the Child,* 11 (1956), 292.
80. White, M. S., Social class, child-rearing practices, and child behavior, *American Sociological Review,* 22 (1957), 704-712.

81. White, B. L. and R. Held, Plasticity of sensorimotor development in the human infant, in J. F. Rosenblith and W. Allinsmith Eds. *The Causes of Behavior: Readings in Child Development and Educational Psychology*, 2nd ed., Allyn and Bacon, Boston, 1966.
82. Widdowson, E. M., Mental contentment and physical growth, *The Lancet CCLX*, 1316 (1951).
83. Wortis, L. J. Child-rearing practices in a low socioeconomic group, *Pediatrics*, 32 (1963), 298-307.
84. Yarrow, L. J., Research in dimensions of early maternal care, *Merrill-Palmer Quart. Behav. and Devel.*, 9 (1963), 101-114.
85. Zemlick, M. J. and Watson, R.I., Maternal attitudes of acceptance and rejection during and after pregnancy, *American Journal of Orthopsychiatry*, 23 (1953), 570.

Temperament and Children at Risk

Stella Chess (U. S. A.)

The early identification of children with a high risk if developing a behavior disorder is obviously crucial for preventive psychiatry. Once a child's vulnerability is recognized, we can take measures to minimize or eliminate environmental stresses that may exceed his adaptive capacity. A timely management program can support the youngster in areas of functioning where he is most susceptible to emotional strain. Yet all too often the assessment of risk comes late, and treatment starts after needless damage has already resulted from a dissonant interaction between the child and his surroundings. Inappropriate handling by parents and teachers may have converted the risk into reality.

There is also an opposite danger. If the psychiatrist too readily assigns a high-risk label, he may produce the iatrogenic stress of unnecessary interventions or he may shield the child from demands that he can master constructively. Not every deviation from normal development represents a risk of disturbance. A behavior pattern can be unusual without being abnormal. Therefore, while one must be alert to every possible clue of vulnerability, one must also avoid trigger-happy diagnoses of pathology.

A child is more likely to be at risk if he has characteristics that make it difficult for him to cope with the demands and expectations usually present in his sociocultural environment. A number of these

***This investigation was supported by Grant MH-03614 from the National Institute of Mental Health.**

characteristics have been delineated in many studies—developmental lags, perceptual deficits, brain damage, physical handicaps, dyslexia, and so on. To these categories of risk, now widely recognized, I would add a less familiar concept: vulnerability associated with traits of temperament.

The term temperament, as used here, refers to the behavioral style of an individual child—the *how* (manner) of his behavior rather than the *what* (content) or *why* (motivation). Every child has a characteristic way of reacting to new persons or situations, for example. Each has a typical level of energy expenditure or an individual threshold of response to sensory stimuli. Temperament, then, is not a pathological state but a normal aspect of psychological functioning.

In a number of studies, my colleagues and I have identified specific attributes in children, beginning with the first few weeks of life [3]. We have also traced the influence of these characteristics on both normal and deviant development [4]. The most extensive of these investigations, the New York Longitudinal Study, has involved a sample of 136 children from middle-class families. Other studies still in progress deal with children from Puerto Rican working-class families, children born prematurely, and children with congenital rubella. In addition, the influence of temperament on the behavior problems of a group of 52 mentally retarded children has been explored [2].

We have found that certain attributes and patterns of temperament are more likely than others to make a child vulnerable to a damaging interaction with his environment. Although temperament in itself neither produces nor prevents a behavior disorder, alertness to its role may suggest preventive programs to decrease the probability of a behavior disorder and to strengthen the chances for optimal adaptation.

Temperament may be assessed in terms of nine categories of reactivity. Their relationship to risk for developing a behavior disorder will be discussed first in terms of the traits considered as independent variables and then in terms of clusters or constellations of traits that constitute vulnerability to stress. The individual categories are now discussed.

Categories of Temperament

ACTIVITY LEVEL

The activity level is the motor component in a child's functioning and the diurnal proportion of active and inactive periods. In general, children with a high activity level present more problems of management than do children of moderate or low activity. They may dash across a room so vigorously that they hurt themselves or knock other children over, leaving behind a trail of broken objects. Energetic motility as a temperamental trait is not to be confused with hyperactivity reflecting abnormal neurological functioning or other pathological conditions. But even though high activity is not abnormal, it may be most inconvenient to parents and teachers. If they constantly react with irritation and scolding, a dissonant interaction is set in motion. Unrealistic demands for restraint of motor activity create a dilemma for the child, who is considered "bad" unless he sits still or moves slowly, a task that is difficult or impossible for him. Punished for his apparently willful infraction of the rules, he may conclude that all attempts to please are futile and he may in fact become habitually disobedient.

Children with a markedly low activity level are easy to care for in infancy. Later, however, this attribute may arouse parental displeasure because it interferes with the household schedule. The child, regarded as dull and inept, may be pressured and teased. An impatient mother may find it easier to dress the slow-moving child herself than to wait for him. With such an approach, his slowness can give way to inertia as he allows others to do things for him.

RHYTHMICITY

Rhythmicity is the regularity and predictability of such functions as hunger-feeding patterns, elimination, and the sleep-wake cycle. This feature of temperament has special pertinence for risk during infancy. Some children manifest such erratic sleep-wake patterns, for example, that their parents find it difficult to keep to their own working schedules. While it is natural and reasonable to attempt a structuring of the cycle, rigidity on the parents' part may exacerbate the problem by creating excessive stress for the child. With regard to feeding habits and toilet training too, the child with biological irregularity is more likely than others to be vulnerable in a culture as clock-conscious as ours.

While the child with great regularity is easier to handle, he may under certain circumstances present another kind of problem. When his parents have to make changes in their schedules, it is difficult to modify his rhythm of functioning. For this child, sudden demands for "flexibility" may be stressful.

APPROACH OR WITHDRAWAL

This represents the nature of the response to a new stimulus, such as an unfamiliar food, toy, or person. Some youngsters move at once into positive interaction with new circumstances, while others retreat from whatever is unfamiliar. The child who initially withdraws from new aspects of his environment may be pressured to accept a new food or school or playmate before he is ready to do so. His temperamental attribute may be mislabeled "negativism" and misinterpreted as obstinacy or a wish to flout his parents. The stressful interaction may intensify the difficulty. Withdrawal from new stimuli makes for greater vulnerability when combined with such temperamental qualities as intensity of response and negative mood, to be discussed below.

ADAPTABILITY

Adaptability is the speed and ease with which current behavior can be modified in response to altered environmental structuring. This category does not refer to the initial response to a new situation but to the possibility of changing a behavior pattern in the direction desired by the parents or others. Many children require repeated exposures to new experiences before they can make a positive adaptation. If given the chance to familiarize themselves with a new bed or a new school routine, they will adapt in time. But if the novel experience is repeated only intermittently, often after a long gap of time, the youngster may manifest his initial withdrawal response on each new exposure.

A child who has learned to adapt to the school experience in general may react negatively for a brief period at the beginning of the new school year or when a change is made in schools or in teaching personnel. A very bright but slowly adaptable child may be misjudged by a teacher as slow to learn. The pressure for speedy adaptation can produce a most stressful learning situation in such a child.

QUALITY OF MOOD

This category considers the amount of pleasant, joyful, or friendly behavior as contrasted with unpleasant, unfriendly behavior or crying. The normal youngster may react positively, negatively, or neutrally to speech stimuli, sensory events, playground experiences, and so forth. If a child's mood is predominantly negative—that is, if he tends to react to difficulties with whining and fussing—he is more likely to provoke the displeasure of parents and peers, increasing the chances for dissonant interaction.

INTENSITY OF REACTION

This measures the energy level of response, irrespective of its quality or direction. Children may be characteristically mild or intense in their expressions of mood. The mild children smile gently to express pleasure, or squeak slightly to communicate displeasure. The predominantly intense children shriek more often than they whine, give belly laughs more often than they smile. An intense 3-year-old child may express his disappointment not with a whimper, but with a bang. The intense reactions of such youngsters are not necessarily an index of how important a particular activity may be for them. Their reactions tend to have an "all or nothing" quality, with little modulation.

Such intensity, when combined with negative mood or initial withdrawal, for example, might be misinterpreted as anxiety or hostility, thus leading to inappropriate intervention. On the other hand, a child with mild reactions may be wrongly regarded as unresponsive or apathetic.

THRESHOLD OF RESPONSIVENESS

This is the intensity level of stimulation required to evoke a discernible response to sensory stimuli, environmental objects, and social contacts.

Some children are exquisitely aware of minor variations in taste, odor, visual, and auditory clues. On the other hand, there are children who may not notice the ringing of a bell while they are busy eating or who seem not to be sensitive to differences of tastes in food.

In our longitudinal study, threshold of responsiveness did not appear to be a significant index of risk. Some investigators, however, have noted the pathological implications of unusual sensitivities [1].

DISTRACTIBILITY

Distractibility is the effectiveness of extraneous environmental stimuli in interfering with or in altering the direction of the ongoing behavior. For the child who is easily diverted by peripheral or chance happenings, task completion may be difficult. This is especially true if the youngster is also nonpersistent—that is, if he finds it hard to return to an activity once it has been interrupted. The child's age also affects the degree to which his distractibility constitutes a vulnerability factor. In early childhood, the failure to finish a job, such as setting the table or putting away toys, is unlikely to provoke parental wrath unless the family places so much value on a "sense of responsibility" that any task left undone becomes the occasion for a lecture or punishment. It is when the child reaches school age that distractibility can become a serious issue leading to an excessively stressful child–environment interaction.

It should be noted that distractibility may also have certain positive consequences, given the right conditions. By making the child responsive to a wide range of stimuli, it may contribute to a high level of alertness and an awareness of the nuances of other people's behavior and feelings.

ATTENTION SPAN AND PERSISTENCE

This represents the length of time a particular activity is pursued, and its continuation in the face of obstacles to maintaining the activity direction. The child with long attention span will stick to a task for an extended period of time. If he is persistent he may or may not stick to the activity uninterruptedly, but if there are interruptions he will keep returning to it.

The child with a short attention span and little persistence may give up an activity too easily at the first sign of failure. Whether he does so silently, noisily, by jumping up actively, throwing an object, or retreating to thumb in mouth and body-rocking, will depend on his other behavioral qualities. In any case, his low attention span and persistence may place him at risk for a harmful interaction, whether at home or in school.

A high degree of persistence may also become a source of stress, depending on specific circumstances. Persistent children are usually selective in the activities they concentrate on, such as: sports, social activities, or reading. Whether their persistence makes for a positive or negative interaction with others hinges on whether the areas of persistence meet the approval of parents, teachers, or peers. A child's persistent interest in reading may delight certain parents who would regard his efforts to get them to buy a new football as "nagging." Thus, persistence most dramatically illustrates the principle that a temperamental quality may evoke either praise or disapproval, according to the values of the sociocultural environment.

Thus far we have been dealing with each of the nine characteristics of temperament as an independent variable. Actually, of course, these attributes do not exist in isolation from one another. Within the living organism they must be examined in terms of their interrelationships. The individual child may be identified by a constellation of traits. Let us look at three major clusters of temperamental traits.

Traits of Temperament in Three Major Clusters

EASY CHILDREN

Some youngsters are preponderantly positive in mood, highly regular, readily adaptable, low or mild in the intensity of their reactions, and unusually affirmative in their approach to new situations. As infants they quickly establish predictable sleeping and feeding schedules, smile at strangers, and readily accept unfamiliar foods. As they grow older, they adapt quickly to changes in school routines, for example. Understandably, these children usually evoke favorable responses in others and tend to experience the world as warm, pleasant, and accepting.

These children would appear to be least at risk for developing a behavior disorder, and as a group they do tend to develop proportionately fewer problems than other youngsters. But under certain conditions behavioral difficulties in "easy children" can derive from their very virtues, particularly their high degree of adaptability. Having faithfully learned the behavioral patterns taught at home, they may be taken aback by conflicting rules and expectations of the peer, school, or recreational group in which they must function a good part of the time. A sharp contradiction between parental and extrafamilial standards of behavior may overwhelm a child who suddenly finds himself the object of bewildering criticism, punishment, or ridicule. Engaging in various defensive maneuvers, he may remain his old self at home, but withdraw or become aggressive outside. His predominantly positive mood may yield to unhappiness, fussiness, and tantrums. He may begin to avoid new situations. Despite high intelligence, he may become a school problem, and despite good coordination he may shun sports.

Identification of the parental demands that lead to socially inappropriate behavior is the key to understanding the risk of behavior problems in these easily adaptable children. In such cases it is not conflict between the parent and child that underlies the development of problems but dissonance between the parent-child unit and the expectations of the wider environment.

DIFFICULT CHILDREN

These youngsters are irregular in their biological functions, have predominantly negative responses to new stimuli, are slow to adapt to environmental change, and have a high frequency of negative mood expressions and intense reactions. As infants, their sleeping and feeding schedules are unpredictable. They initially reject new foods or toys, require long periods of adjustment to altered routines, and fuss more readily than they express pleasure. They respond to frustration with a violent tantrum. In contrast to the "easy children," they make special demands on their parents for unusual consistent and tolerant handling.

Our data clearly indicate that children with the "difficult child" syndrome have the greatest risk of developing a behavior problem. In the New York Longitudinal Study, approximately 70 percent of the children with this temperamental cluster developed behavior problems. Although the difficult children comprised 10 percent of the study sample, they made up 23 percent of the group who were later identified as having behavior problems.

The specific source of stress for the difficult child are the demands for socialization, that is, for altering spontaneous responses and patterns in conformity with the standards of the family, school, or peer group. Such demands may intensify stress to the point of symptom formation when they are made in an inconsistent, impatient, or punitive manner. When the parents can maintain consistent approaches based on an objective view of the child's reactive pattern, he is able to adapt, though slowly, to step-by-step demands for normal socialization. It may take him a long time to learn the rules, but once he does learn them he functions effectively.

There is no evidence that parents of difficult children are essentially different from other parents or that they are responsible for the temperamental characteristics of their offspring. True, parental attitudes and practices that are satisfactory in handling most children are sometimes not adequate to promote adaptation with a minimum of stress in the difficult child. In addition, many parents react to the problems involved in the management of such a child with resentment, guilt, or a feeling of helplessness. A vicious circle is thus formed.

SLOW-TO-WARM-UP CHILDREN

This temperamental type is characterized by a combination of negative, though mildly intense, initial responses to new situations with gradual adaptation after repeated contact with the stimulus. For such a child it is particularly stressful to face insistent demands for an immediately positive response to a new food or a new school. Pressure for quick adaptation typically intensifies the child's tendency to withdraw, and a negative child-environment interaction may be set in motion. But if the parent or teacher recognizes and accepts slow adaptation as part of the child's reactive style and gives him patient encouragement, he will ultimately become interested and involved.

It should again be emphasized that while specific features and patterns of temperament play important roles in the genesis of behavior disorders in childhood, temperament in itself does not produce a psychological disturbance. Rather, deviant development results from the dissonant interaction between a child with given characteristics and the significant aspects of his intrafamilial and extrafamilial environment. Certain qualities of reactivity may place the child at risk, making him unusually vulnerable to stress. But vulnerability does not imply inevitability. Case analyses in our study clearly show that there are children in the nonclinical group with organizations of temperament highly similar to those of children in the clinical groups. Conversely, some children with disorders had temperamental attributes identical with those typifying the nonclinical group as a whole.

It remains true, however, that in our study sample the temperamental traits and constellations identified by the frequency of their association with behavior disorders included: (1) a combination of irregularity, nonadaptability, withdrawal responses, and predominantly negative mood of high intensity; (2) a combination of withdrawal and negative responses of low intensity to new situations, followed by slow adaptability; (3) excessive persistence; (4) excessive distractibility; and (5) markedly high or low activity level.

With recognition of the child's behavioral style, it becomes possible to devise strategies of handling to reduce the chances that the risk of developing a disorder will become a reality. A pathogenic interaction, once identified, can be modified by a preventive treatment program.

One component of such a program is the effecting of environmental change through parent guidance. The goal is to restructure parental management by giving the family a clear picture of the child's temperamental attributes and of the parental behaviors that are creating excessive strain for the child. By offering specific suggestions for changing these behaviors, the clinician can enlist the parents as co-workers in reducing the vulnerabilities of the child at risk.

Bibliography

1. Bergman, P. and S. K. Escalona, Unusual sensitivities in very young children, in *The Psychoanalytic Study of the Child,* Vol. 3., Int. Univ. Press, New York, 1949.
2. Chess, S., *Temperament and behavior disorders in mentally retarded children.* In press, 1969.
3. Thomas, A., H. G. Birch, M. E. Hertzig, and S. Korn, *Behavioral Individuality in Early Childhood,* New York University Press, New York, 1963.
4. Thomas, A., S. Chess, and H. G. Birch, *Temperament and Behavior Disorders in Children,* New York University Press, New York, 1968.

The Mutative Impact of Serious Mental and Physical Illness in a Parent on Family Life

E. James Anthony (U. S. A.)

Alain René Le Sage, an eighteenth-century French novelist, once wrote a story about a lame demon ("a devil on two sticks") who unroofed houses to show what was going on inside. In the investigation that I am about to describe, we, too, have been assuming the role of Diable Boiteux unroofing, in a psychosocial and psychodynamic sense, various houses in the metropolitan area of the city of St. Louis for the purpose of taking a close and intimate look at the lives of the occupying families. Some of the houses were chosen at random to provide us with controls, but others were included because in them a parent figure has currently succumbed to a serious mental or physical disorder necessitating hospitalization. Our primary aim was to discover the ways in which different families dealt with the impact of illness and the changes in organization and function that ensued. We have just completed three years of intensive data collecting and have reached the critical stage of searching for a

*This investigation supported by U.S. P.H.S. MH-12043-01 and RO1-MH-14052-01.

†Academic Lecture delivered at the 19th Annual Meeting of the Canadian Psychiatric Association, Toronto, June 1969 and published in the *Canad. Psychiat. Ass. J.* Vol. 14 (1969).

conceptual model to fit our findings. The emphasis in this presentation is therefore on theory.

Some Previous Perspectives on Illness

There have been several authors within the past 25 years who have investigated the changes in family functioning resulting from a member falling sick. The findings from these studies show differences mainly because the perception of illness and of its mode of operation is different. Curiously enough, there has been little tendency on the part of authors to differentiate between the effects of mental and physical illness, the two being treated as if they exercised a similar influence.

I would like to review several different perspectives on illness starting with illness viewed in a global and popular sense as "trouble" for the family.

ILLNESS VIEWED AS "TROUBLE"

In one of the earliest studies [5], an investigator dealt with the adjustment of low-income families in New York City to a number of stark emergencies, referred to generally as "troubles," the most upsetting of these being illness. He found that when the mother became ill, it created a serious disruption of family routine so that the home became dirtier and more disorderly whereas in the case of the father, illness generally led to a worsening in the family's standard of living and the generation of defeat and disaffection. In these substandard homes, illness in either parent could present as a major crisis. The better the pre-morbid history of the family with regard to organization and integration, the more effectively did it seem to cope with the problem. A number of changes seemed inevitable both inside and outside the family. Within the home, for example, there were changes in status (especially with regard to dominance), in role evaluations, in the strength and direction of feelings between family members, in the amount of sexual activity between the marital partners, in the maintenance of discipline, and in the performance of routine household duties. The extrafamilial effects of illness led to withdrawal of the family from active contact with their social world so that friendships and affiliations were gradually discarded as the family became increasingly absorbed in their "trouble" and disconnected from their environment.

The dramatic shift in the dominance of a sick parent is shown graphically by Figure 1 in which the family is represented by a rectilinear form whose size and shape is governed by the relative dominance of each family member indicated in relation to the positional scale on the left-hand side of the figure. The father, in this case, is represented by the shaded circle.

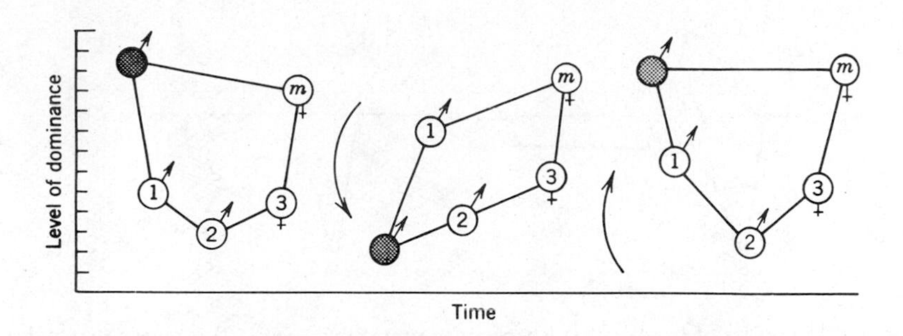

Figure 1 Changes in dominance patterns. (From Koos, 1946.)

When the father becomes incapacitated, his authority diminishes and the family begins to take less notice of his rulings eventually treating him as a relative nonentity, a younger sibling. As he recovers, he begins to regain much of his standing in the family although not quite up to his former level, the episode of illness, if serious, seeming to leave some permanent damage to the power structure of the family.

The amount of interaction in the family may also be affected, both in quality and in quantity. In Figure 2, four different profiles attempt to illustrate four different reactions to the crisis of illness in terms of interactional levels. The family may return to its habitual level, or plateau, at a level below this or, in the case of recurrent illness, may deteriorate to lower levels of interaction. An interesting, if somewhat mystifying, profile is one in which the familial organization (communication and contact) is left better off after the illness than before, suggesting a degree of benefit from the stressful experience.

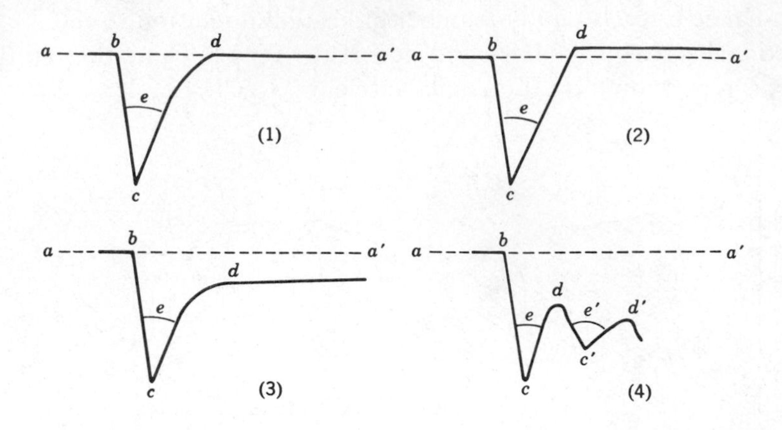

Figure 2 The profiles of trouble. (1) Recovery to pretrouble level; (2) recovery to a higher than pretrouble level; (3) recovery to a lower than pretrouble level; and (4) incomplete recovery. Key: a – a' = normal family interaction; b = onset of trouble; c = depth of trouble; d = point of recovery; and e = angle of recovery. (From Koos, 1946.)

ILLNESS VIEWED AS DEVIANT BEHAVIOR

In another penetrating analysis, Talcott Parsons and Fox developed the view that illness, whether mental or physical, could be considered as a form of deviant behavior, an escape from the pressures of everyday life [9]. The contemporary family, by reason of its small size, its comparative isolation, and its limited services to its members, was extremely vulnerable, the author felt, to the strains of illness, the family as a whole and the patient in particular often tending to exploit it to the fullest extent. The illness provided a specific type of solution for the life problems of each individual and, at the same time, imposed an emotional load on the rest of the family. These solutions and impositions have been schematized by me in Table 1.

It will be noticed that the father, as the primary status-bearer of the family and major contact-member with the outside world, can gain a needed rest from the pressures of breadwinning by becoming ill. In so doing, he claims attention from his wife, who, in turn, withdraws attention from the children causing them to erupt with symptoms of neglect. The mother, as mediator between father and child and as the emotional storm center of the family, may seize

Table 1 The Psychological Impact of Serious Illness on the Precariously Balanced, Emotionally Highly Charged System of the Modern Urban Family*

Family Member	Life Situational Strains	The Illness Solution	The Illness Impact
Father-Husband	As provider, primary status-bearer, classically the "scapegoat" or symbolic target for the hostility of the socializing child.	The sick role offers semi-institutionalized respite from occupational demands and disciplines.	Worsens position of family, makes its adaptive problems more difficult, wife's focus on him withdraws attention from children who must sacrifice part of maternal support.
Mother-Wife	As mediator between father and child, carrying the major socio-emotional responsibility within the family, engendering solidarity and security, excluded generally from status and occupational satisfactions.	The sick role offers escape from heavy "human relations management" responsibilities or a compulsively feministic reaction to exclusion from the man's world.	The most disturbing of all, subjecting husband and children to under-support at a time when major demands are made on them—the greatest single source of danger to the family.
Child-Sibling	As socializer on the tension-ridden path towards maturity in competition with siblings.	The sick role provides escape from growing-up obligations, gains care, concern and close contact, furthers desired infantile regression, and gives advantage over siblings.	Disturbs family equilibrium by making it difficult for mother to meet needs of father and siblings, making rivalry acute.

*From Talcott Parsons and R. C. Fox, 1952.

upon the opportunity afforded by sickness to lay down some of her load of "human relations management." Because of her pivotal role, her illness creates a maximum disturbance in the family leaving both husband and children in a strangely emotional and physical void. "As mother goes, so blows the family" was the way one father and husband described it.

According to these authors, there are two reciprocal problems involved in the process of illness within families. The patient must learn how to be sick and the family members must learn how to respond to his sickness. For both sides the experience has its special difficulties and emotional concomitants. The patient needs to acclimatize himself first to illness and then to wellness and his family must adapt itself to both sets of conditions as they alternate. The adjustment required may tax its resources to the point when illness comes to represent a serious threat to what Jackson refers to as the family homeostasis when the need of the two parties, the sick and the well, to separate becomes imperative and critical.

Becoming sick is not a simple matter because it involves a complex of psychological reactions that both hinder and help the process. At some lower level of consciousness, being sick is equivalent to being guilty and bad and in need of punishment, a type of response more discernible in the child. (Samuel Butler in his story of "Erewhon" seemed well aware of this aspect; when the inhabitants of Erewhon became ill, they were punished with imprisonment.) Being sick also entails shame; shame over being inactive, unoccupied, dependent, childish, needy, and self-absorbed. On the other hand, the regressive and narcissistic gratifications deriving from the sick role and devoted family care also stimulate marked ego enhancements. There is no doubt that it sometimes does the ego a world of good to be sick—to become for a while its own exclusive object of attention and to be insensitive (as Charles Lamb aptly phrased it) "to all the operations of life except the beatings of one feeble pulse" [6]. He goes on, in somewhat sadder vein, to describe the transformation in reverse associated with recovery, the shrinking of the tremendous ego space occupied by the sick man and the gradual dwindling of all the pomp and circumstance connected with illness.

With regard to the family's response, the authors present the proposition that latent dependency needs are endemic in the population and that therefore most families tend to overreact to the passive dependent nature of illness and its inferior childlike status by becoming more sympathetic, supportive, indulgent, and permissive than they need to be. This is because they project their own regressive wishes onto the sick person. Underlying this solicitude, however, are also the less altruistic reactions of envy and jealousy, irritability and impatience and sometimes, beneath the guise of tender, loving care, a lot of sadism to which the chronic patient may respond by becoming even more masochistically entrenched. In the protracted case, both the sick and the well become immersed in a common pool of suffering.

These many observations would seem to support the thesis put forward of "the unique defenselessness of the American urban family when faced with the illness of one of its members."

ILLNESS AS A DISRUPTION OF COMPLEMENTARY FAMILY ROLES

An example of role analysis in the situation of illness has been furnished by Spiegel in his delineation of successive stages in the reestablishment of equilibrium following the imbalance induced by role changes due to illness [13]. There is a significant shift in the complementarity of family roles giving rise to difficulties in relation to role recognition, goals to be achieved, values to be accepted and interpersonal techniques to be employed. At the onset of the illness, habitual roles become nebulous and confused, habitual cues are misinterpreted and misunderstood and once humorous and lighthearted interchanges are taken seriously. This brings into action some counterbalancing mechanisms. Spiegel has described the "natural history" of such a development and I have tried to summarize his views in Table 2.

The family gradually reaches some form of adaptation to the restrictions imposed by the illness and to the unpredictable demands made by the sick person, but not without serious cost to its initial well-being. At first the individual members respond by becoming strongly manipulative in their attempts to restore the *status quo ante* and will try to influence the patient by a variety of persuasions to resume his usual role posture only to have these met by countermanipulations on the part of the patient involving oppositional tactics. When these strategies fall to grief, as they sometimes do, the family may abandon manipulative techniques and resort to a transitional and disarming devise of role reversal. At this time, they en-

Table 2 The Re-equilibration Process in Families Under Stress—Steps in the Restoration of Complementarity of Roles*†

Based on Manipulation		Non-Manipulative	Based on Mutual Insight and Novel Resolution
Role Induction	Counter-Induction or Neutralization	Role Reversal	Role Modification
Coercing Coaxing Evaluating Unmasking Provoking	Defying Witholding Denying Masking Postponing	A transitional process between role induction and role modification involving taking the other's role. It can lead to either induction or modification.	Joking Referral Exploring Compromising Consolidating

*These steps have a temporal order and a kind of internal logic. It is arbitrary and incomplete but has some heuristic value.
†After Spiegel, 1957.

deavor to see and understand the situation from the patient's point of view offering such bridging comments as "I see what you mean," or "I understand how you must feel about it," or "If I were in your place, I imagine I would do the same." In response to this, the patient himself begins to empathize with the family and put himself in their shoes. With this development, a newer and healthier stage of family interaction becomes possible and leads to an adoption of nonmanipulative technique on both sides. Attitudes become flexible, moods humorous, decisions democratic and debatable, and solutions are approached with open-mindedness and the spirit of compromise. The new roles, agreed upon in the family councils, are worked out and worked through with the members trying them on "for size" until they fit the family situation. Ultimately, complementarity is restored, and a new balance is achieved indicating that the disequilibrium of illness is over even though the patient continues to be ill. The difference is that the family is now better able to live with the illness.

ILLNESS AS A CRISIS IN ACCOMMODATION

An analysis of the accommodative processes brought into being by schizophrenic illness was made by Sampson and others in an attempt to trace the connections between the psychotic episode, the family setting in which it occurred, and the adjustments set up within the family [11]. These postulated changes in family life brought about by illness have been summarized in Table 3.

According to these authors, the impact of illness depends to a large extent on the nature of the marital relationship which, in turn, reflects the characteristics of the earlier parent-child relationship. When it is symbiotic (the spouse substituting for the mother), separation or the threat of separation may precipitate a life crisis that undoes the previous precarious accommodation based on dependency. With the homeostasis disturned, a renewed attempt at accommodation is made with increasing involvement and closeness and a rise in the tolerance for deviancy. If this solution fails, the tendency is reversed and progressive detachment from the family takes place until a final breakdown into complete withdrawal becomes inevitable. When the marital union has an autistic pattern, with the partners living together in separate worlds, the crisis is often provoked by some anniversary of a childhood situation involving identification with a parent figure. The accommodative response becomes one of increasing diver-

Table 3 The Impact of Schizophrenic Illness on the Marital Relationship*

Pattern of Marital Relationship	Life Crisis	Accomodative Process†	Pre-Hospital Crisis	Hospitalization
Symbiotic interdependency of mother and patient with spouse as peripheral member of the triad.	Separation	Reciprocal overinvolvement (trigenerational merger or conversion) with high tolerance for deviancy	Rejection of symbiosis with progressive detachment from family.	Transfer of symbiosis to hospital—disengagement from mother—new husband-wife coalition —mother pushed to periphery.
Mutual uninvolvement of patient and spouse ("emotional divorce")—living in separate worlds.	Identification (anniversary reaction)	Reciprocal under-involvement with high tolerance for deviancy.	Further disinvolvement by spouse with progressive detachment from family.	No uniform effect—further disengagement or reconciliation depending on spouse's readiness for re-involvement.

*From Sampson, Messinger, Towne, 1964.
†The family evolves mechanisms for coping with deviant behavior. Professional help is sought only when these mechanisms are experienced as inadequate.

gence until the progressive detachment is recognizable as a psychotic illness. Although the symbiotic and autistic categories represent a simplistic view of the field of psychosis, there is some heuristic advantage to dichotomizing the two types of crisis, stemming from two patterns of marital relationship and producing two forms of accommodation to the illness.

This accommodation may have both a positive and negative side to it. On the positive side, it often allows a crisis to be contained within the family and resolved without recourse to outside help. On the negative side, there is no doubt that treatment often gets postponed until the psychosis is far advanced, the capacity to use help reduced, and the burden on the remaining family members, especially the children, beyond their emotional capacity to bear. The amount of accommodation available to a given family is a complex function of its degree of encapsulation, its tolerance of deviancy, its own internal therapeutic resources, and its system of shared defense mechanisms. To some extent, this represents a summation of the coping mechanisms of the individual members, but the dynamics of interaction may add or subtract from the accommodation process. Curiously, the "straw that breaks the camel's back" may not be a major stress at all but a minor incident that gains heavily in significance because it entails a sudden publicity for the family's most closely guarded secret. For example, a severely psychotic man made life intolerable for his family because of his murderous attacks but they bore with it until a certain day on which he opened the door to the postman and urinated on his shoes!

THE VIEW OF ILLNESS AS A DISCONNECTION

Illness, both mental and physical, can bring about radical changes in the personality and behavior of the patient to the extent of creating a discontinuity between the pre-morbid and post-morbid image presented by the individual. In the case of a psychotic metamorphosis, the younger children especially may experience difficulty in linking up the parent they once knew or thought they knew to the disturbed and disturbing person currently confronting them. This discontinuity is further exaggerated when the sick person himself has blotted out the reality of the past and fabricated an imaginary earlier life for himself. As the patient recovers, the history of his illness frequently undergoes suppression so that a whole set of vivid and vital experiences are denied existence and the children act as if they suffered from an artificial amnesia. This is especially likely to happen when the illness is treated in the family as meaningless, accidental, and too "far out" to be incorporated into the logic of everyday life.

THE VIEW OF ILLNESS AS A CHALLENGE

Whatever one thinks of Toynbee's historical speculations (and you may have grave reservations about them), a useful heuristic framework can be extrapolated from his world view and applied to the micro-society of the family [14]. Table 4 represents my attempt in this direction. Serious illness, either mental or physical, has all the characteristics of Toynbee's challenge. It is something new that confronts the family and in its more serious forms it can be described in such terms as traumatic, pressurizing, and penalizing. The family's response may be as varied and complex as that of society.

This challenge and response formulation would seem to have an adequate explanatory strength for our purpose and, moreover, it contains within it many of the ideas described by the others already mentioned. It allows for three different types of response. In the first, the family undergoes growth and differentiation, thereby becoming a richer, more varied, and better integrated unit. One or two members may manifest latent creative tendencies while others may be driven to imitate them. The illness seems to provide a moratorium on the habitual modes of response and to set up innovations in thinking and feeling not unlike that described by Mann in his *Magic Mountain* [7]. Perspectives are no longer commonplace and bound to reality and the ordinary conventions go by the board especially when the idiosyncrasies of psychosis become equated with a new freedom. The interactions within the family may rise to new levels of sympathy and empathy and the process of individuation may be enhanced.

The second type of response leads to a temporary "breakdown" followed by recovery. During the period of breakdown, there is a loss of productivity, some of the creative urges undergoing recession. Because of the loss of initiative in the parent, the children become less subordinate and this in turn may provoke a dominating response in one or both parents in an attempt to keep control. Family life is less integrated on the inside and more defensive in relation to outsiders. The individual members feel themselves to be victims of

Table 4 Challenge and Response: An analysis of Growth, Breakdown and Disintegration in Social Groups*

Challenge	Response		
	Growth and Differentiation	Breakdown and Rally	Rout and Disintegration
Hard conditions New situations "Blows" Pressures Penalizations	Creativity by minority Imitation of minority by majority Withdrawal-and-return of creative individuals Increasing differentiation	Loss of creative drive and change to domination Withdrawal of allegiance by majority Loss of control over human and physical environment Failure of self-determination Loss of group unity Aggressive reaction to outsiders Appearance of helpful, protective, saving agents	Split in social group Split in individual psyche Deterioration of behavior as seen in: A sense of drift A sense of sin Vulgarization Promiscuity Loss of control or over-control of self A retreat into self Preoccupation with past and future A turning to religion Truancy and self-martyrdom

*After Toynbee

circumstance unable to determine their own destinies. There is some magical expectation that a savior is due to appear and that he will prevent them from slipping further into deterioration. (At this critical point, they may meet up with a therapist activated by rescue fantasies and messianic beliefs who may then garner a rich harvest of "cures.")

The third type of response sees the appearance of a number of disintegrative phenomena. There is a split in the family group so that antagonistic subgroups are set up in conflict with one another and a split within the individual so that he feels divided within himself. As conditions worsen, the prevailing climate is saturated with a sense of drift, of aimlessness, of guilt and shame, of helplessness, hopelessness and finally despair. Daily existence is vulgarized and the members lose their sense of decency and propriety. Promiscuous relationships are sought and severed almost as they begin. Each individual retreats within himself, preoccupied with the past or the future and seemingly totally disinterested in current experiences. As a last resort, some turn to the consolations of religion, appearing to prefer the more esoteric. With each subsequent relapse, the rally is less effective and the rout more likely to begin. According to Toynbee, every social group has its own rhythm of disintegration and the relapse-remission beat may have various sequences. The point at which disintegration occurs will vary from family to family but, once started, its effect is profound and unidirectional. The family structure is gradually blurred with roles becoming undifferentiated and functions increasingly automatized.

It is a common finding that the "natural history" of an illness is modified by the psychosocial setting of the family and is not only different for different families but radically different for the same illness met with in an institution. Illness in the home creates a phenomenological world of its own quite distinct from what is found outside the home. A family is not simply a collection of individuals but a group of dynamically interrelated and interdependent members each with his own degree of contact inside and outside of the family and each with a differing susceptibility to physical and psychological contagion. When a family member is ill, his immediate relatives react to his illness and the patient, in turn, reverberates to the family's response. To some extent, the family is always sick along with its sick member, sometimes physically, sometimes psychologically, and often empathically. In sickness, the individual becomes something special and his relatives, in order of kinship and closeness, suffer with him and share with him in the peculiar preoccupations brought about by pain and suffering.

The Method of "Unroofing"

"Unroofing" is by no means an easy task to accomplish without the wholehearted cooperation of the family underneath. It entails a disturbing invasion of privacy since we set out to observe the solitary and interactional activities of the family members minutely and intimately. The unroofing is done in several ways: we visit the families at a time when they are all together, such as at their meals; we sometimes live with them for a week, participating in their lives to the fullest extent; and we bring them collectively to our research center where they appear in their best clothes and best behavior. We see them individually in prolonged sessions, always focusing on the impact of illness on their lives, the common denominator of their experience, and we meet with them at different times in dyads and triads in order to observe some of the subgroup activity. During the course of our contact we rate them and rank them and, when the investigation has been completed, we reimburse them to the sum of $25 (thanks to the federal government). The fact that we meet with them at a moment of crisis has an important methodological bearing. We have found them at these times to be more susceptible to outside contact, more mobile in their defenses, and less suspicious of the motivations and intentions of the interviewer. The patients in the families being investigated were psychotic (schizophrenic or manic-depressive) and tuberculous. We also have a group of healthy controls who, because they were volunteers, sometimes manifested (20 to 30 percent) a greater measure of psychological ailments than we deemed desirable for our research.

"Unroofing" is a delicate operation and there is no doubt that even the most unobtrusive observer alters the conditions of everyday life for the family. There is also no doubt that habituation to the observer takes place and old habits of behavior gradually reestablish themselves as the stranger reaction subsides. At times it would look as if abnormal behavior was more pronounced as part of an audience response. There are undeniable distortions in this actual living experiment but the advantages of direct and continuous observation far outweigh the disadvantages.

Seeing the families at times of crisis, when their defenses are fluid and their wish to abreact rather than suppress the traumatic experience quite strong, renders them more accessible especially to the technique of focal interviewing, that is, interviewing in depth around a single pressing topic. In this instance, the focus is on the illness and the way it affects the lives, the thoughts, and the feelings of everyone in its vicinity. We have found that this establishes an immediate working bond between the family and the interviewer. This period of illness is often a mystifying time in the life of the family. They are perplexed by the disconnections, discontinuities, and distortions that are brought about, and this stimulates them to circumspect (in Heidegger's terminology) and put things together etiologically and descriptively. We ask them as a family to think aloud and together about their common predicament and to share with us their rational and irrational struggles to understand what it is all about.

The Temporospatium of the Family

Families occupy a certain part of space and time that endows them with their basic characteristics. Within this temporal-spatial niche they spin out their life histories compounded from those of individual family members, and it is this varied assortment that adds a specific quality to the basic historical and socio-cultural characteristics. Accidental features, like illness, also contribute an idiosyncrasy of their own that may stamp the family indelibly with their mark. The mark of chronic illness can be highly distinctive.

Families that shelter a chronic patient begin to create in time a subculture that generates its own pattern of life. Family members, relatives, and friends encapsulate themselves within a social orbit that is mainly populated by individuals showing varying degrees of disorder. In psychotic cultures, not only is there a greater acceptance of eccentric behavior but also an actual fostering of abnormal propensities since it is these divergences that segregate the group and draw its members closer together.

Although to some extent modified by class factors, the families of hebephrenic, paranoid, or schizo-affective schizophrenics to a surprising extent reflect the characteristics of the patient. We therefore find families that are in the main disorganized, suspicious, chaotic, and fluctuating although individual members may offer contrary reactions to these trends. For example, we visited a derelict building badly in need of repair and found two of the children, a boy age 9 and a girl age 7, squatting comfortably on a wall sharing a cigarette. The girl had on no pants and made no postural adjustments to disguise the fact. When asked the whereabouts of the mother, the boy said that "Old Annie" was where she always was, in the back room. "Take care you don't hurt her when you go in," he added, "she lies on the floor by the door." There was a curious warmth in his voice and he might have been speaking of a favorite pet. Annie was a chronic undifferentiated schizophrenic. By way of contrast, a paranoid schizophrenic man turned his home into a beleagured fortress in which the family mounted watches against the enemy and weapon training was rigorously enforced. A great deal of secrecy prevailed and no one was allowed to come and go without an examination of credentials. A child who went out shopping was closely interrogated on his return. One of the children complained bitterly that he even had to report before going to the bathroom! [1]

Within the interpersonal matrix, a great deal of psychopathology can develop insidiously within individuals, especially children, without it becoming recognizable. Abnormal attitudes and behavior are assimilated and symptoms are exchanged with surprising facility. Not infrequently, small psychological epidemics occur.

Some of our tuberculous families have been treated as social isolates because of fears of infection but among the individuals who remain with the social orbit there would seem to be a greater incidence of malingering, hypochondriasis, psychosomatic ailments, and interminable narcissistic preoccupations with the extraordinary things going on inside their bodies.

The temporal and spatial features of the orbit play a decisive role in the dissemination of abnormality. There is a higher frequency of contact with unusual personalities, a greater willingness to interchange on an intimate level of experience, and altogether more time spent in the company of illness-prone people ready to administer remedies, counsel, empathize and sympathize with, and theorize on the nature of things. We have been struck by the frequency of "anniversary reactions" within the orbit as if there were a general expectation that history would inevitably repeat itself and so it does to the satisfaction of the prophets and their naive theories. Children get ill like their parents and follow predictable courses. The density of the orbit is another factor of some importance. Under conditions of undercrowding or overcrowding, there is a tendency for certain family reactions to intensify and proliferate. Manic behavior, for example, in a mother of a large family in a small environment can cause most of the children for a while to become unusually restless and overactive as if they were all participating in some primitive dance ritual designed by the mad maternal choreographer.

For the child living in this orbit, everything seems conducive of the abnormal so that it is invidious to cite a particular event as causal. In assessing the influences at work, we have been especially guided by Mead's concepts of simultaneity and sequence [8]. There is the constant background to the child's life of the things that are always there—the home in which he lives, his regular routines of school-going, churchgoing, shopping, and family outings, the neighbors who visit, or the tradesmen who call—what ecologists refer to as the ecosphere. And then there are the experiences the child undergoes successively through his development and the additional learning that comes with this. These simultaneous and successive influences reinforce each other and ensure that the psychotic influence does not end with the termination of the psychotic attack.

The Three Responses to Illness

GROWTH AND DIFFERENTIATION

As previously indicated, the pre-morbid history of the family has as much prognostic significance for its future integration as the pre-morbid history of the patient has for the outcome of his psychosis. The indices that point to a possible growth experience for the family in the face of illness are roughly similar to those that predict good general adjustment in the adult, namely, a happy childhood for both parents, a satisfactory marital relationship, a good school record for the children, a successful work record for the parents, and a history of adequate coping reactions to the everyday crises of life. The family, with this type of background, responds to difficulties and problems by pooling its resources and working out the most constructive solutions together in open debate, all of which emphasizes the truism that a good family life ensures a good family response to serious illness. In one of our cases, the mother developed a paranoidal illness that began with strong erotic delusions that her doctor was in love with her and was trying to get rid of his wife in order to marry her. In the next phase of the delusional formation, she thought that the doctor's wife had discovered her husband's intentions and had hired some men to take her children away from her. She imagined herself being constantly followed on the streets by these kidnappers and spent a lot of time at the window of her house watching for suspicious-looking characters. She refused to let the children out of her sight and they complained of her constant vigilance and her interference with their play activities. The father had a family council with his three children and discussed their strange situation. From then onward, he conducted what amounted to family therapy sessions as a result of which the understandable exasperation of the children turned into pity for their sick mother. Instead of fighting her paranoia, they discussed the persecution with her, neither contradicting nor acquiescing to its reality. One of the girls wrote a series of poems which were compassionate and tender; another painted a large-scale portrait of the family having a picnic together in happier days. All these creations were presented to the mother on Mother's Day with the sensitive dedication "to the mother who wants to keep us safe." She was in the hospital for the occasion but this proved a turning point in her condition. When we saw the family three months afterwards, they seemed very happy and were on their way to a Californian holiday. The husband reported that his wife had changed in an extraordinary way for the better. She had always been slow to trust people but now she was much less suspicious and controlling. One of the children had become an A student and the family seemed much better integrated than ever before.

Another example of the growth-stimulating effect of illness has to do with a case of tuberculosis. The parents, a Negro couple, had married at 18 after knowing each other for about 4 years. The wife described her husband as shy and quiet and had been drawn to him for these qualities. However, these were also symptomatic of his tendency to withdraw from stressful situations and led him eventually into alcoholism. There were two children, both girls, aged 8 and 9. This is what the wife had to say about the situation.

We were always arguing, mostly about his drinking. Our marriage was on the rocks. Every payday, I would see nothing of him until he had drunk all his money away. The girls and I had to struggle to keep things going. We had been so happy in the first five years that none of us could understand why he wanted to drink so much. When he got T.B., it seemed to bring us all much closer together, even better than when the girls were small. He seemed to realize many things for the first time, how the girls and I had struggled to keep things together in order to help him. He really seemed to come to his senses. He said that being sick allowed him to think, to face reality. It really woke him up. These last two years I have had to be mother and father to the kids. He seemed to change so much for the better. He seemed to become interested in so many things in the world and would often say, 'I never knew that so much went on in the world; I just seem to be hearing it and seeing it for the first time'. He also wanted the kids to see his new world that he had discovered. When we would go to visit him he would take them for long walks around the grounds and point out the trees and flowers. He kept saying that it was not good enough just to be alive; one really had to live. The girls were very surprised. They said that their daddy had never taken them out for walks before, never shown them things and had always been on the bottle. Now he has time for the kids and he has time for me and our marriage is much, much better. It was almost broken up by his drinking but everything was put right by the T.B.

Mother had reported that the older girl had been very concerned when her father was admitted to hospital. Her teacher noted a marked change in her at school. She seemed to become withdrawn and disinterested and her grades deteriorated. Then, said the teacher, she began to report that her father was much better and that she had been out walking with him and that he was going to come home. She seemed to come out of her shell and there was a marked improvement in her attitude and behavior. The little girl's own report confirmed this. She said,

I felt very sad when Dad went to the hospital because I thought he might die. When he became sick, I became very quiet but when he got well I seemed to get well too. I have been doing much better at school since he has been getting better.

BREAKDOWN AND RALLY—THE DYNAMICS OF CHANGE

One of the first reactions of the family to the patient's breakdown is in relation to the changes brought about by illness and the discontinuity with their previous experience of the parent. An adolescent girl said to me: "You cannot believe what it's like to wake up one morning and find your mother talking jibberish." A 10-year-old remarked: "I wake up dreaming or maybe just daydreaming, I don't know what, but her face is coming toward me and she looks good and then suddenly her face begins to change and look mean and horrible like a monster." It is difficult for children to accommodate to this crisis of change especially when the contrast with the pre-morbid personality is marked. Another child said: "Everything goes upside down and we go upside down with it. When Mom goes mental, I go mental also. It's worse if I try to stay the same. Then she really hollers at me."

The child's eye view of the altered parent is full of excuses as he struggles to maintain the benign image that he once had.

> She is quite a nice mother really. She doesn't do anything bad. She doesn't hit or anything. She just sits. She is like a kid mostly. When I give her a lot of candy she just sucks it all up like a vacuum cleaner. She doesn't comb her hair and her dress has spots on it. Sometimes she laughs at me and I am not making any jokes. I say: 'Mom, why are you laughing at me?' and she just laughs more. I don't like it when she laughs like that. It's not like real laughing. She never used to be like this when I was little. She was just ordinary.

Another little boy laid emphasis on the unpredictable world in which he had to live.

> I was sitting at the table, just eating my cereal, and as I was pouring out the milk my hand hit his cup and it went over his lap, and he jumped up and shouted at me and said I did it on purpose and that I was trying to burn him. I wasn't trying to burn him at all, but he said I was trying to kill him and that he knew I hated him. Then he hit me on the head and said I had plans and he knew about them and he'd get me first and I said it was an accident but he just wouldn't listen to me. He wasn't so grouchy last year. He has become so mean.

The child of the tuberculous parent may have to adjust to a sudden restructuring in the pattern of his relationship. A loving parent suddenly becomes a dangerous parent, closeness to whom might lead to death. The children are often drilled at the onset of the illness on the possibilities of infection and the younger ones are apt to misunderstand the reason for this distancing. One particular father was so rigorous in the maintenance of his distance that when he became sputum and culture negative, he went home joyously on a weekend, opened the door of his home, and ran forward to embrace his young son. The child became panic-striken and raced off down the road. Another father would only allow the children to talk to him if they sat at a distance of five feet and had a table fan throwing his breath out of the window. The fear of physical contagion not only interferes with the closeness of the relationship but transforms a well-disposed parent into a dangerous and frightening one.

During the period of illness, these transformations are often represented in dreams. The child is running towards his father and as he gets nearer the father turns into a gorilla or burglar and begins to chase him. This wish to get close and fear of getting close becomes strangely interwoven with the deeper fantasies of the 5 and 6-year--old with Oedipal aspirations and prohibitions.

THE DYNAMICS OF CONTAGION

In a certain number of the cases, a most unusual state of affairs was detected with the mother-child dyad and clearly demanded closer scrutiny. The relationship had all the characteristics of a symbiosis, the child seeming to exist almost completely within the maternal ambience with little or no interposition of any "placental barrier" to impede the free flow of noxious thoughts and feelings between the encapsulated pair. The child's condition in many respects simulated that of the mother, but it could as easily be said that the mother's condition resembled that of the child. It was only a small number of deluded women who provoked such an outcome and, in these instances, the delusional ideas were linked to the safety of the children or, more often, of a particular child, and thereby provoked a primitively protective response, almost as if the mothers were in danger themselves. The children, participating in these situations, were characteristically psychologically undifferentiated, of less than average intelligence, dependent, submissive, suggestible, and deeply involved in the ill parent and in his illness.

CASE 1

A little girl aged 5, living alone with her widowed mother, one day saw a scarecrow in a field adjacent to her home. It waved to her and whistled. She heard it say that it would come and get her. She told her mother who was perturbed by what she heard, and said that when she was small, scarecrows sometimes got free and came into the house and that when they did, you could usually expect a death to take place. The mother warned her to be careful and to keep away from that side of the field. The next day the child came running into the house screaming that the scarecrow had been coming after her and that it was going to kill her mother. The mother immediately rushed out with a broom and the neighbors heard her shouting that she was not going to let any devil get into her house. That night the child had a severe night terror and screamed that the scarecrow was in the room and sitting on her chest. The mother put on the light, barricaded the door with a heavy chair, and took close hold of the child who continued screaming. The next morning, the mother told her neighbor that "they" were not going to get her or her child and that she knew what they were up to. She and the child now slept in the basement, both in a state of great apprehension, and the mother began to have nightmares. She explained to the child that the "scarecrow people" were now devising all sorts of tricks such as dreams to get into the house and kill the occupants. According to the mother, it was the child that they were after and according to the child, it was the mother. Four days later the police broke in and found the pair virtually starving and panic-stricken. The mother was hospitalized with the diagnosis of schizophrenia and the child placed in a residential home. For about four weeks, the child continued to interpret events in her environment in terms of the "scarecrow people" but this then gradually subsided and eventually disappeared [3].

In this transaction, and in several others of similar nature, it was difficult to tell where fantasy ended and delusion began or who was influencing whom. The interplay of fantasy and delusion would lead to the transformation of fantasy into a delusional fantasy which was never systematized because of the cognitive ineptness of the child.

There was sometimes a marked variability of response within the same family, one child accepting the maternal delusions completely and with conviction, another rejecting it out of hand, while a third learned to adapt to a double standard of reality while conforming to realistic expectations outside the home while maintaining an irrational orientation within the family circle. The ego's reality testing often clashed with the needs of object relations, the mother frequently making the acceptance of her delusion a test of loyalty and love. The children were often surprisingly uncritical of evidence offered by the deluded parent, as if they made implicit allowances for her motivation [3].

The possibility of a "mental contagion" that could mysteriously leap the gap between individual minds has generated a great deal of speculation but little direct observation and inquiry into the process involved. The assimilation of a delusional idea is evidently related to an unusual type of reciprocity between two individuals who would forego the tests of reality for the gratifications of mutuality.

Approaching the matter from his own particular theoretical framework, Piaget outlined three stages in the child's construction of reality: an autistic phase dominated by a confusion between self and non-self; an animistic phase during which the child's egocentrism gave him an intensely subjective perspective; and finally, a logical, social development in which the child saw himself as an object among other objects and was able to look at the world objectively [10].

The second of these stages is critical for the further development of the reality sense and requires some important shifts in ways of thinking, of conceiving the world, and of communicating with others. The stage, as a whole, is characterized by a deficiency in thinking logically, coherently, and reversibly. Instead, it is governed by intuitive and magical modes of thought which help to inculcate a naive and primitive conception of the universe loaded with inconsistencies, incompatibilities, inconsequences, and cognitive muddle referred to by Piaget as *syncretism.* It is a world in which inanimate things come to life, the sun and moon follow you around, dreams arrive through your bedroom window, and magical causality rules the world. In an older child, manifesting the same phenomena, the clinician would be alert to a borderline or full psychosis.

It was very understandable that when this sort of developmental magic-phenomenalistic system came into close contact with the psychotic magic-phenomenalistic system of the mother, the two would powerfully reinforce each other (see Figure 3). Piaget was well aware of the similarities between the two magic-phenomenalistic systems and commented that "in their manner of thinking, of perceiving and of reasoning, delusional psychotics recall some of the essential traits of child thought [10].

From these considerations, one could expect that when the thought systems of a deluded mother and of her preschool child impinged on each other, a common pool of paralogical ideas fed from the two unrealistic sources would be set up leading in time to an efflorescence of bizarre ideas in both individuals characteristic of a folie a deux.

THE DYNAMICS OF CONSTRICTION

Under the impact of serious mental illness in its first and unexpected appearance, family life may undergo a marked constriction which manifests itself in a rigidity of operation, a lack of spontaneity of feeling, a narrowness of thinking, and refusal to take chances. The family lives within a wide margin of safety and all hazards are carefully avoided. The individual members behave as if they were walking on eggs and as if any unusual act on their part might release a holo-

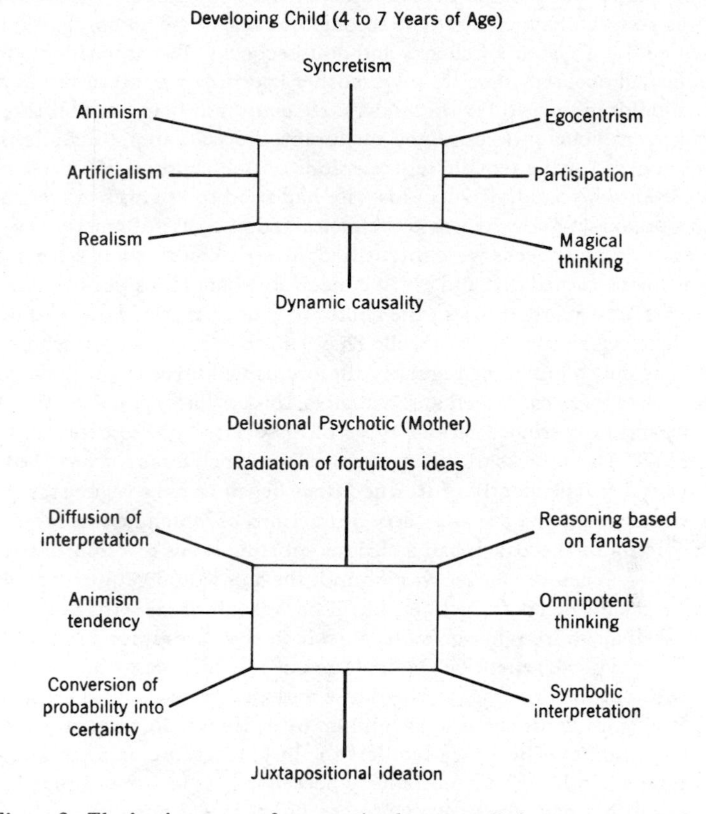

Figure 3 The impingement of one magic-phenomenalistic system on another. (After Piaget.)

caust. The security measures have antecedents in earlier life but are intensified to a pathological degree by the advent of psychosis.

CASE 2

The mother of four children developed an acute psychosis and made a devastating attack on her youngest child, aged 8, who happened to be home from school that day with a sore throat. She chased him around the house attempting to strangle him with the cord from her dressing gown. Fortunately, help arrived in time, and she was removed to hospital. The boy subsequently sent his mother a white rose paid for out of his allowance. It was accompanied by a note of love. Although the mother recovered with a series of shock treatments, she developed no amnesia for the murderous attack. The boy himself was asked by his father not to mention it to the other siblings, but these were all aware that something momentous had happened apart from their mother having become insane.

The father acknowledged that he had always lived with the fear that something dreadful was going to happen and that throughout his life he had prepared for all possible danger by a system of checks and doublechecks. The antecedents to this development had occured when his own mother had run away from the family and left the children to fend for themselves. He could not help but feel that mothers, far from being protective and nurturant, did wild, unpredictable things with little concern for the terrible repercussions on the children. His system of checks had eventually paid off when his wife had tried to kill his son. He had left instructions on exactly how he was to be contacted in a case of emergency. Since the episode, the checks were intensified; electric connections were inspected, gas mains turned off, and every conceivable dangerous point in the house was carefully guarded. When the children went out, their positions were visited to make certain that all was well. They had to report back on where they were and what they were doing regularly. Before using knives or other dangerous implements, they were cautioned and watched. Under this regime, the family members began to experience various types of dissociated phenomena. The middle son had three attacks of "doppelganger" in which a mirror image of his body performed independently of it. The father began to have vague states in which he would go into a daze and carry out actions of which he was later not aware. The victim of the attack had a curious splitting in his reaction to being with his mother. When the father was around, the son would get into bed with his mother and snuggle up against her, but if he was left alone with the mother, he would stay well away from her or work outside in the yard. Prior to the attack, he used to have typical, repetitive Oedipal dreams in which he would be sitting with his mother in the driveway to the house and all of a sudden his father would be driving up in his car as if to run him over. He would wake sweating from these nightmares. The attack had left the boy, therefore, in a particular bind: at a time when he was unconsciously perceiving his father as a murderous attacker, his mother had murderously attacked him. It was not surprising that he developed multiple phobic and counterphobic symptoms coupled with intense feelings of insecurity that were reinforced rather than relieved by his father's many safety measures.

THE DYNAMICS OF CONFUSION

In some of our families, the psychotic parent has continued to stay at home with a severe degree of thought disorder but otherwise socially adjusted.

CASE 3

In the family H, the wife, realizing her husband's utter confusion and his inability to organize himself sufficiently to carry out single household tasks arranged a series of cardboard boxes around the house, the purpose of each being marked carefully on the cover. All his different hobbies, interests, household tools, and so forth were thus categorized, but inevitably by the end of the day he would manage to scramble them, leaving a trail of confusion in his wake. Every day we was confronted with his sorting test, and every day, he failed it lamentably. Not only was he confused himself but was also a source of confusion in others. The eldest daughter was well aware that her father was "nuts" although she was quite fond of him. "He gets excited and can't explain himself. He tries to tell me things and gets all messed up, and I don't know what he's talking about. He is always right on his logic, but it just doesn't work out. At times I seem to get just like him. Perhaps I copy him without knowing it. At 8 I was afraid to talk because I thought I would talk nonsense, and then when I was 13, I went a whole year without saying anything because I couldn't think of anything to say. When I said something, it didn't seem to come out the right way. I can understand my dad's logic, but he can't understand mine." Her adolescent brother was always furious with his father because he couldn't think right, couldn't express himself and ended up making everybody mad and utterly confused. "He's not well even though he lives with us. He just talks and says nothing. He can't explain anything and has problems getting things done. He starts something and can't continue, so it ends in a big mess. He mixed up all my records although I asked him not to touch them. It's very difficult to communicate anything to him. After a while I find myself thinking and talking like him, and I end up not making sense to myself. I think I learn it from him. At times I get so mad that I have to go and run around the block to get it out of my system." A 7-year-old daughter reported: "He doesn't talk like you and I talk. I tell him a lot. He just sits like a log. I'm like that in school. I keep quiet because everybody looks at me. The kids turn round. I would go and try to make him talk, but he can't; so what's the good."

It has been found by various investigators that latent thought disorder, recognizable on testing, is more common among the relatives of schizophrenics, and we have been able to trace elements of this within the children. At times, in a family setting, it would seem as if the members were talking at cross purposes, but in some odd way, understanding one another even at times when the outsider felt that they were all on quite different wavelengths. This capacity to figure out nonsense and neologisms was striking in some of these thought-disordered families.

Rout and Disintegration

THE DYNAMICS OF DETERIORATION

In the relapsing case, the process of disintegration gradually sets in, and splits appear within the individual and within the family group.

Dissociated behavior makes its appearance. The family members begin to lose significant contact with one another and drift apart and away. Vague feelings of shame and guilt dominate affective interchanges, but these also eventually flatten out. Family life becomes coarsened, and the dirt and disorder are no longer noticed. Individuals spend endless time doing nothing or something repetitive and trivial. They review the past perceived unrealistically or plan, also unrealistically, for the future. Religious concerns are often predominant and they may quote the scriptures to explain the significance of their tribulations. As the adults become disengaged, the children get out of control and lead flagrantly delinquent lives.

I refer to this as a pseudo-narcotic state since the disunited family members wander about in a daze as if they were all drugged. The children are grossly underachieving at school, and the teachers complain that they seem to be living in worlds of their own. The fully developed condition is characterized by profound apathy, loss of feeling, impoverished interaction between family members, diminution of sexual desire, and an absence of contact with the outside world. The family gives the impression of being "burned out". An observing neighbor observed one such outcome in the following terms:

> They used to be like one of us. We all went together, and they visited us and we visited them. Then she had her first nervous breakdown and things were a little different, but we still visited. Then she had another and another and I can't count how many but she ended up like a zombi. Then he lost his job and didn't seem to bother getting another and the house just went from bad to worse so we couldn't stand going in any more. Everything just smelt and nobody seemed to care. They didn't want to see anybody. The life's gone out of them and they just hang about doing nothing and they don't even have any feelings about each other.

THE DYNAMICS OF REGENERATION

Where there has been evidence of family strength in the past, the disintegrating process may be halted and even reversed. These initial attempts at salvage may be quite primitive. They may consist of massive denials of deviance, nonrecognition of the illness, naive rationalization of symptoms, and an appeal to specific family mythology, such as "her grandmother had a bit of red Indian blood in her and it sometimes comes out in this way in the children." Next, the illness gets recognized as such and an attempt is made to localize the disturbance by isolating the patient from the rest of the family. If this is fairly successful, the family may then try to reestablish contact with the social environment, at the same time keeping the patient well hidden from public view.

A further step involves the "preparation" of the patient for outside contact. At first, the effort to "normalize" the patient may seem coercive or downright sadistic. He may be criticized, mocked, or teased on every occasion that he shows "nutty" behavior. These techniques are soon dropped since they are rarely effective and are more likely to alienate the patient. At this point, the family may spontaneously discover the rehabilitative instrument of empathy and may begin to identify with the patient's predicament and to see the situation from his unusual perspective. They may even see the funny side of the incongruities of psychosis. The admission of humor into the situation is hopeful even if the jokes remain somewhat grim. It may be finally conceded that the patient's condition, although extreme, can be placed on a continuum along with varying conditions prevalent in the rest of the family ("everyone is sick but some are sicker than others!").

Once again the family group starts to differentiate and integrate and to work and play together as a group. To what extent the latent group capacities of the family help to change the whole course of the illness, it is difficult to say at this point, but clinically, there is no doubt that waning group interactions are regularly associated with disintegration and deterioration, and enhanced group interactions signal the return to health.

The Psychology of Genetic Expectations[1]

The interpersonal matrix of the family with a psychotically ill parent may after a while be made up of psychotic reactions, prepsychotic reactions, parapsychotic reactions like folie a deux, and reactions to psychotic attitudes and behavior. The prepsychotic reactions in the child often have disturbing effects on the family

[1] In a recent paper, Scott and Ashworth [12] discuss the effects of "the shadow of the ancestor" in the transmission of schizophrenia. They attempt to show that psychotic illness in a close relative can affect, *through social influence*, a parent's attitude to their own children.

since they appear to confirm their worst fears. These prepsychotic developments often take the form of micropsychotic episodes that are usually vividly remembered and described by informants since they represent a striking departure from the child's habitual mode of behavior. In microcatatonic.episodes, the child becomes stiff and self-contained, unresponsive to his usual interests, and reluctant to take any initiative or to move except under pressure from others. In microparanoidal episodes there is an upsurge of suspiciousness and a sense of persecution that may develop a loose systematization in the older children. In microhebephrenic episodes there is characteristically silly, inappropriate, and sometimes clownish behavior [2].

In a crude way, certain of the families begin to develop "genetic expectations," and in Figure 4 we can see how these originate. In the

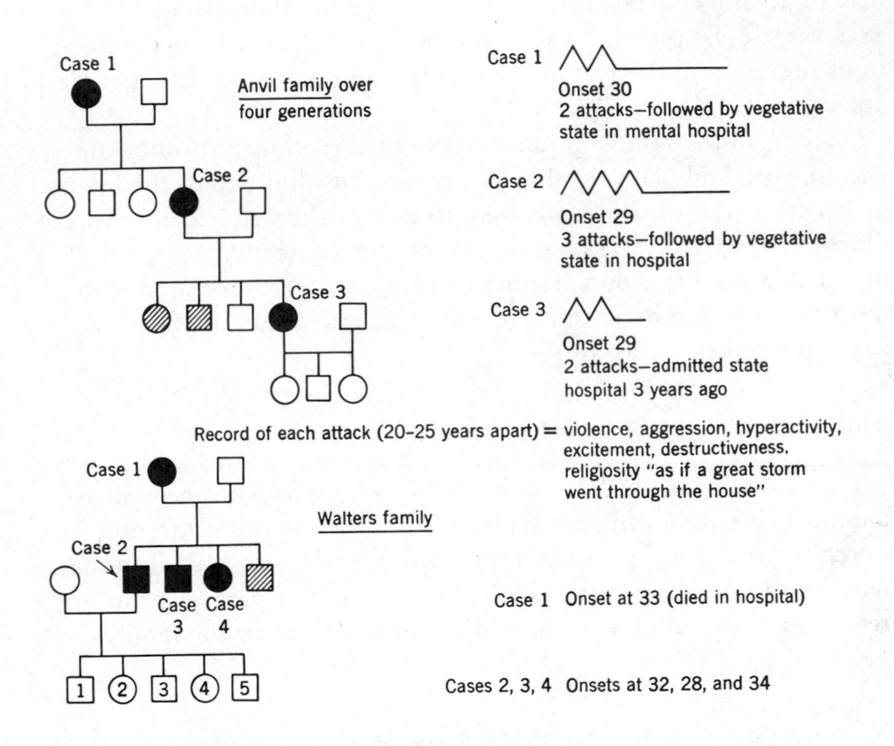

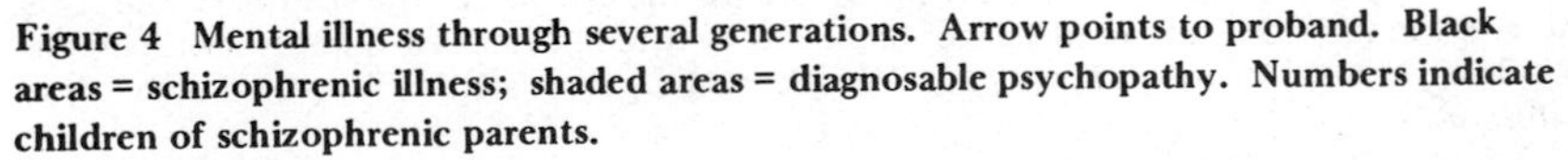
Figure 4 Mental illness through several generations. Arrow points to proband. Black areas = schizophrenic illness; shaded areas = diagnosable psychopathy. Numbers indicate children of schizophrenic parents.

Anvil family, the genetic transmission seems striking and it is not at all surprising that expectations and anticipations were common points of discussion in the family. Relatives spoke of the mother (the proband) "going the same way" and were buttressed in their belief by the extraordinary similarity of the attacks over three generations. The third child, a 7-year-old girl, had already been picked out as the "likely one" and she was made aware of this every time she became angry, upset, or excited which was frequent. When she accidently broke some plates on the table, eyebrows were raised and heads nodded glumly. On her eighth birthday, in the middle of the party, she threw a most turbulent temper tantrum and was uncontrollable for half an hour after which she seemed dazed and confused. An E.E.G. done shortly after showed no abnormality although some reference was made to "choppy" waves. Even in the sibling group, there was a general expectation at all times that the third child would misbehave herself and cause scenes [4].

The same was roughly true with the Walters family where the age of onset was again very much the same. Three of the adults in the second generation had suffered schizophrenic attacks. The proband was still in the hospital with a florid paranoid schizophrenia. The oldest boy was a wary, suspicious person who treated the interview like a third-degree examination. He was very reluctant to give any information and even asked for a lawyer to be present so that he would not incriminate himself. He examined the forms used in the research very carefully and declared that he was not going to give "evidence." He insisted that his father had lots of enemies and that it was always necessary to take proper precautions. Relatives reported: "He's his father again—he's going to crack up like him. He's already half a nut!" In contrast, the youngest boy was cheerful, amiable, and disbelieving. He viewed his father's illness simply as an interference with his freedom to play freely with his peers. The second child, a girl, thought her father was "a very sick man, but if he stayed at home, he would make us all sick like him." She feels frightened when he is around, not of him, but "of the stories he tells." Whereas the older boy was deeply and almost inextricably caught up in his father's psychosis, the younger children seemed to be able to stand outside it.

Theory-Making and Disease

Bergson called attention to the universal human propensity for myth making. All families have a tendency to theorize on their experiences and this may take place at various levels of sophistication. At more primitive levels, it encourages the development of magical thinking, superstition, prejudice, stereotypy, and simple-minded categorization. In the more culturally advanced families, psychological knowledge and subtlety may generate comprehensive and self-consistent etiological theories that, on closer examination, also incorporate many of the primitive components duly disguised.

The implicit aim behind this theorizing is to reestablish a predictable environment for the family and to make "meaningful connections," in Jasper's sense of the term, between the past, present, and the future. When the family has developed a reasonable set of explanations to account for the psychotic visitation or the presence of a physical disease, they appear to become more stabilized.

The general theory of disease evolved by the family serves to explain the various phenomena to the family itself and to the public with which it comes in contact. In addition, each individual member reserves his own idiosyncratic formulation based on his conscious and unconscious fantasies and fears. Our experience has been that these theories and part-theories play an important part in assimilating the incongruities of illness and in helping the family to accommodate to them. They provide all unusual expression and behavior with a flexible frame of reference which then allows the family to live more comfortably with the diseased person and the social milieu. They are also powerful in generating an expectational set regarding the impact of the illness; if the theories veer towards contagion, other members will "catch" the illness; if they favor modeling, there are those who will "learn" the sick role; if they postulate inherited factors, ancestral attributes will be carefully searched for in the predisposed.

These are, therefore, some of the clinical factors that have emerged through our process of "unroofing" together with some of the concepts that we have developed to explain them so that we, like the families we research, can live at peace with our peculiar findings.

Bibliography

1. Anthony, E.J., A clinical evaluation of children with psychotic parents, *Amer. J. Psychiat.*, 126:2, August 1969.
2. Anthony, E.J., The developmental precursors of adult schizophrenia. *J. Psychiat. Res.*, 6(1968) (Suppl. 1) pp. 293-316. Also in *The Transmission of Schizophrenia*, D. Rosenthal and S. Kety, Eds., Pergamon Press, New York, 1968.
3. Anthony, E.J., Folie a Deux—A Developmental Failure in the Process of Separation-Individuation, in *Festschrift in Honor of Margaret Mahler*, International Universities Press, New York, in press.
4. Anthony, E.J., A Clinical and Experimental Study of High Risk Children and Their Schizophrenic Parents, in *Genetic Factors in Schizophrenia*, A.R. Kaplan, Ed. Charles C. Thomas, Springfield, Ill., in press.
5. Koos, Earl L., *Families in Trouble*, King's Crown Press, New York, 1946.
6. Lamb, Charles, *The Collected Essays of Charles Lamb*, E.P. Dutton, New York, 1929.
7. Mann, Thomas, *The Magic Mountain*, Knopf, New York, 1927.
8. Mead, Margaret, *Continuities in Cultural Evolution*, Yale University Press, New Haven, 1964.
9. Parsons, T. and R. Fox, Illness, therapy, and the modern urban American family, *J. Social Issues*, 8(1952), No. 4, pp. 31-44.
10. Piaget, J., *The Language and Thought of the Child*, Harcourt, New York, 1926.
11. Sampson, H., S.L. Messinger and R.D. Towne, *Schizophrenic Women; Studies in Marital Crisis*, Atheron Press, New York, 1964.
12. Scott, R.D. and P.L. Ashworth, The shadow of the ancestor: a historical factor in the transmission of schizophrenia, *Brit. J. Med. Pyschol.*, 42 (Part 1) (1969), pp. 13-32.
13. Spiegel, John P., The Resolution of the Role Conflict Within the Family, in *The Patient and the Mental Hospital*, Greenblatt, Levinson and Williams, Eds., Free Press of Glencoe, Illinois, 1957.
14. Toynbee, Arnold J., *A Study of History*, Oxford University Press, London, 1934-1961.

Sex Differences in Children's Responses to Family Stress

M. RUTTER (U. K.)

Several studies, using a variety of different methods, have clearly demonstrated a strong association between chronic parental illness and psychiatric disorder in the children. The evidence that this association is not fortuitous but represents the sometimes harmful consequences for the child of chronic illness, especially mental illness, in the parent was reviewed previously [126]. Since then there have been a number of largely confirmatory studies [161], which will not be considered here. Rather, it seems more appropriate to consider the possible mechanisms involved in the association and more particularly to examine sex differences in children's responses to parental mental illness.

Not all parental illnesses lead to deviant development in the children nor, when there are harmful consequences, are all children equally affected. The earlier studies suggested that parental mental disorder was most likely to be followed by behavioral disturbance in the children when the parent exhibited long-standing abnormalities of personality. The clinical "seriousness" of the illness in terms of neurosis or psychosis was probably not important but the involvement of the child in the symptoms of the parental illness did seem to be crucial. Children in families where both parents were ill or where the parental illness was accompanied by break-up of the marriage seemed to be especially at risk. It was noted that long-standing mental disorder was often associated with hostility and discord between husband and wife and sometimes this discord might have more impact on the child than the mental illness itself. Circumstantial evidence indicated that the effect was not primarily genetic, but rather that abnormalities in family relationships might constitute the main adverse influence on the child.

A Prospective Study of the Families of Psychiatric Patients

A prospective study was designed to test this hypothesis. A group of families in which one parent had a psychiatric disorder are being followed over a 4-year period, but the data presented here refer entirely to the findings in the first year.[1] The sample consists of the families of *all* patients living in the old Borough of Camberwell in London [160] who spoke colloquial English at home, had one or more children under the age of 15 years, and who were *newly* referred to a psychiatric clinic during the course of a 10-month period – some 200 families in all. The original 10-month sample contained fewer men than women and there were few psychotics, so an additional sample of another 50 or so families were added, consisting of consecutive referrals in these categories. For present purposes the samples have been combined.

The refusal rate in the study was low – under 5 percent. Both the husband and wife were seen separately by different interviewers for interviews of 2 to 3 hours, sometimes extending to 2 sessions. Information was systematically obtained on the patient's disorder, the social context of the symptoms, and their impact on the family, the health and behavior of the spouse and children, many aspects of family life and activities (including contacts with kin and friends, leisure pursuits, and the distribution of household tasks and child-care activities), the nature and extent of parent-child interaction, and the relationships between different members of the family.

Some information was obtained on all children but detailed information was obtained for only 2 children in each family (chosen at random). Information on the children's behavior at school was obtained by means of a questionnaire completed by teachers [127].

[1]This investigation is being carried out in conjunction with Dr. Philip Graham, Mr. Quinton, Mr. Ziffo, Mrs. George, Miss Rowlands, Miss Tupling, and Miss Osborne. It is supported by a grant from the Association for the Aid of Crippled Children, New York.

Similar questionnaires were also completed for two other children in the same class (matched for age and sex). This was done in such a way that the teacher did not know who were the study children and who the controls. Considerable attention was paid to the standardization of interviewing methods, and on attaining high reliability and validity. In this we were reasonably successful [28, 129]. For present purposes the teachers' questionnaire is used as the only measure of the children's psychiatric state, as it provided the harshest test of associations between the family situation and child psychiatric disorder, our main concern [126]. On the questionnaire, the children's behavior is being assessed outside the home by teachers generally unacquainted with details of the child's family life, thus allowing no serious possibility of contamination of results.

The questionnaire has been shown to be a reasonable index of psychiatric disorder [127, 131] although, like any questionnaire, it is rather a crude index. As well as providing an overall assessment of the presence or absence of psychiatric disorder, it can be scored to differentiate neurotic disorders from antisocial disorders.

RESULTS OF STUDY

Two types of comparison can be made: (1) between children in the patient's families and children in the general population, in other words *"case versus control"* comparisons (this shows the difference between the children of patients and other children of the same age, sex, and school class); (2) *within sample* comparisons. In this case the comparison involves children all of whom have a parent under psychiatric care and it shows which children in which type of family develop disorder in relation to parental mental illness. As we are primarily concerned in determining what aspects of the situation lead to the development of psychiatric disorder in some children of patients (but not others), it is the second comparison which will be discussed first.

WITHIN-SAMPLE COMPARISONS

The diagnosis of the parental illness and the sex of the ill parent bore no relation to the likelihood of the children developing psychiatric disorder. The *clinical* characteristics of the parental disorder seemed largely irrelevant in this context, except that for boys (but not girls) the rate of child disorder was higher when a parent had an antisocial personality. The *social* impact of the illness on the family bore some relation to the rate of disorder in the children but by far the most important variable was the *quality of family relationships.*

Table 1 Marriage Rating and Teacher Questionnaire Designation of Boys

Marriage Rating	Teacher Questionnaire: Neurotic		Antisocial		Total Deviant		Total Number
	Number	Percent	Number	Percent	Number	Percent	
Good	1	(4)	0	(0)	1	(4)	23
Fair/Poor	5	(7)	11	(15)	21	(30)	71
Very Poor	6	(10)	27	(47)	37	(63)	59

Table 2 Marriage Rating and Teacher Questionnaire Designation of Girls

Marriage Rating	Teacher Questionnaire: Neurotic		Antisocial		Total Deviant		Total Number
	Number	Percent	Number	Percent	Number	Percent	
Good	2	(13)	2	(13)	4	(27)	15
Fair/Poor	9	(12)	12	(16)	23	(31)	74
Very Poor	7	(14)	10	(20)	17	(33)	51

For example, Tables 1 and 2 show child disorder in relation to the parental marriage rating. This is a highly reliable rating based on many factors including the frequency of quarreling, the amount of warmth between husband and wife, the hostility and criticism expressed by each about the other, and the quality of husband-wife interaction in household activities and leisure pursuits. The marriage rating bore *no* relation to the rate of disorder in girls, but in boys the worse the parental marriage the higher the rate of antisocial disorder in the sons. It can be seen from Table 3 that this association applied whether or not the parent had a personality disorder, but the rate of disorder was most high when there was *both* a parental personality disorder *and* a poor marriage.

Thus, boys were found to be more susceptible to the adverse effects of marital discord. This conclusion holds when specific aspects of the marriage, such as frequency of quarreling, are considered. Again the more the parents quarreled, the more likely were the boys to show antisocial disorder. In girls there was no difference. There was the same finding also when parental structure was considered. "Broken homes" were associated with antisocial disorder in boys, but not in girls. The same applies to admission to a children's home or to foster care; this was associated with an increased risk of antisocial disorder in boys, but in girls there was no such effect. Similar findings emerged from a consideration of the parent-child relationship. When parents showed very little warmth to their children, the rate of antisocial disorder was increased for sons but not daughters.

Table 3 Personality of Patient, Marriage Rating, and Boys' Teacher Questionnaire Designation

	Marriage Rating								
	Good			Fair/Poor			Very Poor		
Personality of Patient	Number Deviant	Percent	Total Number	Number Deviant	Percent	Total Number	Number Deviant	Percent	Total Number
Abnormal	1	(29)	7	7	24	(76)	31	41	40
Normal	0	(0)	16	13	(29)	45	6	(33)	18

In summary, discord and disruption in the home were consistently and strongly associated with antisocial disorder in boys, but not in girls. No consistent associations were found between family characteristics and neurosis in either boys or girls.

Family Disturbances and Antisocial Behavior

The finding that disturbance of family relationships is associated with antisocial disorder in boys is in keeping with numerous other prospective studies which have all shown family discord to be a powerful predictor of later disturbance in the children [36, 42, 49, 91, 117, 145]. It is striking that of all the family variables, it is discord, quarreling, unhappiness, and disruption which are most strongly and consistently associated with disorder in the child. Methods of child-rearing and types of disciplinary techniques are much less important in this respect [13, 30, 112]. Extremes may adversely affect children but, on the whole, patterns of child-rearing seem to be less influential on children's psychological development than are the quality of relationships in the home.

Unfortunately very few studies have examined findings separately according to the sex and diagnosis of the children. Some investigations have shown differences in the family background of neurotic and antisocial children [76, 88] but with a few notable exceptions [87]; the family characteristics of neurotic children have been less systematically investigated than those of delinquents, and those of girls have been much less studied than those of boys.

CAUSE OR EFFECT

The association between family discord and antisocial behavior is a strong one, but which leads to which and how it does so need also to be considered. In a thoughtful review of this issue, Bell [16] concluded that some of the parent-child correlations reported in the literature represent the effects of children on parents rather than the other way round. Robins [123], too, has provided a very useful discussion of the problems in differentiating causes from consequences when examining the social correlates of psychiatric disorder.

Nevertheless, although the children's characteristics undoubtedly influenced the parent-child interactions in the present study, it seems probable that the main effect was in the direction of parent to child, if only because the method of sampling was deliberately chosen so that in most cases the parental disorder extended the child's disorder.

Even if one can assume that the family situation was in some way part of the causative mechanisms involved in the genesis of the child's difficulties, this still leaves open the question as to whether the main effect was genetic or psychosocial in origin. The fact that the associations between parental discord and antisocial disorder in the child were found in a group of families in *all* of which a parent exhibited psychiatric disorder, makes a genetic explanation less likely. However, the issue can only be finally resolved by a comparable study of adopted or fostered children – a strategy used with great force in relation to schizophrenia [81, 124].

Sex Differences in Response to Family Stress

Perhaps the most novel aspect of the findings of this study concerns the large and consistent sex differences. All varieties of family discord and disruption – whether between the mother and father or between a parent and child – were strongly associated with antisocial disorder in boys but not in girls. Whether the explanation of these findings may lie in the methods used needs first to be considered.

Is the Sex Difference Due to Methodological Biases? (1) Is the sex difference peculiar to children's behavior at school? The findings refer entirely to disorder measured on the teachers' questionnaire. There is ample evidence from several studies (Rutter and Graham [130]; Rutter et al. [131]) that children behave differently at home and at school. It cannot be assumed that the same sex differences will follow a consideration of children's behavior at home (although preliminary findings suggest that the pattern is broadly similar).

(2) Can teachers perceive deviance in girls as well as in boys? If teachers were not as perceptive of psychiatric problems in girls as in boys, the questionnaire would not differentiate as well in girls, and associations with other variables would necessarily be more apparent in boys. But this is not the case. In other situations associations are stronger for girls than for boys (see below) and validity studies have shown no sex difference in teachers' perception of disorder.

(3) Is sex difference due to diagnostic differences? In this study, as in others, the diagnosis of the children's disorder was crucial. Family discord was related to antisocial disorder but not to neurosis. However, this cannot account for the sex difference in that it remains even when diagnosis is held constant. It could be suggested that diagnostic differences may be less reliable or less valid for girls than for boys, at least on the teachers' questionnaire, but this has not been found in this study or in previous investigations. Furthermore, sex differences were large even when total deviance was examined without reference to diagnosis.

It may be concluded that the sex difference cannot be accounted for in terms of the methods used and some other explanation must be found.

Does the Same Overall Family Situation Constitute a Different Stimulus for Girls than it Does for Boys? That the same overall family situation may constitute a different *stimulus* for girls than it does for boys is implicit in what is known about sex differences in parent-child interaction (see below). What is apparently the same situation may in practice be different for different children. Thus, the child who has greater contact with the disturbed parent or who has to take over more responsibility in the home when one parent is ill may be subject to greater stress than his sib who is less involved in the family difficulties. In the same kind of way the degree and type of stress will alter according to the nature of the child's relationships with the ill parent and with the strength and scope of the child's relationships with other adults. So far, only minor sex differences in these respects have been found and nothing has emerged which could account for the main findings.

Do Boys and Girls Respond to Different Family Stresses? Alternatively, it may be that, although boys and girls experience much the same stresses, they are adversely affected by different stresses. For example, it could be that whereas boys are susceptible to family discord, girls might be susceptible to undue restrictiveness. Surprisingly, there has been little investigation of this question. The few studies that have examined it – for example, Becker et al. [14] with respect to adjustment, Bronfenbrenner [25] with respect to leadership, and Hetherington [70] with respect to sex role behavior – have all suggested that there may be important differences in the ways boys and girls respond to family situations.

So far as the present study is concerned, the chief variables examined to date have involved family relationships. There are many other variables still to be studied and it may be that girls will prove to be more vulnerable than boys to some of them.

Are Girls More Permanently Affected by Stressful Events in Early Childhood? If girls were affected more permanently by stressful events in *early* childhood, they would necessarily be less liable to respond with new disorders to *current* family stresses. The present study findings are inconclusive in this respect but such evidence as there is seems to be against the hypothesis. The hypothesis would only be applicable if the family discord in the patient's families was of very recent duration, but in most cases it seemed to have been quite long-standing. It has already been noted that parent-child separations, which had usually occurred when the children were young, were much more strongly associated with disorder in boys than in girls. It was also found that when the parental illness was of over 5 years' duration, disorder occurred slightly more often in the sons than in the daughters.

Other longitudinal studies [12, 134] offer very limited evidence on the point but, as with this study, what little there is seems against the hypothesis.

Are Boys Generally More Susceptible to Sociofamilial Discord or Disruption? Finally in this connection it may be that the results reflect a general tendency for boys to be more susceptible than girls to the ill-effects of psychosocial stress. There is remarkably little evidence on this point. Most of the studies of reactions to acute stress have been solely concerned with men [75]. This applies particularly to the effects of stresses associated with battle and with other aspects of war. However, there are a few reports of civilian reactions to bombing. Contrary to the general belief that women are emotionally less stable than men, it was noted that among people attending British hospitals or clinics with emotional shock from air raids, men considerably outnumbered women (Gillespie [60]; Wilson [159]). These findings must be interpreted with caution in view of the selected nature of the samples studied and the absence of information on the age, sex, or other characteristics of the population at risk. On the other hand the sex differences reported were quite large and they are especially striking as in ordinary circumstances neuroses and depression are much more common in women than in men [2, 136].

Similar findings derive from a consideration of mortality following bereavement. It is widely recognized that recent bereavement may precipitate mental illness, particularly depression [116]. In this, women appear to be at least as susceptible as men, but the sex differences reported are of dubious validity in view of the fact that the studies involved selected hospital patients in whom decisions about referral and admission may well have biased the sex distribution. This criticism does not apply, however, to community-based studies of deaths following bereavement, which have shown that bereavement produces a markedly increased mortality among those recently widowed. There are several possible explanations for this finding [164], but a consideration of the timing (the deaths most commonly occur in the 6 months following bereavement) and other circumstances suggest that the deaths following bereavement are at least partially due to emotional stress. The risk of death has been found to be considerably greater for widowed men than for widowed women and also greater for bereaved boys than for bereaved girls [120]. Confirmation of this finding is needed, but the evidence to date suggests the greater vulnerability of the male in this context.

Studies of family pathology in relation to delinquency have nearly all concerned boys. An exception is a recent study of approved schoolgirls by Cowie and his colleagues [35], which showed an exceptionally high incidence of various forms of family breakdown. Of course, approved schoolgirls are a highly selected sample but Monahan's figures [102] showed that broken homes were more frequent in delinquent girls than delinquent boys even in first offenders. Toby [154] suggested on this basis that, relatively speaking, broken homes are more strongly conducive to delinquency in girls than in boys and pointed out in support that in cultures where there is a high rate of broken homes the rate of female delinquency is also higher – for example, among American Negroes. Possibly this may also apply to children of West Indian immigrants where the rate of antisocial girls referred to Child Guidance Clinics may be higher than in children born to English parents [65].

This apparently contradicts the findings of the present study, but interpretation depends on the likelihood of police bringing charges against girls, on the level of response to other factors, and on the base rate of delinquency in boys and in girls. A better test would be to examine the association the other way round – namely to look at delinquency rates in boys and girls from broken homes. Curiously, this has not been done. Yarrow [163], in his excellent review of the effects of separation experience, pointed out that scarcely anyone had looked for sex differences. This is a regrettable state of affairs and the issue of sex differences in children's responses to family disruption needs further investigation. At the moment the delinquency findings are impossible to interpret. It may be that in spite of the present findings, girls are generally more susceptible to the ill effects of family disruptions. However, taking into account the very much lower rate of delinquency in girls, it seems at least as likely that girls are *less* susceptible – it could be that they withstand the stresses of family discord and disruption much better than boys and it is only with very severe family pathology that they become delinquent.

Studies of foster children are also relevant in this context. Unfortunately, they suffer from the bias created by the fact that boys are more readily taken into foster care than are girls. Also the findings refer to *adult* adjustment rather than to the effects in childhood. However, it appears from Murphy's study [107, 108] that boys are more affected than girls by family pathology (alcoholism, mental disorder, and criminality), parental rejection, and by the amount of support given during the foster-care period. In contrast, he found that the adult outcome of girls was more influenced by the child coming from a home where the mother was unmarried or where the parents had separated prior to placement. This last finding was not confirmed by Meier [97, 98], who found a nonsignificant trend in the opposite direction.

With regard to other family stresses there is next to no evidence on sex differences. Weinstein and Geisel [157] argued that boys were more susceptible to family disturbances, but Baruch and Wilcox [11] reported the opposite. Both studies are open to substantial criticism so the results are inconclusive. Little is known about sex differences in response to school stresses, but there is some evidence that boys are at least as susceptible as girls to the effects of a good or bad relationship with the teacher [61].

The evidence is surprisingly meager and to some extent contradictory but when considered in relation to the clear-cut findings of the present study it seems that boys may be more vulnerable to the adverse effects of family discord and disruption.

Possible Mechanisms in the Development of Sex Differences

Surprisingly little attention has been paid to sex differences in most of the leading theories of child development. However, it may be useful to consider briefly some of the suggested mechanisms of development which give rise to possible explanations of known sex differences.

PSYCHOANALYTIC THEORY

In keeping with the prejudices of his time, Freud [52-54] regarded women as the inferior sex. He attributed this inferiority to the supposed overwhelming importance of penis envy in development and to a presumed greater complexity of the Oedipal phase in girls. In his view, the development of boys and girls was similar up to the onset of this phase. However, Freud's account of female development was never as well worked out as that of male development [3], and in many ways it is the least tenable and most forced aspect of his theorizing [144, 133]. There is doubt concerning many of his hypotheses about children's sexual knowledge [34, 144]. Although penis envy undoubtedly occurs, whether it has the overwhelming importance for later development that he claimed is very dubious. Even Deutsch [40], who accepted the bulk of Freud's teaching on this topic, maintained that it was most unlikely that penis envy had any primary role in the formation of feminine personality. Erikson [43] followed Freud in maintaining the importance of penis envy but like Deutsch thought that experiential factors were also important. Boys and girls do differ in their identification and attachment to parents, but Freudian theory leads to no clear prediction as to which sex should be the psychologically weaker (and certainly it offers no clues as to why the *male* should be weaker).

ATTACHMENT BEHAVIOR

Bowlby [21], especially, has pointed to the importance of the development of bonds between parent and child and he has suggested that much psychiatric disorder stems from disruption or distortion of such bonds [20]. Animal studies offer some support for this notion in that long-lasting psychological damage has been shown to follow *profound* social deprivation in early infancy [68]. However, social isolation may have to be very severe to have persisting effects [99] and contact with peers seems to be at least as important as contact with parents [69].

There appear to be sex differences in early mother-infant interaction both in humans [62, 106] and in nonhuman primates [77, 100]. On the whole, female infants are more dependent than males and there is more mother-daughter interaction, but sex differences vary according to the age of the infant. Although there is some suggestion that mother-daughter attachment may be stronger than mother-son, any conclusions based on this must also take into account father-infant interaction. Unfortunately, next to nothing is known about this in the human, but in animals other than the human, father-infant interaction seems to show sex differences only after infancy [101]. At least in older (human) children, cross-sex effects may also be relevant. There is some evidence that parents tend to be more affectionate and lenient with a child of the opposite sex and more reserved and strict with one of their own sex. Conversely, they tend to interact more with children of the same sex [23, 24, 41, 125]. At present, the findings on attachment behavior are too complex and too scanty to allow clear predictions on sex differences in susceptibility to psychological stress, although there are suggestions that early sex differences in parent-child interaction may play an important role in children's development.

CHILD REARING

Most of the outstanding studies of parental behavior have made little or no comment on sex differences. Unfortunately it is usually not clear whether this is because sex differences were looked for and not found or whether no systematic examination of sex differences was made. This applies, for example, to the Newson's [109, 110] careful and informative study of the upbringing of children in an English city. Sears et al. [135] found some differences in the ways that mothers treated boys and girls and D'Andrade [37] and Barry et al. [10] showed some consistency across cultures in sex differences regarding parents' training and expectations of the two sexes. Parental behavior, as reported by children, also varies according to the sex of the child but there are complex sex-age interaction effects [63]. Similarly, care-taking patterns for Kibbutz infants also showed sex-age interaction effects. In general, mothers attend more frequently to boys when they are young and fathers to boys when they are older [59].

However, most of the differences are surprisingly small, it is unclear to what extent the parental differences derive from biological differences in the children's behavior towards their parents (this issue is discussed in some of the papers on mother-infant interaction mentioned above), and the findings are of little help in explaining sex differences in response to family discord.

SUGGESTIBILITY AND CONFORMITY

Insofar as the patients' families provided deviant social pressures, sex differences in conformity and suggestibility might be relevant. In adults, studies have been quite consistent in showing that women are more liable than men to change their expressed attitudes following propaganda or social influences of other kinds [74, 82], but this seems not to be the case for young girls [1] except possibly with peer group pressures [73], so this does not get us much further, particularly in view of the weak association between altered attitudes and altered behavior [86].

IMITATION AND IDENTIFICATION

Bandura has argued for the importance of social reinforcement in learning and has suggested that imitation and identification play an important part in the development of behavior patterns both normal and abnormal. Over the last decade he and his colleagues have carried out a series of most ingenious experiments which have greatly advanced our understanding of these mechanisms [5-8]. On the whole, boys have been found to imitate aggressive behavior more readily than do girls but there are no consistent sex differences in the imitation of other kinds of behavior [47]. Thus, sex differences in the tendency to imitate as such cannot be invoked to account for sex differences in response to family discord.

CONDITIONABILITY

Eysenck and others [44, 45, 50] have theorized extensively on the role of conditioning in the development of psychiatric disorder. Put crudely, it has been suggested that antisocial disorders are due to a failure to acquire the necessary conditioned reflexes [46, 79], Hence, personality differences associated with conditionability have been postulated. Unfortunately, this attractive notion is set back by the finding that the same person responds differently to different types of conditioning [39, 51]. It seems that conditionability is probably not a general characteristic – there is eye-blink conditionability, heart-rate conditionability, G.S.R. conditionability, and so on, but they intercorrelate quite poorly. Furthermore, although there is some preliminary evidence that measures of conditioning may correlate with responses to treatment in phobic patients [96], they do not account for differences in the *acquisition* of phobias [94]. Sex differences in conditioning have been reported [19, 38, 119, 141] but the differences have been quite small and not always in the same direction. The concept of conditionability does not help in explaining sex differences in response to stress.

PHYSIOLOGIC RESPONSES TO STRESS

It would be instructive if physiologic measures gave a good indication of emotional disturbances in response to stress. Unfortunately, the association between autonomic and behavioral measures is too indirect and too variable from individual to individual [80, 84, 85] for this line of reasoning to be very productive. Sex differences in autonomic function and in response to stimulation have been reported [15, 17, 19, 89, 158] but they seem to vary according to which autonomic measure is used [119] and such (usually quite small) differences as have been found are very difficult to interpret and allow no ready prediction regarding sex differences in emotional responses to stress.

TEMPERAMENTAL DIFFERENCES

Particularly since Gesell's emphasis on behavioral differences between infants [58], there has been a tendency to explain children's responses to stress in terms of constitutional differences in temperament or in vulnerability. Thomas and his colleagues [150, 151] have carried this concept furthest in relation to temperamental differences and have produced some evidence to suggest that such differences in children may go some way towards explaining differences in their development of behavioral disorders [128, 151]. However, although there are differences between boys and girls in a wide range of cognitive and behavioral attributes [90, 149], so far there is no evidence that differences in temperamental characteristics can account for the major sex differences in child psychiatric disorder.

SEX DIFFERENCES IN RESPONSE TO BIOLOGICAL STRESS

A better understanding of sex differences in response to psychological stresses may come from a broader consideration of sex-linked susceptibilities to biological stresses. Here, the findings are remarkably clear cut. Although boys are larger than girls at most ages [57] and also stronger than girls in muscle power [64], there is sound evidence that they are more vulnerable to almost any kind of physical hazard.

Boys suffer more from the effects of complications of pregnancy and childbirth [29, 138], they more often get and more often die from infections in childhood [152, 156], they are more likely to suffer impairment of growth after radiation, as shown following Hiroshima, Nagasaki [66], and the Marshall Islands disaster [33], and they die younger [93]. In fact, apart from auto-immune conditions (and, of course, disorders of the female sex organs), in nearly all cases where there is a sex difference, it is the male who gets the disease earlier in life and who more often dies from the disease [18, 32].

It has sometimes been thought that this sex difference might be due to greater sociocultural pressures and strains which our culture lays upon male shoulders. That this is most unlikely to be the case was neatly shown by Madigan [93] in his comparison of Roman Catholic Brothers and Sisters who had entered a religious community in early adult life and who were engaged in teaching or administration. Although the men and women led closely similar lives, the women outlived the men by several years, as in the general public. Even more striking is the finding that male rats appear to show greater behavioral deficits following malnutrition than do female rats [9].

Why this should be so is not known but it is likely that the sex difference in maturation is one factor. Girls are more mature than boys at all ages up to maturity. The difference, due to the Y chromosome [147] is as much as several weeks even at birth, is one year at the time of starting school, and almost two years at puberty [48, 146]. The sex difference is even more marked with *disorders* of development (such as delays in language) than it is with normal development [131].

The reason for supposing that the greater immaturity of boys is a partial cause of their greater vulnerability rests on the fact that, in general, immature organisms are more susceptible to damage than are mature ones and on the observation that the sex difference in morbidity varies according to age [148]. Thus, it has been reported that cerebral palsy is commoner in boys when the birth is full-term but not when it is premature [92]. Similarly, radiation affects the growth of boys more than girls if the exposure to radiation is during childhood [66], but not if it is during foetal life [162]. In fact, sex differences in relation to prenatal stress generally are nothing like as consistent as those for postnatal stress [78]. There is also some suggestion that the sex difference in infantile mortality is less marked for premature births than it is for mature births, although there are other possible explanations for this [29].

However, slower development cannot be the whole explanation as not only do girls reach physical maturity earlier than boys but also they live considerably longer. The male grows up more slowly, gets more illnesses, and dies sooner! As if to compensate for this biological weakness of the male, there are about 125 boys for every 100 girls conceived.

Some people have suggested that the male inferiority may be due to his having 4 to 5 percent less chromosomal material [32]. Also, although the major sex differences in body chemistry and composition are not apparent until near puberty [114], it seems that there may be some sex differences even in infancy [115]. How these relate to the greater vulnerability of the male is quite unknown. However, whatever the reason, there can be no doubt that in terms of susceptibility to physical stresses the male is the weaker sex. It may well be that the presumed greater male susceptibility to psychological stress is also biologically determined and related to this susceptibility to physical stresses.

Why Is Adult Neurosis Commoner in Women?

If it is accepted that the evidence points towards the male being psychologically as well as physically more vulnerable, the question immediately arises as to why adult neurosis is so much commoner in women than in men and why the sex distribution for child psychiatric disorder is the reverse of that for adult psychiatric disorder [4]. In this context it is appropriate to return to the findings of the present study to consider case versus control comparisons.

PROSPECTIVE STUDY – CASE VERSUS CONTROL COMPARISONS

Up to this point the findings have entirely referred to within-sample comparisons, but as mentioned earlier a second type of comparison is also possible. For each child in a patient's family, questionnaires were completed for two control children of the same age and sex in the child's school class (the teacher not being informed who were cases and who controls).

Table 4 shows the rates of deviance in the children of patients and in the control children. Psychiatric disorder was over twice as

Table 4 **Teacher Questionnaire Findings for Cases and Controls (Matched for age, sex, and school class)**

	Male Patients				Female Patients			
	Boys		Girls		Boys		Girls	
	Number	Percent	Number	Percent	Number	Percent	Number	Percent
Cases								
Normal on Q.	51		50		53		55	
Deviant on Q.	24	(32)	24	(32)	29	(35)	24	(30)
Total	75		74		82		79	
Controls								
Normal on Q.	106		123		120		145	
Deviant on Q.	44	(29)	22	(15)	43	(26)	13	(8)
Total	150		145		163		158	

common in the daughters of patients as in the control girls (30-32 percent versus 8-15 percent), regardless of whether the patient was the father or mother. In sharp contrast, the rate of disorder in the sons of patients was only slightly (and nonsignificantly) above the rate in the control boys. In the controls, as in virtually all previous studies [131], the rate of disorder was twice as high in boys as in girls. In the cases, on the other hand, disorder was equally common in the two sexes. The case-control difference applies at all ages for girls but at no age was there a significant difference for boys.

Table 5 **Diagnosis on Teacher Questionnaire for Cases and Controls**

	Boys				Girls			
Questionnaire Diagnosis	Cases		Controls		Cases		Controls	
	Number	Percent	Number	Percent	Number	Percent	Number	Percent
Normal	104		226		105		268	
Deviant	53		87		48		36	
Neurotic	12	(8)	38	(12)	20	(13)	17	(6)
Antisocial	33	(21)	43	(14)	26	(17)	15	(5)
Mixed	8	(5)	6	(2)	2	(1)	4	(1)
Total	157		313		153		304	

Table 5 shows that the increased rate of disorder in the cases was due more to an increase in antisocial disorder than to neurotic disorder. The slight case-control difference for boys was entirely accounted for by an increase in antisocial disorders and the large difference for girls was somewhat more marked for antisocial disorder than neurosis, although both were increased.

These findings appear paradoxical in that the within-sample differences applied largely to boys whereas the case versus control differences applied largely to girls. The possible reasons for this reversal of sex difference need to be discussed.

Are There Any Biases in the Methodology? Most of the methodological problems have already been considered but a possible bias arising out of the way in which controls were selected (from among children in the same school class) needs to be mentioned. The lack of difference between cases and controls with respect to boys (but not girls) could be explained if there was a very strong tendency to place all troublesome boys in the same class but no such tendency for girls. If this happened there should be a higher correlation between the questionnaire scores of boy-cases and boy-controls than between girl-cases and girl-controls, but this was *not* found. This finding makes it most unlikely that streaming could have created any substantial bias but, as a further check, a fresh control group is being selected at random from the general population rather than by school class.

Is the Difference Between Cases and Controls Different in Kind from that Found Within Cases? If the differences *between* the patients' families and the control families were *qualitatively* different from those found *within* the group of patients' families, this might explain the contrasting sex ratio in the two comparisons.

Within the cases, child disorders were mainly associated with family discord and persistent parental antisocial behavior. Thus, if the case-control comparison differed in kind, the difference must have involved some other variable. It seems unlikely that there was a *qualitative* difference between patients and non-patients in the presence of psychiatric disorder (although there was probably a quantitative difference) in view of the high rate of psychiatric disorder found in people not attending psychiatrists [136]. There were too few psychotics for this to constitute the difference. If the difference did not lie in the presence of psychiatric disorder, it is not at all clear what differences there could have been between cases and controls which were not also present within cases.

It seems unlikely that this suggestion provides an adequate explanation of the sex differences but the matter requires further exploration by a detailed comparison of patients' families and families in the general population – a study now in progress.

Are Different Mechanisms Involved in the Development of Disorder in Boys and Girls? It could be that different mechanisms are involved in the pathogenesis of psychiatric disorder in boys and girls. In boys disorder seemed to arise in large part as a response to family discord. In girls some other mechanism may be responsible, and it is suggested that it may be largely genetic. In other words the effects of parental mental disorder are predominantly genetic in girls and predominantly environmental in boys.

At first sight this seems rather an unlikely hypothesis and admittedly there is no direct evidence in support. Nevertheless, previous longitudinal studies have suggested that different mechanisms may be important in the development of boys and girls. For example, the study of children seen at the Judge Baker Clinic who later developed schizophrenia [155] showed that certain symptoms were antecedents of schizophrenia in boys but not in girls [55]. On the other hand, maternal psychopathology was associated with schizophrenia in girls but not in boys [56]. Of course, whether these differences reflect genetic or environmental effects cannot be determined from the data. Studies of psychological development in normal children [26, 27, 72, 80, 104, 105] have also shown that different factors are predictive in boys and in girls.

There are precedents, then, for the suggestion that different factors may be important in the psychological development of boys and girls. The first half of the hypothesis – that boys develop antisocial disorder in response to family discord – carries with it the corollary that they must be more susceptible than girls in this respect. As we have seen, there is some evidence in support of this view. The second half of the hypothesis – that girls (who are daughters of psychiatric patients) develop psychiatric disorder through genetic mechanisms – has a similar corollary, that the genetic effect must affect girls more than boys.

The difficulty in this half of the hypothesis lies in corollary – why should genetic factors have a greater effect on girls than boys? This brings us back to the earlier question as to why adult neurosis and depression are commoner in women whereas there is a very much smaller sex difference for neurosis in girls [131]. If it assumed that the sex difference in adult disorders is genetically determined (a point to be returned to), then a genetic effect on the children is likely to affect girls more than boys.

So far this suggestion fits in with the situation in the present study. Most of the parents had neurosis or depression and it could be that the rate of disorder in girls was increased by the addition of adult-type neurosis. The rate in boys would be increased only to a small extent due to adult neurosis and depression being largely female disorders.

This implies that adult neurosis differs from child neurosis (because the sex ratio is different) and there is good evidence in support of this suggestion. Robins [122] clearly showed in her long-term follow-up study that there is little continuity between child neurosis and adult neurosis. It is evident that most neuroses in childhood are short-lived and it is probable (although less well demonstrated) that most adult neuroses begin in adult life rather than in childhood. But as Pritchard and Graham [118] found, some child neuroses do persist into adult life. Apart from certain types of phobia [95], we do not yet know how to distinguish child neuroses which remain confined to childhood, from those which arise in childhood and continue into adult life and those neuroses which start for the first time after reaching maturity.

A consequence of these findings is that the genes hypothesized to cause the increased rate of disorder in the daughters of patients must do so by increasing their susceptibility to those adult-type neuroses which have their origins in childhood. This suggestion can be tested by determining if the disorders in the daughters are unusually persistent. If they are not, serious doubt would be cast on the hypothesis. Evidence on this should become available in a few years' time.

There are two further predictions based on the hypothesis which allow some preliminary testing of its validity. Firstly, if the effect on girls is largely genetic then there should not be a sex difference with parental disorders (such as schizophrenia) which occur with approximately the same frequency in both sexes. There were too few schizophrenics in the present sample to test this but the preliminary findings from a similar but larger study of schizophrenics by Dr G. W. Brown and his colleagues has shown in the children of schizophrenics just what is predicted. There was no sex difference in case versus control comparisons in his study [27a].

Secondly, there is another implication of the hypothesis which can be tested. It will be recalled that the excess of disorder in the girl-cases over the girl-controls was largely in terms of antisocial disorder but the parents mainly had neurosis or depression. This implies that antisocial disorder in girls is genetically associated with adult neurosis.

Unlikely though this seems on first consideration, there is some evidence in support. The Robins [122] follow-up study of children attending a child guidance clinic showed that most children of both sexes (74 percent of boys and 68 percent of girls) had been referred for antisocial problems, there being no appreciable sex difference in this. But in adult life only 10 percent of the boys compared with 44 percent of the girls were neurotic. In boys antisocial behavior in childhood led to sociopathy in the adult, in girls it more often led to neurosis, particularly "hysteria". There was a similar tendency in the Pritchard and Graham [118] study but the numbers were too small to assess the significance of the sex difference.

It may also be relevant to note that, apart from the children of mentally ill parents, the only other situation where the rate of psychiatric disorder is as high in girls as in boys is when the children have some neuro-epileptic disorder [111, 132]. This parallel suggests that there may be a biologic effect on susceptibility to psychiatric disorder.

It may be concluded that the hypothesis that the effects of parental mental illness on girls is largely genetic remains plausible but requires further testing before it can be regarded as more than speculative.

Is the Sex Difference in Adult Neurosis and Depression Genetically Determined? The hypothesis just discussed rests on the assumption that the sex difference in adult neurosis and depression is genetically determined. There is evidence that hereditary factors play some part in susceptibility to neurosis and depression [139], but whether genetic influences determine the sex difference in rates of these disorders is unknown. It seems that concordance rates in twins for hospital-treated neurosis are similar for men and women but in one study it was found that only in female pairs were identicals more alike than fraternals in "neuroticism" [137]. The role of genetics in sex differences for adult neurosis and depression requires further investigation.

Is the Sex Difference in Adult Neurosis and Depression Socially Determined? Apart from genetics, there are several other possible explanations of the sex difference, the most likely of which concerns differences in men's and women's social role. This is partly determined by society's attitude towards the two sexes, and in most cultures the inferiority of the female is taken for granted. Because she is assumed to be inferior, social pressures may make her so.

The Bible is quite clear that man is the basic model, woman being just an afterthought created from one of man's ribs, and in the Christian church, even today, woman is allowed only an inferior position. Arabs commiserate when a woman gives birth to a daughter, and orthodox Jewish men give thanks in their prayers that they were not born a woman.

In the English language masculinity is taken to mean "virile, vigorous, powerful" in contrast to feminine which is used as an "epithet denoting simplicity, inferiority, weakness" [113]. Even the heroes in children's stories are more than twice as likely to be male as female [31a]. There have been emotive protests against the biological injustice of these cultural stereotypes [103] but they are deeply entrenched.

As a consequence, in nearly all societies women tend to occupy a subordinate position. Often they are discouraged from taking a job outside the home and, if men do allow them to work, they are frequently expected to take simpler, less arduous, more lowly paid jobs. Although the pattern in our culture is changing and is in any case variable, in marriage, too, women frequently have to take second place in decision making and in other aspects of dominance and control [31, 143, 153]. They often pay the bills but they less often control the purse strings. Perhaps most important of all as well as bearing children, they usually have to take the main responsibility in child-rearing.

To what extent these social differences constitute a stress of protection is not clear. However, some estimate may be obtained by comparing the effects of marriage on health in men and women. In men the position is quite straightforward; the married state carries with it a considerably lower rate of mental and physical illness and a lower death rate [2, 121, 136]. In part this may be due to handicapped men not marrying, but the differences between married men and divorced or widowed men (who also have higher rates of death and illness) suggests that the married state may also act as some sort of safeguard against physical and mental illness.

The position for the female is quite different. In women, and especially in young women, the differences are small and may sometimes even be in the opposite direction [142]. Thus, in Shepherd's general practice study [136] married men had significantly lower rates of psychiatric disorder than single men, but in women there was no significant difference and the rate was actually slightly lower in the single than in the married. Similarly, Hinkle and Wolff [71] in a study of health and people's life situation found that the healthiest group consisted of middle-aged women with a full-time job who had never sought marriage – a minority group in our society but apparently a particularly healthy one.

These findings refer to mental health, but similar results have come from studies of "happiness." Whereas single men report themselves as unhappy much more often than do married men, there is little difference in the happiness of married women and single women [22, 67]. The matter requires further investigation but it seems that whereas men may be protected by marriage; for women, child-rearing, housekeeping, and the role of the passive marriage partner may sometimes constitute a stress. The implication is that our culture creates greater stresses for women than for men and that this may be part of the explanation for adult neurosis and depression being commoner in the female.

Conclusions

The evidence on sex differences discussed in this chapter highlights the need to investigate the mechanisms involved in children's responses to parental mental disorder. There are important gaps in our knowledge of the topic but it appears that boys and girls may react very differently to family stress. The findings already available are sufficient to indicate the need to take into account in our daily clinical practice the obvious but sometimes overlooked fact that "boys and girls are different."

Bibliography

1. Abelson, R. P. and G. S. Lesser, The measurement of persuasibility in children in C. I. Hovland and I. L. Janis, Eds., *Personality and Persuasibility,* Yale University Press, New Haven, 1959.
2. Adelstein, A. M., D. Y. Downham, Z. Stein, and M. W. Susser, The epidemiology of mental illness in an English city, *Social Psychiatry,* 3 (1968), 47.
3. Baldwin, A. L., *Theories of Child Development,* John Wiley, London, 1968.
4. Baldwin, J. A., Psychiatric illness from birth to maturity: an epidemiological study, *Acta Psychiat. Scand.,* 44 (1968), 313.
5. Bandura, A., D. Ross, and S. A. Ross, Imitation of film-mediated aggressive models, *J. abn. soc. Psychol.,* 66 (1963a), 3.
6. Bandura, A., D. Ross, and S. A. Ross, Vicarious reinforcement and imitative learning, *J. abn. soc. Psychol.,* 67 (1963b), 601.
7. Bandura, A., J. E. Grusec, and F. L. Menlove, Vicarious extinction of avoidance behaviour, *J. Pers. soc. Psychol.,* 5 (1967a), 16.
8. Bandura, A., J. E. Grusec, and F. L. Menlove, Some social determinants of self-monitoring reinforcement systems, *J. Pers. soc. Psychol.,* 5 (1967b), 449.
9. Barnes, R. H., Experimental animal approaches to the study of early malnutrition and mental development, *Federation Proceedings,* 26 (1967), 144.
10. Barry, H., M. K. Bacon, and E. L. Child, A cross-cultural survey of some sex differences in socialization, *J. abn. soc. Psychol.,* 55 (1957), 327.
11. Baruch, D. W. and J. A. Wilcox, A study of sex differences in preschool children's adjustment co-existent with interparental tensions. *J. genet. Psychol.,* 64 (1944), 281.
12. Bayley, N. and E. S. Schaefer, Correlations of maternal and child behaviours with the development of mental abilities: data from the Berkeley Growth Study, *Mon. Soc. Res. Child Dev.,* 29 (1964), 6, No. 97.
13. Becker, W. C., Consequences of different kinds of parental discipline in M. C. and L. W. Hoffmans, Eds., *Review of Child Development Research Vol. 1.,* Russell Sage Foundation, New York, 1964.
14. Becker, W. C., D. R. Peterson, Z. Luria, D. J. Shoemaker, and L. A. Hellmer, Relations of factors derived from parent-interview ratings to behaviour problems of five-year-olds, *Child Develop.,* 33 (1962), 509.
15. Beintema, D. J., *A Neurological Study of Newborn Infants,* Clinics in Developmental Medicine No. 28, Wm Heinemann, London, 1968.
16. Bell, R. Q., A reinterpretation of the direction of effects in studies of socialization, *Psychol. Rev.,* 75 (1968), 81.
17. Bell, R. Q. and N. S. Costello, Three tests for sex differences in tactile sensitivity in the newborn, *Biol. Neonat.* (Basel), 7 (1964), 335.
18. Bentzen, F., Sex ratios in learning and behaviour disorders, *Amer. J. Orthopsychiat.,* 33 (1963), 92.
19. Berry, J. L. and B. Martin, G.S.R. reactivity as a function of anxiety, instructions, and sex, *J. abnorm. soc. Psychol.,* 54 (1957), 9.
20. Bowlby, J. Childhood bereavement and psychiatric illness in D. Richter, J. M. Tanner, Taylor Lord, O. B. Zangwill, Eds., *Aspects of Psychiatric Research,* Oxford University Press, London, 1962.

21. Bowlby, J., *Attachment and Loss, Vol. 1: Attachment,* Hogarth Press, London, 1969.
22. Bradburn, N. M. and D. Caplovitz, *Reports on Happiness,* Aldine, Chicago, 1965.
23. Brim, O. G., The parent-child relations as a social system: I. Parent and child roles, *Child Develop.,* 28 (1957), 343.
24. Bronfenbrenner, U., Towards a theoretical model for the analysis of parent-child relationships in a social context, in J. C. Glidewell, Ed., *Parental Attitudes and Child Behaviour,* Chas. C. Thomas, Springfield, Ill., 1961a.
25. Bronfenbrenner, U., Some familial antecedents of responsibility and leadership in adolescents in L. Petrullo and B. M. Bass, Eds., *Leadership and Interpersonal Behaviour,* Holt, New York, 1961b.
26. Bronson, W. C., Early antecedents of emotional expressiveness and reactivity control, *Child Develop.,* 37 (1966), 793.
27. Bronson, W., Adult derivatives of emotional expressiveness and reactivity-control: developmental continuities from childhood to adulthood, *Child Develop.,* 38 (1967), 801.

27a. Brown, G. W., personal communication, 1969.

28. Brown, G. W., and M. Rutter, The measurement of family activities and relationships – a methodological study, *Human Relations,* 19 (1966), 241.
29. Butler, N. R. and D. G. Bonham, *Perinatal Mortality*, E. & S. Livingstone, London, 1963.
30. Caldwell, B. M., The effects of infant care in M. L. and L. W. Hoffman, Eds., *Review of Child Development Research,* Vol. 1, Russell Sage Foundation, New York, 1964.
31. Carstairs, G. M., The changing role of women, *The Listener,* LXVIII (1962), 947.

31a. Child, I. L., E. H. Potter, E. M. Levine, Children's textbooks and personality development: an exploration in the social psychology of education, *Psychol. Mon. 60,* Whole No. 279 (1946).

32. Childs, B., Genetic origin of some sex differences among human beings, *Pediat.,* 35 (1965), 798.
33. Conard, R. A., C. E. Huggins, B. Cannon, A. Lowrey, and J. B. Richards, Medical survey of Marshallese two years after exposure to fall-out radiation, *J. Amer. Med. Assoc.,* 164 (1957), 1192.
34. Conn, J. H., Children's reactions to the discovery of genital differences, *Amer. J. Orthopsychiat.,* 10 (1940), 747.
35. Cowie, J. C., V. Cowie, and E. Slater, *Delinquency in Girls,* Wm. Heinemann, London, 1968.
36. Craig, M. M. and S. J. Glick, *A Manual of Procedures for Applications of the Glueck Prediction Table,* University London Press, London, 1965.
37. D'Andrade, R. G., Sex differences and cultural institutions in E. E. Maccoby, Ed., *The Development of Sex Differences,* Tavistock Publications, London, 1967.
38. Davidson, P. O., R. W. Payne, R. B. Sloane, Introversion, neuroticism and conditioning, *J. abn. soc. Psychol.,* 68 (1964), 136.
39. Davidson, P. O., R. W. Payne, R. B. Sloane, Conditionability in normals and neurotics, *J. exp. Res. Pers.,* 3 (1968), 107.
40. Deutsch, H., *The Psychology of Women, Vol. 1,* Research Books Ltd., London, 1947.

41. Devereux, E. C., U. Bronfenbrenner, and G. J. Suci, Patterns of parent behaviour in the United States of America and the Federal Republic of Germany: a cross national comparison, *Int. soc. Sci. J.*, 14 (1963), 2.
42. Douglas, J. W. B., J. M. Ross, and H. R. Simpson, *All our Future: a Longitudinal Study of Secondary Education*, Peter Davies, London, 1968.
43. Erikson, E. H., *Childhood and Society* (2nd Ed.), W. W. Norton & Co., New York, 1950.
44. Eysenck, H. J., *The Dynamics of Anxiety and Hysteria*, Routledge and Kegan Paul, London, 1957.
45. Eysenck, H. J., Classification and the problems of diagnosis in H. J. Eysenck, Ed., *Handbook of Abnormal Psychology*, Basic Books, New York, 1960a.
46. Eysenck, H. J., Learning theory and behaviour therapy in H. J. Eysenck, Ed., *Behaviour Therapy and The Neuroses*, Pergamon, London, 1960b.
47. Flanders, J. P., A review of research on imitative behaviour, *Psychol. Bull.*, 69 (1968), 316.
48. Flory, C. D., Sex differences in skeletal development, *Child Develop.*, 6 (1935), 205.
49. Forssman, H. and I. Thuwe, One hundred and twenty children born after application for therapeutic abortion refused, *Acta Psychiat. Scand.*, 42 (1966), 71.
50. Franks, C. M., Conditioning and abnormal behaviour in H. J. Eysenck, Ed., *Handbook of Abnormal Psychology*, Basic Books, New York, 1960.
51. Franks, C. M. and V. Franks, "Conditionability" as a general factor of man's performance in different conditioning situations. *Paper in Abstracts. Vol. 1*, p. 331 of XVIII Internat. Congr. Psychol., Moscow, 1966.
52. Freud, S., Three contributions to the theory of sex, *Nerv. Ment. Dis. Mon. Series* 1930, No. 7 (1905).
53. Freud, S. Some psychical consequences of the anatomical distinction between the sexes, *Standard Edition*, 19 (1925), 243.
54. Freud, S., *New Introductory Lectures on Psychoanalysis*, Hogarth Press, London, 1933.
55. Gardner, G. G., The relationship between childhood neurotic symptomatology and later schizophrenia in males and females, *J. nerv. ment. Dis.*, 144 (1967a), 97.
56. Gardner, G. G., Role of maternal psychopathology in male and female schizophrenics, *J. cons. Psychol.*, 31 (1967b), 411.
57. Garn, S. M., Body size and its implications in L. W. and M. B. Hoffman, Eds., *Review of Child Development Research*, Vol. 2, Russell Sage Foundation, New York, 1966.
58. Gesell, A., Early evidences of individuality in the human infant, *Scientific Monthly*, XLV (1937), 217.
59. Gewirtz, H. B. and J. L. Gewirtz, Visiting and caretaking patterns for kibbutz infants: age and sex trends, *Amer. J. Orthopsychiat., 38 (1968)*, 427.
60. Gillespie, R. D., *Psychological Effects of War on Citizen and Soldier*. Norton, New York, 1942.
61. Glidewell, J. C., M. B. Kantor, L. M. Smith, and L. A. Stringer, Socialization and social structure in the classroom in L. W. and M. L. Hoffman, Eds., *Review of Child Development Research*, Vol. 2, Russell Sage Foundation, New York, 1966.

62. Goldberg, S. and M. Lewis, Play behaviour in the year-old infant: early sex differences, *Child Develop.*, 40 (1969), 21.
63. Goldin, P. C., A review of children's reports of parent behaviours, *Psychol. Bull.*, 71 (1969), 222.
64. Goss, A. M., Estimated versus actual physical strength in three ethnic groups, *Child Develop.*, 39 (1968), 283.
65. Graham, P. J. and C. E. Meadows, Psychiatric disorder in the children of West Indian immigrants, *J. Child Psychol. Psychiat.*, 8 (1967), 105.
66. Greulich, W. W., C. S. Crismon, and M. L. Turner, The physical growth and development of children who survived the atomic bombing of Hiroshima or Nagasaki, *J. Pediat.*, 43 (1953), 121.
67. Gurin, G., J. Veroff, and S. Feld, *Americans View Their Mental Health*, Basic Books, New York, 1960.
68. Harlow, H. F. and G. Griffin, Induced mental and social deficits in Rhesus monkeys in S. F. Osler and R. E. Cooke, Eds., *The Biosocial Basis of Mental Retardation*, Johns Hopkins Press, Baltimore, Md., 1965.
69. Harlow, H. F. and M. K. Harlow, Effects of various mother-infant relationships on Rhesus monkey behaviours in B. M. Foss, Ed., *Determinants of Infant Behaviour IV*, Methuen, London, 1969.
70. Hetherington, E. M., The effects of familial variables on sex typing, on parent-child similarity and on imitation in children in J. P. Hill, Ed., *Minnesota Symposium on Child Psychology, Vol. 1*, Univ. of Minnesota Press, Minneapolis, 1967.
71. Hinkle, L. E. and H. G. Wolff, Health and the social environment in A. H. Leighton, J. A. Clausen, and R. N. Wilson, Eds., *Explorations in Social Psychiatry*, Tavistock Publications, London, 1957.
72. Honzik, M. P., Environmental correlates of mental growth: prediction from the family setting at 21 months, *Child Develop.*, 38 (1967), 337.
73. Iscoe, I., M. Williams, and J. Harvey, Modifications of children's judgements by a simulated group technique: a normative developmental study, *Child Develop.*, 34 (1963), 963.
74. Janis, I. L. and P. B. Field, Sex differences and personality factors related to persuasibility in C. I. Howland and L. L. Janis, Eds., *Personality and Persuasibility*, Yale Univ. Press, New Haven, 1959.
75. Janis, I. L. and H. Leventhal, Human reaction to stress in E. Borgatta and W. W. Lambert, Eds., *Handbook of Personality Theory and Research*, Rand McNally, Chicago, 1969.
76. Jenkins, R. L., Psychiatric syndromes in children and their relation to family background, *Amer. J. Orthopsychiat.*, 36 (1966), 450.
77. Jensen, G. D., R. A. Bobbitt, and B. N. Gordon, Sex differences in social interaction between infant monkeys and their mothers in J. Wortis, Ed., *Recent Advances in Biological Psychiatry*, Vol. IX, Plenum Press, New York, 1967.
78. Joffe, J. M., *Prenatal Determinants of Behaviour*, Pergamon, London, 1969.
79. Jones, H. G., Behaviour therapy and conditioning techniques in E. Miller, Ed., *Foundations of Child Psychiatry*, Pergamon, London, 1968.
80. Kagan, J. and H. A. Moss, *Birth to Maturity*, John Wiley, New York, 1962.
81. Kety, S., D. Rosenthal, P. H. Wender, and P. Schulsinger, The types and prevalence of mental illness in the biological and adoptive families of

adopted schizophrenics, in D. Rosenthal and S. S. Kety, Eds., *Transmission of Schizophrenia,* Pergamon, London, 1968.

82. King, B. T., Relationships between susceptibility to opinion change and child-rearing practices in C. I. Hovland and I. L. Janis, Eds., *Personality and Persuasibility,* Yale Univ. Press, New Haven, 1959.
83. Kreitler, H. and S., Children's concepts of sexuality and birth, *Child Develop.,* 37 (1966), 363.
84. Lacey, J. I., The evaluation of autonomic responses: toward a general solution, *Anu. N.Y. Acad. Sci.,* 67 (1956), 123.
85. Lacey, J. I. and R. van Lehn, Differential emphasis in somatic response to stress, *Psychosom. Med.,* 14 (1952), 71.
86. Leventhal, H., S. Jones, and G. Trembly, Sex differences in attitude and behaviour change under conditions of fear and specific instructions, *J. exp. Soc. Psychol.,* 2 (1966), 387.
87. Levy, D., *Maternal Overprotection,* Columbia Univ. Press, New York, 1943.
88. Lewis, H., *Deprived Children,* Oxford Univ. Press, London, 1943.
89. Lipsitt, L. P. and N. Levy, Electrotactual threshold in the neonate, *Child Develop.,* 30 (1959), 547.
90. Maccoby, E. E., Ed., *The Development of Sex Differences,* Tavistock Publications, London, 1967.
91. McCord, W. and J. McCord, *Origins of Crime,* Columbia Univ. Press, New York, 1959.
92. McDonald, A. D., Cerebral palsy in children of very low birth weight, *Arch. Dis. Childhd.,* 38 (1963), 579.
93. Madigan, F. C., Are sex mortality differentials biologically caused? *Milbank Mem. Fund Quart.,* 35 (1957), 202.
94. Marks, I. M., *Fears and Phobias,* Wm. Heinemann, London, 1969.
95. Marks, I. M. and M. G. Gelder, Different ages of onset in varieties of phobia, *Amer. J. Psychiat.,* 123 (1966), 218-221.
96. Martin, I., I. M. Marks, and M. G. Gelder, Conditioned eyelid responses in phobic patients, *Behav. Res. Ther.,* 7 (1969), 115.
97. Meier, E. G., Current circumstances of former foster children, *Child Welfare,* 44 (1965), 196.
98. Meier, E. G., Adults who were foster children, *Children,* 13 (1966), 16.
99. Meier, G. W., Other data on the effects of social isolation during rearing upon the adult reproductive behaviour in the Rhesus monkey (Macaca-Mulatta), *Animal Behaviour,* 13 (1965), 228.
100. Mitchell, G. D., Attachment differences in male and female infant monkeys, *Child Develop.,* 39 (1968), 611.
101. Mitchell, G. D., Paternalistic behaviour in primates, *Psychol. Bull.,* 71 (1969), 399.
102. Monahan, T. P., Family status and the delinquent child: a reappraisal and some new findings, *Social Forces,* 35 (1957), 250.
103. Montagu, A., *The Natural Superiority of Women* (2nd Ed.), Collier-Macmillan, London, 1968.
104. Moore, T., Language and intelligence: a longitudinal study of the first eight years. Part I. Patterns of development in boys and girls., *Hum. Develop.,* 10 (1967), 88.

105. Moore, T., Language intelligence: a longitudinal study of the first eight years. Part II Environmental correlates of mental growth, *Hum. Develop.*, 11 (1968), 1.
106. Moss, H. A., Sex, age, and state as determinants of mother-infant interaction, *Merril-Palmer Quart.*, 13 (1967), 19.
107. Murphy, H. B. M., Natural family pointers to foster care outcome, *Mental Hygiene*, 48 (1964a), 380.
108. Murphy, H. B. M., Foster home variables and adult outcome, *Mental Hygiene*, 48 (1964b), 587.
109. Newson, J. and E., *Infant Care in an Urban Community*, Allen & Unwin, London, 1963.
110. Newson, J. and E., *Four Years Old in an Urban Community*, Allen & Unwin, London, 1968.
111. Nuffield, E. J. A., Neuro-physiology and behaviour disorders in epileptic children, *J. ment. Sci.*, 107 (1961), 438.
112. Oleinick, M. S., A. K. Bahn, L. Eisenberg, and A. M. Lilienfeld, Early socialization experiences and intrafamilial environment, *Arch Gen. Psychiat.*, 15 (1966), 344.
113. Onions, O. T., Ed., *The Shorter Oxford English Dictionary* (Third Ed.), Clarendon Press, Oxford, 1959.
114. Owen, G. M. and J. Brozek, Influence of age, sex and nutrition on body composition during childhood and adolescence in F. Falkner, Ed., *Human Development*, W. B. Saunders, Philadelphia and London, 1966.
115. Owen, G. W., L. J. Filer, M. Maresh, and S. J. Fomon, Sex-related differences in body compositions in infancy in F. Falkner, Ed., *Human Development*, W. B. Saunders, Philadelphia and London, 1966.
116. Parkes, C. M., Recent bereavement as a cause of mental illness, *Brit. J. Psychiat.*, 110 (1964), 198.
117. Power, M. J. and Shoenberg, Children before the courts in one community. Mimeographed Report, 1967.
118. Pritchard, M. and P. Graham, An investigation of a group of patients who have attended both the child and adult department of the same psychiatric hospital, *Brit. J. Psychiat.*, 112 (1966), 603.
119. Purchit, A. P., Personality variables, sex difference, G.S.R. responsiveness and G.S.R. conditioning, *J. esp. Res. Pers.*, 1 (1966), 166.
120. Rees, W. D. and S. G. Lutkins, Mortality of bereavement, *Brit. med. J.*, (1967), 13.
121. Registrar-General, *Statistical Review of England and Wales for the Two Years 1946-1947.* Test. Vol. 1. Medical, H.M.S.O., London, 1951.
122. Robins, L. N., *Deviant Children Grown Up*, Williams and Wilkins, Baltimore, 1966.
123. Robins, L. N., Social correlates of psychiatric disorders: can we tell causes from consequences, *J. Health Social Behaviour*, 10 (1969), 95.
124. Rosenthal, D., P. H. Wander, S. S. Kety, F. Schulsinger, J. Welner, and L. Ostergaard, Schizophrenics offspring reared in adoptive homes in D. Rosenthal, D and S. S. Kety, Eds., *Transmission of Schizophrenia.* Pergamon, London, 1968.
125. Rothbart, M. K. and E. E. Maccoby, Parent's differential reactions to sons and daughters, *J. Pers. soc. Psychol.*, 4 (1966), 237.
126. Rutter, M., *Children of Sick Parents*, Oxford Univ. Press, London, 1966.

127. Rutter, M., A children's behaviour questionnaire for completion by teachers' preliminary findings, *J. Child Psychol. Psychiat.*, 8 (1967), 1.
128. Rutter, M., H. G. Birch, A. Thomas, and S. Chess, Temperamental characteristics in infancy and the later development of behavioural disorders, *Brit. J. Psychiat.*, 110 (1964), 651.
129. Rutter, M. and G. W. Brown, The reliability and validity of measures of family life and relationships in families containing a psychiatric patient, *Social Psychiatry*, 1 (1966), 38.
130. Rutter, M. and P. Graham, Psychiatric disorder in 10 and 11 year old children, *Proc. Roy. Soc. Med.*, 59 (1966), 382.
131. Rutter, M., J. Tizard, and K. Whitmore, Eds., *Education, Health and Behaviour,* Longmans, Green, London, 1970a.
132. Rutter, M., P. Graham, and W. Yule, *Neurological Disorders in Childhood: A Study of a Small Community,* Wm Heinemann, London, 1970b.
133. Slazman, L., *Developments in Psychoanalysis,* Grune and Stratton, New York, 1962.
134. Schaefer, E. S. and N. Bayley, Maternal behaviour, child bahaviour and their intercorrelations from infancy through adolescence, *Mon. Soc. Res. Child. Dev.*, 28 (1963), 3, No. 87.
135. Sears, R. R., E. E. Maccoby, and H. Levin, *Patterns of Child Rearing,* Peterson, Evanston, Ill., 1957.
136. Shepherd, M., B. Cooper, A. C. Brown, G. W. Kalton, *Psychiatric Illness in General Practice,* Oxford Univ. Press, London, 1966.
137. Shields, J., Psychiatric genetics in M. Shepherd and D. L. Davies, Eds., *Studies in Psychiatry,* Oxford Univ. Press, London, 1968.
138. Singer, J. E., M. Westphal, and K. R. Niswander, Sex differences in the incidence of neonatal abnormalities and abnormal performance in early childhood, *Child. Develop.*, 39 (1968), 103.
139. Slater, E., Genetical factors in neurosis, *Brit. J. Psychol.*, 55 (1964), 265.
140. Sontag, L. W., Physiological factors and personality in children, *Child Develop.*, 18 (1947), 185.
141. Spence, K. W. and J. T. Spence, Sex and anxiety differences in eyelid conditioning, *Psychol. Bull.*, 65 (1966), 137.
142. Srole, L., T. S. Langner, S. T. Michael, M. K. Opler, T. A. C. Rennie, *Mental Health in the Metropolis,* McGraw-Hill, New York, 1962.
143. Susser, M. W. and W. Watson, *Sociology in Medicine,* Oxford Univ. Press, London, 1962.
144. Suttie, I. D., *The Origins of Love and Hate,* Kegan Paul, Trench, Trubner & Co., London, 1935.
145. Tait, C. D. and E. F. Hodges, *Delinquents, Their Families and the Community.* Chas. C. Thomas, Springfield, Ill., 1962.
146. Tanner, J. M., Ed., *Human Growth,* Pergamon, London, 1960.
147. Tanner, J. M., A. Prader, H. Habich, and M. A. Ferguson-Smith, Genes on the Y chromosome influencing rate of development in man: skeletal age studies in children with Klinefelter's (XXY) and Turner's (XO) syndromes, *Lancet,* 2 (1959), 141.
148. Taylor, D. C., Differential rates of cerebral maturation between sexes and between hemispheres: evidence from epilepsy, *Lancet,* 2 (1969), 140.
149. Terman, L. M. and L. E. Tyler, Psychological sex differences in Carmichael, Ed., *Manual of Child Psychology* (2nd Ed.), Chapman and Hall, London, 1954.

150. Thomas, A., H. G. Birch, S. Chess, M. E. Hertzig, and S. Korn, *Behavioural Individuality in Childhood,* N.Y. Univ. Press., New York, 1963.
151. Thomas, A., S. Chess, and H. G. Birch, *Temperament and Behaviour Disorders in Children,* N.Y. Univ. Press, New York, 1968.
152. Thompson, D. J., H. M. Gezon, T. F. Hatch, R. R. Rycheck, and K. D. Rogers, Sex distribution of staphylococcus ameus colonization and disease in newborn infants, *New Eng. J. Med.,* 269 (1963), 337.
153. Titmuss, R. N., *Essays on the Welfare State,* Allen & Unwin, London, 1958.
154. Toby, J., The differential impact of family disorganization, *Amer. Social Rev.,* 22 (1957), 505.
155. Waring, M. and D. Ricks, Family patterns of children who became adult schizophrenics, *J. nerv. ment. Dis.,* 140 (1965), 351.
156. Washburn, T. O., D. N. Medearis, and B. Childs, Sex differences in susceptibility to infections, *Pediat.,* 35 (1965), 57.
157. Weinstein, E. A. and P. N. Geisel, An analysis of sex differences in adjustment, *Child Develop.,* 31 (1960), 721.
158. Weller, G. M. and R. Q. Bell, Basal skin conductance and neonatal state, *Child Develop.,* 36 (1965), 647.
159. Wilson, H., Mental reactions to air-raids, *Lancet,* 1 (1942), 284.
160. Wing, L., C. Bramley, A. Hailey, and J. K. Wing, Camberwell cumulative psychiatric case register Part 1. Aims and methods, *Social Psychiatry,* 3 (1968), 116.
161. Wolff, S. and W. P. Acton, Characteristics of parents of disturbed children, *Brit. J. Psychiat.,* 114 (1968), 593.
162. Wood, J. W., R. J. Keehn, S. Kawamoto, and K. G. Johnson, The growth and development of children exposed in utero to the atomic bombs in Hiroshima and Nagasaki, *Amer. J. Publ. Health.,* 57 (1967), 1374.
163. Yarrow, L., Separation from parents during early childhood in L. W. Hoffman and M. L. Hoffman, Eds., *Review of Child Development Research,* Vol. 1, Russell Sage Foundation, New York, 1964.
164. Young, M., B. Benjamin, and C. Wallis, The mortality of widowers, *Lancet,* 2 (1963), 454.

Separation and Loss within the Family

JOHN BOWLBY AND C. MURRAY PARKES (U. K.)

Probably all of us today are keenly aware of the anxiety and distress that can be caused by separations from loved figures, of the deep and prolonged grief that can follow bereavement, and of the hazards to mental health that these events can constitute. Once eyes are opened, it is seen that many of the troubles we are called upon to treat in our patients are to be traced, at least in part, to a separation or a loss that occurred either recently or at some earlier period in life. Chronic anxiety, intermittent depression, attempted or successful suicide are some of the more common sorts of troubles that we now know are traceable to such experiences. Furthermore, prolonged or repeated disruptions of the mother-child bond during the first five years of life are known to be especially frequent in patients later diagnosed as psychopathic or sociopathic personalities.

Evidence for these statements, especially that relating to the much increased incidence of loss of a parent during childhood in samples of patients with these troubles when compared to control samples is reviewed elsewhere [3, 6]. A point we particularly want to emphasize is that, although losses occurring during the first five years are probably especially dangerous for future personality development, losses that occur later in life are potentially pathogenic also.

Although today a causal linkage between psychological disturbance and a separation or loss that occurred at some time during childhood or adolescence, or later, is well attested, both statistically and clinically, there remain very many problems in understanding both the processes at work and also the exact conditions that determine whether outcome is good or bad. Yet, we are not wholly ignorant. Our plan in this paper is to give special attention to the ways in which we may be able to help our patients. Whether they are young or old, and whether the loss is recent or long passed, we believe we can now discern certain principles on which to base our therapy.

We shall start by describing grief and mourning as they occur in adults and work thence to childhood.

Grief and Mourning in Adult Life

There is now a good deal of reliable information about the way in which adults respond to a major bereavement. It stems from a number of sources, notably the records of Lindemann [13] and Marris [15], amplified by a recent and still largely unpublished study [17, 18].[1] Though the intensity of grief varies considerably from individual to individual and the length of each phase also varies, there is none the less a basic overall pattern.

In an earlier paper [4], it was suggested that the course of mourning could be divided into three main phases, but we realize now that this numbering omitted an important first phase, which is usually fairly brief. What were formerly numbered phases 1, 2, and 3 have therefore been renumbered phases 2, 3, and 4. The four phases now recognized are:

1. Phase of numbness that usually lasts from a few hours to a week and may be interrupted by outbursts of extremely intense distress and/or anger.
2. Phase of yearning and searching for the lost figure, lasting some months and often for years.

[1] Information was obtained from a fairly representative sample of 22 widows between the ages of 26 and 65 during the year following loss of a husband. Each widow was given not less than five long clinical interviews at 1, 3, 6, 9, and 12½ months after bereavement. Good rapport was obtained, and much gratitude was expressed for the understanding given. In ten cases the husband's death had been sudden; in three it was rapid; and in nine it had been foreseen by at least a week.

3. Phase of disorganization and despair.
4. Phase of greater or less degree of reorganization.

PHASE OF NUMBING

The immediate reaction to news of a husband's death in our study varied very greatly among the widows and also from time to time in any widow. Most felt stunned and in varying degrees quite unable to accept the news. A case in which the phase lasted rather longer than usual was that of a widow who reported that, when told of her husband's death, she had remained calm and "felt nothing at all" – and was therefore surprised to find herself crying. She consciously avoided her feelings, she said, because she feared she would be overcome or go insane. For three weeks she continued controlled and relatively composed, until finally she broke down in the street and wept. Reflecting on those three weeks, she later described them as having been like "walking on the edge of a black pit."

Many other widows reported how the news had altogether failed to register with them at first. Nevertheless, this calm before the storm was sometimes broken by an outburst of extreme emotion, usually of fearfulness, but often of anger, and in one or two cases of elation.

PHASE OF YEARNING AND SEARCHING FOR THE LOST FIGURE

Within days or a week or two of the loss a change occurs and the bereaved begins, though only episodically, to register the reality of the loss: this leads to spasms of intense distress and tearfulness. Yet, almost at the same time, there is great restlessness, preoccupation with thoughts of the lost person combined often with a sense of his actual presence, and a marked tendency to interpret signals or sounds as indicating that the lost person is now returned. For example, hearing a door latch lifted at 5 p.m. is interpreted as husband returning from work, or a man in the street is misperceived as the missing husband.

Some or all of these features were found to occur in the great majority of the widows interviewed. Since the same features are also reported by several other investigators, there can be no doubt that they are a regular feature of grief and in no sense abnormal.

When evidence of this sort was reviewed some years ago [4], the view was advanced that during this phase of mourning the bereaved is seized by an urge to search for and to recover the lost figure. Sometimes the person is conscious of this urge, though often he is not:

sometimes a person willingly falls in with it, as when he visits the grave or visits other places closely linked with the lost figure, but sometimes he seeks to stifle it as irrational and absurd. Whatever the attitude a person may take toward this urge, however, he nonetheless finds himself impelled to search and, if possible, to recover.

This view was advanced in 1961. So far as we know, it has not been called in question, though we doubt whether it is yet widely accepted. However that may be, the further evidence now available shows it to be well supported.

The following is taken from a recent paper [17] in which evidence for the search hypothesis is set out:

> Although we tend to think of searching in terms of the motor act of restless movement toward possible locations of the lost object, [searching] also has perceptual and ideational components . . . Signs of the object can be identified only by reference to memories of the object as it was. Searching the external world for signs of the object therefore includes the establishment of an internal perceptual "set" derived from previous experience of the object.

An example is given of a woman searching for her small son who is missing: She moves restlessly about the likely parts of the house scanning with her eyes and thinking of the boy; she hears a creak and immediately identifies it as the sound of her son's footfall on the stair; she calls out, "John is that you?" The components of this sequence are:

(a) Restless moving about and scanning the environment;

(b) Thinking intensely about the lost person;

(c) Developing a perceptual "set" for the person, namely a disposition to perceive and to pay attention to any stimuli that suggest the presence of the person and to ignore all those that are not relevant to this aim;

(d) Directing attention toward those parts of the environment in which the person is likely to be;

(e) Calling for the lost person.

> It is emphasized that each of these components is to be found in bereaved men and women; in addition some grievers are consciously aware of an urge to search.

Two very usual features of mourning which were interpreted in our earlier papers as being a part of this urge to search are weeping and anger.

The facial expressions typical of adult grief, Darwin concluded (1872), are a resultant, on the one hand, of a tendency to scream like a child when he feels abandoned and, on the other, of an inhibition of such screaming. Both crying and screaming are, of course, ways by means of which a child commonly attracts and recovers his missing mother, or some other person who may help him find her; and they occur in grief, we believe, with the same objectives in mind – either consciously or unconsciously.

The frequency with which anger occurs as part of normal mourning has, we believe, habitually been underestimated – perhaps because it seems so out of place and shameful. Yet there can be no doubt about its very frequent occurrence especially in the early days. Both Lindemann and Marris were struck by it. It was evident, at least episodically, in 18 out of the 22 widows studied by Parkes, and in 7 of them it was very marked at the time of the first interview. Targets of this anger were a relative (four cases), clergy, doctors, or officials (five), and in four cases the dead husband himself. In most such cases the reason given for the anger was that the person in question was held either to have been in some part responsible for the death or to have been negligent in connection with it, either toward the dead man or to the widow.

Among the four widows who expressed anger toward their dead husband was one who burst out angrily during an interview nine months after her loss: "Oh Fred, why did you leave me? If you had known what it was like, you'd never have left me." Later, she denied she was angry and remarked, "It's wicked to be angry." Another widow also expressed angry reproach against her husband for his having deserted her.

Some degree of self-reproach was also common, and usually centered on some minor act of omission or commission associated with the last illness or the death. Although there were times when this self-reproach was fairly severe, in none of this series of widows was it as intense and unrelenting as it is in subjects whose grief persists until finally it becomes diagnosed as a depressive illness [16].

In the earlier paper [4], it was pointed out that anger is both usual and useful when separation is only temporary: it then helps overcome obstacles to reunion with the lost figure; and, after reunion is achieved, the expressions of reproach toward whoever seemed responsible for the separation make it less likely that a separation will occur again. Only when separation is permanent is the anger and reproach out of place.

> It was concluded; there are therefore good biological reasons for every separation to be responded to in an automatic instinctive way with aggressive behaviour: irretrievable loss is statistically so unusual that it is not taken into account. In the course of our evolution, it appears, our instinctual equipment has come to be so fashioned that all losses are assumed to be retrievable and are responded to accordingly.

The hypothesis that many of the features of the second phase of mourning are to be understood as aspects not only of yearning but of actual searching for the lost figure is central to our whole thesis. It is intimately linked, of course, to the picture of attachment behavior that one of the authors has advanced [7]. Attachment behavior, it is argued, is a form of instinctive behavior that develops in humans, as in other mammals, during infancy, and has as its aim or goal proximity to a mother-figure. The function of attachment behavior, it is suggested, is protection from predators. While attachment behavior is shown especially strongly during childhood when it is directed toward parent figures, it nonetheless continues to be active during adult life when it is usually directed toward some active and dominant figure, often a relative but sometimes an employer or some elder of the community. Attachment behavior, the theory emphasizes, is elicited whenever a person (child or adult) is sick or in trouble, and is elicited at high intensity when he is frightened or when the attachment figure cannot be found. Because, in the light of this theory, attachment behavior is regarded as a normal and healthy part of man's instinctive makeup, it is held to be most misleading to term it "regressive" or childish when seen in older child or adult. For this reason, too, the term "dependency" is regarded as leading to a seriously mistaken perspective: for in everyday speech to describe someone as dependent cannot help carrying with it overtones of criticism. By contrast, to describe someone as attached carries with it a positive evaluation.

This picture of attachment behavior as a normal and healthy component of man's instinctive equipment leads us also to regard separation anxiety as the natural and inevitable response whenever an attachment figure is unaccountably missing. It is in the light of this hypothesis, we believe, that the panic attacks to which bereaved people are known to be prone can best be understood. They are apt to come on during the early months of bereavement, especially when the reality of loss happens to have been brought home to the bereaved.

Both our own small-scale but intensive study and also a larger survey reported by Maddison and Walker [14] suggest that most women take a long time to get over the loss of a husband. By whatever psychiatric standard they are judged, less than a half are themselves again at the end of the first year. Of the 22 widows interviewed by Parkes, 2 were judged still to be grieving a great deal and 9 more were intermittently disturbed and depressed. Only 4 seemed by the end of the first year to be making a good adjustment. Insomnia and a variety of minor aches and ailments were extremely common. In the survey undertaken by Maddison and Walker, one-fifth of the widows were still in very poor health and disturbed emotional state at the end of a year.

We emphasize these findings, distressing though they are, because we believe that clinicians sometimes have unrealistic expectations of the speed with which someone should get over a major bereavement. It is possible that some of Freud's theoretical formulations may have been a little misleading in this regard. For example, an oft-quoted passage from *Totem and Taboo* runs thus: "Mourning has a quite precise psychical task to perform: its function is to detach the survivor's memories and hopes from the dead"[9]. When judged by this criterion, it must be recognized, most mourning is unsuccessful. Freud himself was alive to this, however. Thus, in a letter of condolence to Binswanger he writes:

> Although we know that after such a loss the acute state of mourning will subside, we also know we shall remain inconsolable and will never find a substitute. No matter what may fill the gap, even if it be filled completely, it nevertheless remains something else. And actually this is how it should be. It is the only way of perpetuating that love which we do not want to relinquish [10].

The widows interviewed by Parkes a year after bereavement echoed these words. Over half of them still found it hard to accept the fact that their husband was dead: most of them still spent much time thinking about the past and still sometimes had a sense of their husband's nearby presence. In none of these widows had memories and hopes become detached from the dead.

In our own studies and also in those of Maddison and Walker it has been found that the younger a woman is when widowed the more intense her mourning and the more disturbed is her health likely to be at the end of 12 months. By contrast, if a woman is already over 65 when her husband dies, the blow is likely to be much less disabling. It seems as though the ties are already beginning to loosen. This quite marked difference in the intensity and length of mourning may perhaps provide a clue to understanding what happens following a loss during childhood.

Grief and Mourning in Childhood

Some years ago one of the authors [2] emphasized that young children not only grieve but that they often do so for much longer than was sometimes supposed. In support of that view he quoted some of the observations of his colleagues – Robertson [19] and Heinicke [11][2] – of the persistent grieving for mother of 1- and 2-year-old children in residential nurseries, and also accounts of children in the Hampstead Nurseries during the war. These studies seem to make it clear that in those circumstances very young children grieve overtly for a missing mother for at least some weeks, crying for her or indicating in other ways that they are still yearning for her and expecting her return. The notion that grief in infancy and early childhood is short-lived does not bear scrutiny in the light of these observations. In particular the account given by Freud and Burlingham [8] was cited of a boy aged 3 years and 2 months whose grief clearly persisted for some time though in muted form. We repeat that account now because we believe it contains so much of relevance. On being left in the nursery Patrick had been admonished to be a good boy and not to cry – otherwise his mother would not visit him.

> Patrick tried to keep his promise and was not seen crying. Instead he would nod his head whenever anyone looked at him and assured himself and anybody who cared to listen that his mother would come for him, she would put on his overcoat and would take him home with her again. Whenever a listener seemed to believe him he was satisfied; whenever anybody contradicted him, he would burst into violent tears.
>
> This same state of affairs continued through the next two or three days with several additions. The nodding took on a more compulsive and automatic character: My mother will put on my overcoat and take me home again.
>
> Later an ever-growing list of clothes that his mother was supposed to put on him was added: She will put on my overcoat and my leggings, she will zip up the zipper, she will put on my pixie hat.

[2]See also a later study by Heinicke and Westheimer [12].

When the repetitions of this formula became monotonous and endless, somebody asked him whether he could not stop saying it all over again. Again Patrick tried to be the good boy that his mother wanted him to be. He stopped repeating the formula aloud, but his moving lips showed that he was saying it over and over to himself.

At the same time he substituted for the spoken words gestures that showed the position of his pixie hat, the putting on of an imaginary coat, the zipping of the zipper, etc. What showed as an expressive movement one day, was reduced the next to a mere abortive flicker of his fingers. While the other children were mostly busy with their toys, playing games, making music, etc., Patrick, totally uninterested, would stand somewhere in a corner, moving his hands and lips with an absolutely tragic expression on his face.

A good deal of controversy followed Bowlby's early papers; and we suspect it will be some time yet before all the problems raised are clarified. Of the many issues debated there are only two that we want to comment on here. The first concerns the usage of the term mourning; the second concerns the similarities and differences between childhood mourning and adult mourning.

In the earlier papers it was thought useful to use the term "mourning" in a broad sense to cover a variety of reactions to loss, including some that lead to a pathological outcome and also those that follow loss in early childhood. The advantage of this usage is that it then becomes possible to link together a number of processes and conditions that evidence shows are interrelated – much in the way that the term "inflammation" is used in physiology and pathology to link together a number of processes, some of which lead to a healthy outcome and some of which miscarry and result in pathology. The alternative practice is to restrict the term mourning to a particular form of reaction to loss, namely the one "in which the lost object is gradually decathected by the painful and prolonged work of remembering and reality testing" [20]. A danger of that usage, however, is that it may lead to expectations of what healthy mourning should be like which are wholly at variance with what we now know actually occurs in many people. Furthermore, if the convention of a restricted usage is preferred, we find outselves faced with the necessity of finding, and perhaps coining, some new term; for I believe it essential, if we are to discuss these matters productively, that we have some convenient word by which to refer to the whole range of processes that are brought into action when a loss is sustained. On this occasion we shall use the term "grieving" in this sense, since it has already been employed by prominent analysts in a rather broad way and there is no dispute that very young children grieve.

In addition to having concentrated attention on a central area of psychopathology, the controversies of recent years have had a number of other effects that must be welcome to everyone. They have shown how little we yet know about how children of all ages, including adolescents, respond to a major loss and about what factors are responsible for outcome being more favorable in some cases than in others; secondly, they have stimulated valuable research.

We have already emphasized how very difficult it is even for grown-ups to grasp fully that someone near to them is dead and will not return. For children it is clearly much more difficult still. Wolfenstein [20] has reported on the responses of a number of children and adolescents who had lost a parent and who had come into analysis, many of them within a year of the bereavement. Among points that struck her group of observers was that "sad feelings were curtailed; there was little weeping. Immersion in the activities of everyday life continued. . . ." Yet gradually the analysts treating them became aware that overtly or covertly these children and adolescents were "denying the finality of the loss" and that expectation that the lost parent would return was still present at a more or less conscious level. The same long-persisting expectations are recorded by Barnes [1] as occurring in two nursery school children who lost their mother when they were aged 2½ and 4 years respectively. Again and again these children continued to express the hope and expectation that mother would return.

When in due course, through the help of analysts or others, these children gradually became aware that mother would, in fact, not return, they responded, as did the widows described above, with panic and anger. Ruth, a 15-year-old described by Wolfenstein, remarked some months after her mother had died, "If my mother were really dead, I would be all alone . . . I would be terribly scared." At another time it is recounted how Ruth, in bed at night, would sometimes feel desperate with "frustration, rage and yearning. She tore the bedclothes off the bed, rolled them into the shape of a human body, and embraced them."

Thus, although there certainly are differences between the way a child responds to loss and the way an adult does, there are also very basic similarities.

There is, moreover, one further similarity to which we wish to draw attention. Not only child but adult also, we believe, needs the assistance of another trusted person if he is to recover from the loss. In discussing the responses of children to loss, and how best to help them, almost every writer has emphasized how immensely important it is that a child have available a single and permanent substitute to whom he can gradually become attached. Only in such circumstances can we expect a child ultimately to accept the loss as irremediable and then to reorganize his inner life accordingly.[3] The same is true, we suspect, for adults, although in adult life it may be a little easier to find support in the companionship of a few others as well. This leads to two interrelated and very practical questions: What do we know of the factors that aid or hinder healthy mourning? How can we best help a mourner?

Conditions that Aid or Hinder Healthy Mourning

It is now generally agreed among psychiatrists that, if mourning is to lead to a more rather than a less favorable outcome, it is necessary for a bereaved person – sooner or later – to express his feelings. "Give sorrow words," wrote Shakespeare, "the grief that does not speak knits up the o'erwrought heart and bids it break."

Yet, though so far we can all agree, for someone unable to express his feelings and for someone else trying to help him do so, the questions remain: how give sorrow words? what are the feelings to be expressed? and what is stopping their expression?

There is now evidence that the most intense and most disturbing effects aroused by loss are fear of being abandoned, yearning for the lost figure, and anger that he cannot be found – effects linked, on the one hand, with an urge to search for the lost figure and, on the other, with a tendency to reproach angrily anyone who seems to the bereaved to be responsible for the loss or to be hindering recovery of the lost person. With his whole emotional being, it seems, a bereaved person is fighting fate, trying desperately to turn back the wheel of

[3]How unsatisfactory any other arrangement is was poignantly expressed by Wendy, the 4-year-old described by Barnes [1]. When her father enumerated the long list of people who knew Wendy and loved her, Wendy replied sadly, "But when my Mummy wasn't dead I didn't need so many people – I needed just one."

time and to recapture the happier days that have been suddenly taken from him. So far from facing reality and trying to come to terms with it, a bereaved person is locked in a struggle with the past.

Plainly, if we are to give the kind of help to a bereaved person that we should all like to give, it is essential we see things from his point of view and respect his feelings – unrealistic though we may regard some of them to be. For only if a bereaved person feels we can at least understand and sympathize with him in the tasks he sets himself is there much likelihood that he will be able to express the feelings that are bursting within him – his yearning for the return of the lost figure, his hope against hope that miraculously all may yet be well, his rage at being deserted, his angry, unfair reproaches against "those incompetent doctors," "those unhelpful nurses," and against his own guilty self; if only he had done so and so, or not done so and so, disaster might perhaps have been averted.

Whether we are in the role of friend to a recently bereaved person or of therapist to someone who has suffered a bereavement many years ago and has failed in his mourning, it seems to be both unnecessary and unhelpful to cast ourselves in the role of a "representative of reality": unnecessary because the bereaved is, in some part of himself, well aware that the world has changed; unhelpful because, by disregarding the world as one part of him still sees it, we alienate ourselves from him. Instead, our role should be that of companion and supporter, prepared to explore in our discussions all the hopes and wishes and dim unlikely possibilities that he still cherishes, together with all the regrets and the reproaches and the disappointments that afflict him. Let us give two examples.

In an earlier paper [5], the case was described of Mrs. Q., a woman of about 35; her father had died unexpectedly following an elective operation, and at a time when her therapist (J.B.) was abroad. For a year she had kept her feelings and her ideas to herself, but on the anniversary of the loss the true picture came out.

During the weeks following her father's death, she now told me, she had lived in the half-held conviction that the hospital had made a mistake in identity and that any day they would 'phone to say he was alive and ready to return home. Furthermore, she had felt specially angry with me because of a belief that, had I been available, I would have been able to exert an influence on the hospital and so enabled her to recover him. Now, twelve months later, these ideas and feelings persisted. She was still half-expecting a message from the hospital, and she was still angry with me for not approaching the authorities there. Secretly, moreover, she was still making arrangements to greet her father on his return. This explained why she had been so angry with her mother for redecorating the flat in which the old people had lived together and why too she had continued to postpone having her own flat redecorated: it was vital, she felt, that when at last her father did return he should find the places familiar."

Now there was no need for her therapist to intervene on behalf of reality: others had already done so and she knew well enough what view of the world was held by her relatives and friends. What she needed was the chance to express the yearning, the hopes and the bitter anger that her relatives and friends could *not* understand. She described how the previous week she had thought she had seen her father looking into a shop window and how she had crossed the road to inspect more closely the man in question. She described her fury with the staff nurse who had given her the news of her father's death and how she had felt inclined to throw her on the concrete floor and bash her brains out. She described how she felt her therapist had failed her by being away just when she most wanted him; and she described much else besides that, in the cold light of day, she herself knew was unrealistic and unfair. What she needed from the therapist, and we hope found, was someone who could understand and sympathize with her *unrealism* and her *unfairness.* As the months rolled by, her hopes and her anger faded and she began to reconcile herself to the reality of loss.

The same role was played with a boy of 16, whom we shall call Bill. He had first been seen by a psychiatrist (J.B.) at a clinic when he was 4 years old because things were going badly in his foster home. The history was uncertain but we gathered that Bill's mother was a prostitute who had placed her son in a foster home when he was 2 years old and had then disappeared. Bill presented great problems and the foster parents refused to keep him. Special foster care was arranged and, later, treatment in a residential establishment for seriously disturbed children. A few times a year he was seen at the clinic by the same psychiatrist and in that way we provided some continuity. Now at 16 he was due to leave school soon.

In that interview Bill told the psychiatrist of his plan to go to America to find his mother. He had already been to a steamship company and was arranging to work his passage over. He was quite an intelligent boy and his plans for transport seemed practicable. Yet you can imagine the psychiatrist's astonishment! Here was a boy who had last seen his mother when he was 2 and had never heard from her since, who had no idea where she might be, and who was not even sure of her name. Plainly the scheme was a wild-goose chase. Yet, the psychiatrist held his tongue. This was Bill's world and Bill's plan, and he was confiding it to his therapist; it was not the latter's role to debunk it. In fact a whole session was spent discussing the plan. Bill believed his father was an American serviceman and he presumed his mother had returned with him after the war. His plans for crossing the Atlantic were looked at again and the methods whereby he might earn enough on the other side to continue his search. No queries were raised by the psychiatrist, but Bill was invited to come back for a further talk in a week or so. He came back. He described how he had been thinking a great deal about the plan but was beginning to have doubts. Perhaps it would be difficult to locate his mother; and perhaps, even if he were successful, she might not be too welcoming. After all, he reflected, he would be a stranger to her. Once again, given a chance to explore in sympathetic company all the feelings and plans that he had nursed secretly for years, the patient's own sense of realism was sufficient.

Naturally in other patients, especially older ones who have suffered a loss years earlier during childhood or adolescence, to help them recover their lost feelings, their lost hopes of reunion and their anger at being deserted, can be a long and technically difficult task. But the overall aims remain the same.

Yearning for the impossible, intemperate anger, impotent weeping, horror at the prospect of loneliness, pitiful pleading for sympathy and support — these are the feelings that a bereaved person needs to express, and sometimes first to discover, if he is to make progress. Yet, these are all feelings that are apt to be regarded as unworthy and unmanly. At best to express them may seem humiliating; at worst it may be to court criticism and contempt. No wonder such feelings so often go unexpressed, and may later go underground.

This leads us to the question why some people find it harder — often much harder — to express their feelings of grief than others do.

Our own belief is that a main reason why some find expressing grief extremely difficult is that the family in which they have been brought up, and with which they still mix, is one in which the attachment behavior of a child is regarded unsympathetically as something to be grown out of as quickly as possible. In such families crying and other protests over separation are apt to be dubbed babyish, and anger or jealousy as reprehensible. In such families, moreover, the more a child demands to be with his mother or his father the more he is told that such demands are silly and unjustified; the more he cries or throws a tantrum the more he is told he is babyish and bad. As a result of being subjected to such pressures he is likely to come to accept these standards for himself; to cry, to make demands, to feel angry because they are not met, to blame others, will all be judged by him as unjustified, babyish, and bad. So, when he suffers serious loss, instead of expressing the kinds of feelings that every bereaved person is filled with, he is inclined to stifle them. Furthermore, his relatives, products of the same family culture, are likely to share the same critical outlook toward emotion and its expression. And so the very person who most needs understanding and encouragement is the one least likely to receive it.

A vivid illustration of this process of internalization of reproachful controls is provided by the case of Patrick, the 3-year-old boy in the Hampstead Nursery described earlier. Patrick, you will remember, had been admonished to be a good boy and not to cry – otherwise his mother would not visit him. It seems likely that this was typical of her attitude toward his expressions of distress. It is therefore not surprising that he strove to stifle all his feelings and, instead of expressing them, developed a ritual that became increasingly divorced from the emotional context in which it had originated.

Avoidance of mourning is one important pathological variant of grief but it is not, we believe, the only one. There are many bereaved adults seeking help from psychiatrists who show little evidence of the inhibition of emotion that has been described above. On the contrary, as is documented in a previous paper [16], these people are showing all the features of grief in a severe and protracted form. The problem here is not one of why the patient is unable to express grief but why she (and it is usually a woman) is unable to get over it. It may be, of course, that even in these cases there is some as yet unrecognized component of grief that is being inhibited; but there are three characteristics which seem to distinguish these chronic grief reactions and which may suggest an alternative explanation.

In the first place the patient's attachment to her lost spouse is usually found to have been an extremely close one, with a great deal of the self-esteem and role identity of the survivor dependent on the continued presence of the spouse. Such patients are likely to report having experienced great distress even during brief temporary separations in the past. Secondly, the patient has no close relationship with another family member toward whom she can transfer some of the ties which bound her to her husband. Her intense relationship with him seems to have been so exclusive that even those family members who exist have drifted away, so that after bereavement the survivor has found no person and no interests to distract her from her grief. Finally, the marriage relationship is likely to have been an ambivalent one, perhaps because the husband resented the possessiveness of his wife. At all events the survivor usually finds some source of self-reproach and castigates herself for having failed to be a better wife or for having allowed her husband to die. The grief of such people often seems to contain an element of self-punishment, as if perpetual mourning had become a sacred duty to the dead by means of which the survivor could make retribution.

The treatment of such patients is likely to prove difficult as they often seem to relish the opportunity to repeat, yet again, the painful drama of their loss. While there is no general agreement as to the value of psychotherapy for them, much can be done to help reestablish their commitment to the world. Family, local clergy, or the befriending service of an organization such as Cruse or Samaritans, can be mobilized to act as a bridge; while a memorial service, a holiday with friends, or even the redecoration of the home can be a turning point, a *rite-de-passage,* out of the role of "mourner" to the new role of widow.

Seen in this light, bereavement becomes a family problem. Therefore, we need to know what changes occur in the dynamic structure of a family when a leading member dies. Relevant information is emerging from a study of young Boston widows and widowers currently in progress. Apart from emotional problems the most immediate problem is one of roles. Who, for example, is to take over the roles of a dead husband? Some of them, such as the management of household affairs, commonly devolve upon the surviving widow. Others remain unfilled: thus many widows sleep with a pillow or bolster in bed beside them. A young widow will usually try to perceive her dead husband as a continuing help in decision making, and to make his wishes and preferences the ground for much of her own behavior. When decisions must be made that fall outside the field of this "internal referee," she will most often turn to her husband's brother as the person closest to the husband in culture and blood. Similarly, a widower tends to regard his sister-in-law as the most helpful member of his wife's family and to seek her help in making decisions about children and household affairs.

As time passes, however, these role assignments fade and are followed often by a gradual disintegration of the extended family. The widow or widower no longer looks to the spouse's family as a source of support and, instead, develops a greater degree of self-reliance, despite the loneliness and internal family strains that this entails. Friends and children then become an important source of affirmation as the widow or widower develops a tougher stance and tackles the world afresh.

The ability of a widow or widower to cope with these fresh roles and responsibilities clearly depends partly on her personality and previous experience and partly on the demands made by and the support she finds in the family environment. Children may be a burden or a blessing, so may in-laws; and the woman without experience of a job outside the home has many hurdles to negotiate. It is not surprising that a significant proportion of widows fail to find any satisfying mode of living. When asked 13 months after bereavement how they felt, 74 percent of the young Boston widows agreed that "you never get over it."

A study that illustrates the part that friends and relatives play in influencing the outcome of bereavement has been carried out by Maddison and Walker [14]. They studied two groups of widows, each of 20 subjects who had agreed to be interviewed, and matched as far as possible on the usual sociological variables. One group had been selected because at the end of 12 months they all seemed, on the basis of their health records, to have reached a fairly favorable outcome; the other group were selected because their health records suggested that outcome had not been favorable. Interviews confirmed that the health record is in fact a good index of how a person is coping with the emotional problems of bereavement.

During the course of long semi-structured interviews, the interviewer inquired who had been available to the widow during her first 3 months of widowhood, and in regard to each whether she had found them helpful, unhelpful, or neutral. In addition, questions were directed to finding out whether the widow had found it easy or difficult to express her feelings with each person mentioned, whether or not they had encouraged her to dwell on the past, whether they had been eager to direct her attention to problems of the present and future, and whether they had offered practical help. Since the object of the inquiry was to find out only how the widows themselves recalled their dealings with others, no attempt was made to check how their accounts may have tallied with those of the people they had been in contact with.

When the replies of the two groups of widows were compared, the following differences stood out. First, widows whose condition after 12 months was unfavorable reported that they had received too little encouragement either to express their grief and anger, or to talk about their dead husband and the past. They complained that, instead, people seemed to have made expression of feeling more difficult by insisting that she pull herself together or control herself, that anyway she was not the only one to suffer, that she would be wise to face the problems of the future rather than dwell unproductively on the past. By contrast, widows with a fairly good outcome reported how the people they had been in contact with had made it easy for them to cry and to express the intensity of their feelings; and they described what a relief it had been to be able to talk freely and at length about past days with their husband and the circumstances of his death.

How are we to interpret these findings? An obvious explanation, and perhaps the most likely, is that the attitude of these friends and relatives caused the widow to suppress or avoid expression of grief and that the pathological outcome had occurred as a consequence of this. Alternatively, the widow may have attributed to her friends and relatives her own fear of expressing feeling and blamed them for her own incapacity. Or both processes may have occurred together.

Yet the forms of pathological outcome described by Maddison and Walker are not all attributable to inhibition or avoidance of grief; there were several widows who showed the chronic grief syndrome described above. In these cases it is possible that the experiences the widows reported reflect a breakdown in communication such that the family were not seen as sympathetic and helpful. Lacking their understanding and support, the widow may well have found it difficult to find an inducement to start again, to commit herself to a new investment in the world with all the dangers of further disappointment and loss. Instead, it seems she had tended to look backwards, to search repeatedly for the husband she could find only in memory, and to condemn herself to persistent grief.

This brings us to our final point. We are uneasy about some of the theory that is presented in the psychoanalytic literature and about some of the language that is used in clinical discussion. For example, it is not unusual to find the weeping of grown-ups after a disastrous loss referred to as "a regression," or the strong longing for the company of another person, an urge to cling, described as being the expression of "infantile dependence." Not only do we believe such theorizing to be mistaken on scientific grounds but it plainly represents an attitude which, if carried over to clinical work, can only reinforce the tendencies of a bereaved person to feel guilty and ashamed of the very feelings and behavior we believe it will help him most to express.

There are other words and concepts that we believe lead to the same difficulties. "Magical thinking" and "fantasy" are terms to be used with extreme caution. A fantasy is by definition something wholly unrealistic; so that to refer to a child's hopes and expectations of her dead mother's return as a "wishful fantasy" is, in our eyes, to do them less than justice. Mrs. Q's belief that her father might still be alive was, we believe, likely to be mistaken, as she herself suspected, but it was not absurd. Mistakes are made occasionally, and missing people do return when least expected. The ideas of Bill, the 16-year-old boy who hoped to find his mother, were probably misconceived but given certain premises it was a legitimate enough plan. By avoiding such loaded terms as "denial of reality" and "fantasy" and using, instead, phrases such as "disbelief that X has occurred," "belief that Y may still be possible," or "making a plan to achieve Z," it seems to us that we are able to see the world more as our patients see it and to maintain that neutral and empathic position from which, we know from experience, we are best able to help them.

Bibliography

1. Barnes, M. J., Reactions to the death of a mother, *Psychoanal. Study of Child.*, 19 (1964), 334–357.
2. Bowlby, J., Grief and mourning in infancy and early childhood, *Psychoanal. Study of Child.*, 15 (1960), 9–52.
3. Bowlby, J., Childhood mourning and its implications for psychiatry, *Amer. J. Psychiat.*, 118 (1961a), 481–498.
4. Bowlby, J., Processes of mourning, *Internat. J. Psychoanal.*, 42 (1961b), 317–340.
5. Bowlby, J., Pathological mourning and childhood mourning, *J. Amer. Psychoanal. Assn.*, 11 (1963).
6. Bowlby, J., Effects on behavior of disruption of an affectional bond, in *Genetic and Environmental Influences on Behavior*, ed. J. M. Thoday and A. S. Parkes, Oliver & Boyd, Edinburgh, 1968.
7. Bowlby, J., *Attachment and Loss: Vol. 1, Attachment*, Hogarth Press, London; Basic Books, New York, 1969.
8. Freud, A. and Burlingham, D., *War and Children*, International Universities Press, New York, 1943.
9. Freud, S., *Totem and Taboo*, Standard Edition, 13, Hogarth Press, London, 1902–1913.
10. Freud, S., Letter to Binswanger in *Letters of Sigmund Freud* (1929), ed. E. L. Freud. Hogarth, London, 1961.
11. Heinicke, C. M., Some effects of separating two-year-old children from their parents: A comparative study, *Human Relations*, 9 (1956), 105–176.
12. Heinicke, C. M. and Westheimer, I. J., *Brief Separations*, Longmans, Green & Co., London, International Universities Press, New York, 1966.
13. Lindemann, E., Symptomatology and management of acute grief, *Amer. J. Psychiat.*, 101 (1944).
14. Maddison, D. and Walker, W. L., Factors affecting the outcome of conjugal bereavement, *Brit. J. Psychiat.*, 113 (1967), 1057–67.
15. Marris, P., *Widows and their families*, Routledge & Kegan Paul, London, 1958.
16. Parkes, C. M., Bereavement and mental illness, *Brit. J. Med. Psychol.*, 38 (1965), 1–26.
17. Parkes, C. M., Separation anxiety: an aspect of the search for a lost object, in *Studies of Anxiety*, ed. M. H. Lader. *British J. Psychiatry, Special Publication No. 3* (1969).
18. Parkes, C. M., The first year of bereavement: A longitudinal study of the reaction of London widows to the death of their husbands, *Psychiatry*, in press.
19. Robertson, J., Some responses of young children to loss of maternal care, *Nurs. Times*, 49 (1953), 382–6.
20. Wolfenstein, M., How is mourning possible? *Psychoanal. Study of Child*, 21 (1966), 93–123.

Unemployment and Family Life

C. VEIL, C. BARAT, M. GIRAULT, AND M. SABLIÈRE (FRANCE)

Eric, a 17-year old boy, heavy-set, continually hungry and a compulsive eater, nonpragmatic except for his obsessive preoccupation with the subway, films, and television, enters a psychiatric hospital as an outpatient and is immediately taken in charge by a team of specialists. This team investigates the many different aspects of his situation, particularly his family problems and, among other things, undertakes therapy with his mother. After several months of study and treatment, the team discovers that the father is unemployed, a fact which had been recorded when the boy entered the institution. In retrospect, the team recognized that the father's unemployment had played a determining role in Eric's illness.

Thus even well-informed persons in specialized teams can neglect certain phenomena such as unemployment and regret their neglect afterwards. Unemployment is a fact which is not usually envisaged nor systematically taken into consideration (no importance being attached to it) but, as we shall see, its effects often prove to be of primary importance in family life.

One should state from the beginning that it is difficult to be clear and systematic in this domain. In fact, family life is far from identical in all civilizations and even in different areas of the same civilization. To speak of "family life" in general may be convenient but simplistic. In the same way, work and its absence (unemployment) take on forms and are invested with meanings which we are obliged to condense despite and beyond their diversity.

Review of French Surveys of Unemployment

For reasons which are well understandable, we shall first rely upon French sociological surveys (enlarging our investigation further on). Let us remember that in France there exists a legal system of protection against unemployment, that the legislator considers unemployment to be a personal misfortune, and that the community strives to alleviate its inevitable economic consequences. Among other arrangements, there exists an obligatory insurance system, not for everyone however, and a system of allowances subject to restrictive terms of distribution. This system works out in such a way that some families are very well protected while others are much less so or practically not at all.

In a survey made in Marseilles by the Center of Social and Nutritional Research, Carrere [4] reports on the distribution of unemployed persons within the family: the person unemployed is the father in 45 percent of the cases, the mother in 34 percent, the children in 16 percent (boys 11 percent, girls 5 percent), another member of the family—grandfather, grandmother, brother-in-law—in 5 percent of the cases.

As to their family situation: 52.5 percent are married, 24.5 percent are bachelors, 11.5 percent are widowers, 11.5 percent are divorced or separated. The marital status of the unemployed population differs considerably from that of the totality of the actively employed population. Thus, the survey on the working forces in the countries of the European Economic Community, made in 1960 [9, p.50], reveals that the proportion of bachelors, which is 31 percent for all the countries put together, reaches 58.2 percent among the unemployed population. The matrimonial status reveals a selective character but, as Ledrut points out:

> the selective character of the matrimonial status is not simple. There is an effect which results from the status of bachelor or widower or divorcee, and it has an influence above all on men. But there is also an effect which results from family responsibilities. Bachelors with family responsibilities have a lower unemployment rate than married men without responsibilities [9].

The selective effect of the bachelor status makes itself felt particularly among men and among young people.

The latter are the most vulnerable. With the exception of young bachelors, particularly if they are not heads of households and if they live with their family, the vulnerability or risk of losing a job is the same for the unemployed of diverse statuses and of diverse family responsibilities; married men with dependents do not seem to be less vulnerable than bachelors without dependents. In an article which appeared in a daily newspaper, Dumont [7] emphasizes that adolescents are the first victims of collective lay-offs; often they have little training, having stopped their studies to begin working at an early age. Those who pursued their high school studies received no technical training, the school having no knowledge how to prepare the child and the adolescent for industrial life. Frequently, the parents are opposed to their child's following a professional training course; unfortunately, they prefer work which is better paid immediately. Many employers reject young men who would be leaving in several months for military service. However, young men want to work and feel the need to assume responsibilities. For them, unemployment constitutes a delay or a failure in the accomplishment of their legitimate aspirations and may sometimes have disastrous consequences, such as postponing their admission to the adult world and maintaining their submissive and dependent status in the family—consequences which are at the very least irritating and sometimes catastrophic.

A great number of workers fear unemployment.

> In his work a man depends upon his trade and his employment. The security of the household depends on their stability. When a man loses one or the other he risks seeing his family deprived of all resources. An accident can make him unfit for his trade, a disagreement with his employer can make him lose his job. Thus, the fear of unemployment is very great among many of those who were interviewed. In our first survey of 132 households, 34 percent feared unemployment [3].

In Carrere's survey [4], the occupations of the unemployed are summarized in the following way: the women are occupied at home in most cases, 7.7 percent are looking for work, and 12.9 percent do temporary work (domestic work, for example). As for the men, 31.6 percent are solely looking for work, 14.3 percent admit to an occasional job, 7.1 percent help with the housework, 13.6 percent remain idle.

The living conditions of the unemployed are marked by privations and, in a general way, poverty. Expenses, and above all "miscellaneous expenses" (those which increase along with a rise in the standard of living) are reduced. Food restrictions are the first to be felt: the nutrition of the unemployed and their families, though sufficient in quantity, is unquestionably deficient in quality (animal proteins, calcium) and unbalanced.

Family responsibilities do not seem to be an obstacle to the geographical or professional mobility of the unemployed. Those who have responsibilities or heavy expenses do not retreat before the problems caused by a transfer or the risk of a new kind of work.

Many unemployed persons feel shameful, rejected, socially inferior, or discredited; the intensity of the feeling varies in relation to the family status and social integration. Men who have a family life tend to feel less shame than those who do not. The inclination to feel ashamed is high among divorced women, whereas it scarcely exists among married women. Ladrut presents the relationship between family ties and the shame of the unemployed person in the following way:

> Work is more important for the personality where there is a family responsibility. This effect can only be compensated for by strong work attachments; the responsibility of men who are heads of family doubtless brings with it a greater sensitivity to shame, but the local social ties, notably family ones, certainly diminish the effects that this responsibility can have on the personality [9].

It is to be expected that unemployment will be a source of family disorganization, especially if the head of the family suffers a loss of prestige because of it. The unemployed person sometimes reacts aggresively against the society which has allowed him to lose status, and sometimes he reacts with a feeling of humiliation and a sense of abandonment.

> Family solidarity can arrest this loss-of-prestige phenomenon by attributing the responsibility for the unemployment to society or to the employer, which implies a more social and less institutional perception of employment. The more the mere fact of holding a job affects regard for the personal merits of the head of the family, the more his prestige is affected by the loss of that job. The perception varies according to the social milieu.
>
> When much less importance is attached to social opinion, symbolized by an unknown quantity, a shifting can occur towards another form of shame or humiliation. Though it strengthens the defenses of the personality, family life can also weaken them. As a matter of fact, we can observe an inverse connection between social humiliation and family humiliation, between the shame of telling a stranger that one is unemployed and the shame felt within the family because of the attitude of the family milieu. In other words, there is an inverse correla-

tion between family condemnation and the discredit and loss of prestige thus revealed on the one hand, and, on the other, social shame . . . Everything depends on the values of this family milieu and on its attitude towards the employment world and towards society as a whole [9].

Before attempting to make any general statement, it is necessary to be certain that the phenomena observed in the city are to be found in the rural community, and that the sociocultural differences, though marked from one country to another, do not profoundly change the nature or the depth of the ties between unemployment and family life.

In his psychosocial study of the hat-makers in the valleys of the Aude, Moscovici remarks that:

> Unemployment is selective; it is not a blind force which strikes just anyone or any part of the community. It makes the poor even poorer, the old even older and those who just barely manage to live more insecure [10].

In describing the consequences of being unemployed, he records that this condition leads to irreversible after-effects: social cohesion is destroyed and passive behavior appears. Chronic unemployment means indefinite waiting. Now, this waiting in expectation, as Fromm puts it, is a situation in which

> In terms of his inner experience, man no longer feels that he is in active control of his own capacities and wealth, but tends rather to look upon himself as a diminished 'thing', dependent on powers outside himself, into which he has projected his essential living being.

At the same time as his working, social, and family life comes apart at the seams, the unemployed person finds himself little by little reduced to his elementary needs. The reactions are catastrophic: he can no longer go to the cafe, his social ties weaken and, in this emergency, his self-devaluation increases. The unemployed man identifies himself with the most pejorative images of himself held by others, and this brings his reactions close to those usually held by weak minority groups. He clings to mythical beliefs that drive him deeper into defeat. The more he succumbs, the more does his thinking take on a magical quality until he shows a marked tendency to a naive personification of the evil that besets him in a way analogous to the psychological mechanism of regression.

Moscovici [10] also observes that the unemployed often benefits from financial aid given by his family, larger than he usually gets but, all things considered, little enough, and often limited to a mere attempt at face saving. In France, even in the poorest regions unemployment attacks first the individual and only subsequently his family group.

A Review of Surveys in Other Countries

The situation is completely different in Pakistan, according to the economist Islam [8], who has written about an agricultural region which is underdeveloped and overpopulated. We are struck by the fact that work there is not, in fact, a personal affair; it concerns an entire family, in which a varying number of persons are active. When there is a great deal of work, everyone participates, including women and children. The rest of the time there is partial or seasonal unemployment (or both at the same time) and quite often disguised unemployment (that is to say, a decrease in money received for the same amount of work done: for example, the active members of the family are all at work, but they must work for a longer time in order to receive the same final return obtained within a shorter time when work is more abundant). The working members of the family are relatively priviledged; they eat better and more often than the nonworking members. Except for this reservation, the family tie is so strong that it can bar the acceptance of employment; offers of work somewhere else can be inacceptable for the simple reason that they would force the worker away from his group. What is more, the observer risks being confused by certain behavior; he should be aware of the fact that the persons concerned do not ascribe to the same norms or standards of employment (and thus of underemployment) as he does.

These norms are difficult to grasp, and their subtlety of operation is well described in Bourdieu's sociological survey:

> Given a similar work-load, the country people of the Kabyle region are prone to declare themselves unemployed if they consider their activity insufficient, whereas the farmers and shepherds of Southern Algeria prefer to say that they are employed [3].

It would appear that the persons interviewed by Bourdieu react differently to the same circumstances, but they all regard themselves as subject to the "the categorical duty to work," even if it be for an almost worthless return. The social entourage and the family expect each one to do what he can. In a developing society such as Algeria at the end of the colonial era, the family also evolves: though traditionally only the men in an extended family work away from home, there is a general movement towards narrowing the family down to the conjugal couple; at the same time, the women are working more and earning more both in absolute and in comparative terms. It is therefore understandable that prostitution should develop, paradoxically enough as a modern form of feminine labor. Bourdieu also subtly observes how two types of logic—traditional and capitalist—are telescoped, engendering in certain workers who are reduced to pseudo-work a need to assert that their production is real.

Several of Bourdieu's notes deal with the reinforcement or the resurgence of a magical mode of thought: "I live according to Barak," says one unemployed person, and many respondents explain that their unemployment is at least partially due to the obscure will of a mysterious "One."

UNEMPLOYMENT IS A PSYCHOLOGICAL DISASTER.

It prohibits "the elaboration of a rational program for living." For the underoccupied sub-proletariat nothing is solid, nothing is sure, nothing is permanent; time becomes precarious and, like space, discontinuous.

> Unemployment causes a systematic disorganization in behavior, attitude and ideology, and this, first and foremost, in an urban world where the non-obtainment of a steady income threatens the social function of the head of the family, his authority within it and his respectability outside it . . . The father, the brothers, the cousins and sometimes even the wife and children are obliged to provide for the needs of the group so that the normal functions are then reversed: the most drastic and scandalous situation is that in which the men are dependent on their wives [3].

It is surprising to find comparable expressions of this state of affairs among authors who have studied radically different societies. For example, Tausky and Piedmont [15] note that widespread public opinion in the United States regard the job possibilities as so great that persons without work or badly paid can have only themselves to blame; the unemployed are self-disparaging and, moreover, manifest many psychiatric disturbances. The authors suggest that the more the culture is individualistic and egalitarian, the more severe is the blow to the self-esteem of those who have difficulty in searching for, finding, and keeping a job.

In Socialist countries unemployment does not exist as such. The employment categories also are simplified, at least on first inspection. A person who remains without work must necessarily be either ill or asocial, that is to say that he is given either maximum assistance or equally maximum reprobation or rejection. However, the basic reality is less schematic, and we would like to discover more shades of opinion about this.

Williams [19] reports on a pilot project successfully carried out by the Office for Cooperation and Economic Development, in five highly industrialized countries (Western Germany, the United States, the Netherlands, the United Kingdom, Sweden). Special counselors were appointed to help those who had been idle for a long time or who frequently changed their jobs. These counselors proved to be both enlightened and effective, and helped to establish the fact that the people concerned often suffered from various handicaps or had serious personal and familial difficulties.

The form and nature of these difficulties can vary a great deal, and the analysis is very instructive. It will come as no surprise that out of 47 unemployed males in whom mental disturbances were found to exist, 41 were bachelors (or living alone). As was to be expected, too, the young people who sustained job failures often received poor support from their families. There was also a frequent concurrence between the date of marital break-up and the start of unemployment. On the other hand, it would be difficult to imagine finding a man who had ceased to work the day that his wife entered prison for the reason that he was forced to stay at home to take care of the children. An example of the unsettling effect of family disruption on employability is demonstrated by the following case:

> Man aged 36 who has worked in 16 different places during the past five years. He finished his apprenticeship as an automobile mechanic and works today as an unskilled laborer, a coal-delivery man, digger, or house painter. He is in good health and has not suffered any serious illnesses. He is ready to accept any kind of manual labor.
>
> His frequent changes of jobs are a direct result of his family situation. He has three children. Seven years ago his wife left him to live with someone else. He was awarded custody of the children and at one time he took care of them alone for more than six months, the children then being one, two and three years of age. A social agency has found him a maid for whom he has to pay 35 DM per month, the rest being paid by the agency. She is an aged widow who has raised several children, and she fulfills her task to the satisfaction of her employer. The

local official charged with supervising the care of the children, certifies that the maid maintains the home adequately.

If he changes jobs often, it is because he tries to find well-paid work in order to provide for the needs of his three young children.

He is a good worker. For years he has been trying to obtain a permanent position in a local steel mill, and the placement counselor has at last succeeded in having him hired as a crane operator there. He is now pleased with his wages and will probably make every effort to keep his job [19].

Williams [19] calls attention to the general problem of mothers: their responsibilities often keep them from accepting proposed jobs or force them to quit those they hold; or restrict them to discreditable types of work. (In this context, a recent survey done by the National Institute of Demographic Studies seems to show a certain evolution in French society. Employers as well as labor unions are loath to go beyond the alternative of all or nothing: mothers should work full time or else be restricted to household tasks. But, according to Roux, 57 percent of married women have expressed the desire to work part-time, at least during certain periods in their career. The author adopts the position that he is in favor of part-time work (or temporary work) for married women of less than 45 years of age, and perhaps later work full-time when their children are grown. It is interesting to note furthermore that the husbands, of whom 47 percent are opposed to full-time work for their wife, would accept by 58.8 percent that she work half-time; for temporary work, the percentages go respectively to 37.1 and 44.1 percent [12].

To sum up what we have said: the unemployed man, in difficulty due to a situation imposed upon him and which is not of his making, is often humiliated by society's behavior towards him. He feels ashamed, socially inferior, and discredited, and this all the more so if he is an executive or a white-collar worker. These feelings are often accompanied by a withdrawal into himself and a kind of isolated loneliness when he cannot compensate for his sense of inferiority by finding something else on which to concentrate his energies. "Shame is always due to a feeling of failure, not necessarily of fault" (Sartre in *Being and Nothingness*). The head of the family is humilated when he cannot meet his responsibilities, and is sometimes led to face-saving pretense, like the man who set out every day from home at his usual office hours and wandered around the city until mealtime so as to avoid letting his family discover that he had lost his job and, as he imagined, his prestige and authority in the home.

We frequently run into an attitude of negation and flight in the face of the reality of unemployment: refusal to be called unemployed and to consider one's self as such, going sometimes so far as refusal to register at the unemployment office and to collect unemployment compensation. A survey which appeared in "Elle" [14] very well illustrates this attitude of negation in a family where the father, a high executive, became unemployed.

> From his very first week of idleness, quietly, by unspoken accord, we banished the word 'unemployment' from our vocabulary. In fact, they wanted to exploit him; they proposed hardly two-thirds of his last salary under the pretext that he was unemployed. That's it, unemployed. They had the nerve to call him that.

There are also certain men who overwork and systematically brush aside everything which could distract them from their work, to which they dedicate themselves excessively, investing all their energies in it; this can lead to real catastrophies and personal breakdowns when a work stoppage or unemployment interrupts their activities.

On the other hand, there are individuals who are comfortably ensconsed in unemployment. The "tramps," very well studied by Vexliard [16, 17, 18], who number about 6000 in Paris, not only do not look for work but refuse to work. Tramps rarely become so deliberately. For example, it occurs when a job is lost. The unemployed tramp suddenly becomes aware of the distance separating him from his old world, and he experiences a feeling of self-depreciation against which he then reacts by rejecting this world and by making a reevaluation of himself. A return to the old way of life then becomes impossible. He leads an aimless existence, rejects any idea of work or of family life, and becomes accustomed to frustration without conflict. Being a tramp means the lowering of the threshold of resistance to desocialization; normally this threshold is high when needs and desires are ethical, highly developed, refined, complex, and demanding.

The "hippies" with their long hair contest the consumers' society, looking for an escape in drugs, in a marginal, irresolute, or evasive way of life, refusing all constraint.

Completely different from the tramp or the hippy, the "professionally unemployed man" is rarely met with during the various sociological surveys. Confronting the reality of the honest and hardworking unemployed person without resources who wishes to work, a myth has been created of the unemployed individual who is such by profession: this is only an alibi born of the collective conscience, which in this way tries to escape from any culpability for the situation. However, the idea of a social pathology of unemployment, although far from embracing the mass of the unemployed, should not be rejected. A minority of the unemployed do turn out to deviate greatly from the statistical norm and to be characterized by psychological maladjustment, practical inadequacy, and sociological lack of adaptation [13].

In addition to the failure it implies, the very fact of being unemployed is burdened with diverse psychological consequences: creation of stereotypes, emotional regression, and secondary benefits drawn from defeat. Living through the experience of loss of work followed by a prolonged lack of work provokes a kind of social regression, the unemployed person exchanging his role of worker for that of a person on relief; he regularly puts up with a series of frustrations and refusals and, having acquired the habit of being unemployed, he runs the risk of no longer being able to extricate himself. Thus, we might speak of a "poisoning" caused by work stoppage.

The drama of the individual must also be placed in its social context. In covering this subject, we have seen that certain constants, cutting across the diversity of social organizations, are found everywhere. We have seen, too, that family and social pressures act upon and influence the unemployed person in rather diverse ways. In order to see this more clearly, it will be necessary to go further into detail.

In any given country, unemployment is more or less tolerable depending on the milieu. In certain social strata, like those occupied by white-collar workers, that have not been directly effected by unemployment, unemployment represents a calamity from which it is necessary to preserve the children at any price, by insisting that they follow a "safe" career such as that of a civil servant. Security and stability of employment become then the first criteria in the choice of a job. Elsewhere, unemployment may be seen differently, for example as an epiphenomenon of work itself: an unskilled worker knows that he risks being unemployed one day or another. There are other social sections where unemployment was rare until recently, but where it is gradually becoming more common; such is the case with executives, who in the past were not exposed to this sort of risk.

Whether foreseen or not, unemployment always upsets people's lives. It is usual, at least in industrial civilizations, to measure a man's worth by the pay he receives. The position of each man within modern society is located according to his purchasing power. To what can the unemployed person then lay claim? Even if it be true that the unemployment of some is inevitable so as to allow for employment of the greater number, how can we accept the fact that fortune strikes so unjustly? It is more reassuring to believe that it is the most stupid, the most incapable and the laziest who are victims of lay-offs and are faced with closed doors. The unemployed person finds himself, *ipso facto*, doubly depreciated.

There is a third kind of devaluation. With a few exceptions, in most of present-day societies, it is the father who is the head of the family and responsible for earning the money necessary for its upkeep. If the mother and children work, this brings in what is called "supplementary income." The father's unemployment brings about a loss of social status which can have the gravest consequences for him (since he ceases to conform to the image of the sire and nourisher) and for the entire family group whose socioeconomic situation as well as their affective and emotional interrelations will be profoundly disturbed.

The mother's unemployment can also have immediate and grave consequences. This is likely to happen, for example, when the mother is in sole care of the children and is housed by her employer. The resulting lack of resources, and especially of housing, may force her to separate from her children and get them placed in temporary homes by social agencies. Complete family disruption may occur since dispersal of the children cannot always be avoided, the younger ones being placed with foster parents and the older ones put in institutions.

Segregated thus by society as a whole within a special status, it is not surprising that the unemployed person conceives of himself as different, as not belonging. We have already seen that the family group, sometimes the cause of unemployment and often changed by it, may become highly disturbed in its external relationships and shaken in its internal cohesion as a consequence. Bake has noted that along with a separation of the immediate family from the rest of the family group, there also exists a general dislocation of the group as a whole [1]. What is true in New Haven also holds true in Paris, in the

Aude country, and even in Algiers, but there are some important qualifications to be added regarding the rural areas of developing countries. It remains no less true than elsewhere that all adults who do not ostensibly work are obliged to justify themselves. If justification is not given, or not accepted, the adult ceases to be considered as such. The mother, or the eldest daughter, can get away with it, but the son and, above all, the father cannot escape from facing a severe challenge to his honor.

The series of articles by Servan-Schreiber already quoted from previously [14], report the reactions of a woman to her husband's long period of unemployment. This document brings to light a sequence of phases and we ourselves can verify that the evolution as described is indeed inevitable and widespread. (1) The denial of what is obvious: "From his very first week of idleness, quietly, by unspoken agreement, the word 'unemployment' is banished from the family's vocabulary." (2) Next comes the violent invasion of reality at the level of the family budget, and sooner or later someone will have "the nerve" to violate the taboo; the fact of unemployment obtains recognition. (3) This is followed by efforts not to repudiate the past (we will not sell the car even if we are unable to use it). (4) Sooner or later, there is an eruption of domestic squabbles and a growing difficulty of communication between husband and wife. (5) There is a growing alienation from external ties, the family keeping aloof from their friends. (6) The internal dynamic "arrangements" begin to alter, the wife falling back on the protection of her own mother, and the husband attempting to perform household tasks. About the latter, the woman is, to say the least, torn: she understands that her husband is trying to revamp his self-image by making himself "useful," but she is humiliated for him (and for herself), and weeps to see him using the vacuum cleaner. (7) Little is said of the changes in the children; they are mainly envisaged as potential victims of the circumstance who must be protected at all costs.

The Dynamic Impact of Unemployment on the Children

It is on this last point that the Servan-Schreiber account calls for criticism. Actually, the child of an unemployed person is involved in a drama of the most serious importance to his future. In a penetrating analysis in depth Dolto has this to say:

> At the time of oedipal castration, the specific character of the father as castrator takes on an anal component, particularly if, during parental transactions, the child is witness to a love relationship directly tied to the presence or absence of money conflicts [6].

The stress of unemployment may therefore bring about an "analization" (anal repression) of the Oedipus complex with the production of symptoms.

For example, if, at this Oedipal stage, the love tie between the parents is not of a nature that transcends money problems, the child may begin to commit thefts. These acts compensate for the intolerable narcisistic injury that he sustains not only because of his actual impotence in the face of his incestuous wishes but also because he is under threat from a father whom he regards as discredited by the mother. Identification with the father for the boy and with the mother for the girl under these circumstances becomes meaningless, and the motivation for the theft is to relieve narcissistic distress. Such pilfering may have oral compensatory aims (candy) or may symbolize, in a fetishistic way, the seductive power of an idealized Oedipal object, and its effect is to reinforce the imaginary power of the child, although, unhappily, it may also serve to exclude him from competing in a more creative and culturally acceptable fashion.

The employment failure of the father, the child's model for identification, signifies also a collapse of his symbolic power and this, in the absence of an adequate paternal surrogate, may provoke serious somatic or mental disturbances in the character development of the child should unemployment coincide with the Oedipal crisis. It may lay the basis for anal and genital passivity which, at puberty, may take the form of homosexuality, or to a diffuse passive-aggressiveness leading eventually to juvenile delinquency.

In fact, any social mishap that in the eyes of the family places the father at a special disadvantage as a protagonist in the Oedipal struggle, (which normally is resolved because the father's power and prestige compensates the son for the internal prohibitions and deprivations he must endure) may lead to the development of character disturbances.

To treat children, during their latency period, who have undergone this type of experience after a fairly normal pre-Oedipal development, requires either an analysis of the desymbolizing phallic effects of Oedipal castration or the treatment of an obsessional neurosis whose function is to repudiate the genital symbolism which the father has proved inadequate to sustain.

Conclusion

In conclusion, we must once again emphasize that situations can be as different and as varied on the level of reality as on the level of fantasy. There are many kinds of unemployment; of societies, of families, and each individual situation is unique. Nevertheless, it is a general rule that the unemployed person appears first of all as a defeated victim whose fall drags down with him the entire family group. In this connection we can evoke the remarks made by Bessaignet about a different problem—migration: the position of the migrant as such and even the factors in him that separate him from others (his color, for example) in the final analysis, count less than the problems specific to the society which receives him (for example, the proclivities to sociological, technological, and industrial evolution) [2]. Any thorough understanding of a social problem and any solution to it, must be made by way of the total society. Unemployment is a function of the unemployed individual, to be sure, but also of almost everything around him as well.

Unemployment can be interpreted as the modality of a vast system of socioeconomic and instinctive-affective exchanges. Food deprivation, which is such a generalized and striking feature of it, may call into being an interplay of both external and internal (oral, and to a lesser extent, anal) pressures, a game in which the unemployed are the ultimate losers.

Which brings us to our last question: is the person a loser by chance or has he himself been somehow responsible for the sequence of events which has reduced him to this sorry predicament? An immediate response tends to excuse him: can we reproach him for being old or young, of being the offspring of a poor family or the citizen of a poor country? In this latter case, he has only the choice between unemployment or exile; and, if he chooses exile, he risks remaining unemployed, the last to be hired and the first to be fired [11]. A second possible answer involves the family. The everyday types of unemployment, whether due to technological or personal reasons can be catastrophic for the family as a whole, but even under the gravest conditions, the destructive effect can be offset by the resilience of the family. The tendency of a particular individual not to encounter unemployment but to remain unemployed is dependent upon the quality of his family life. It is not the rigid, hidebound, dictatorial family which protects its members best; nor the disunited, slipshod, disordered one; both of these types may be, in part, responsible for chronic employment failure. It is the family whose members are the most united in their feelings and the freest in their actions and interactions that is most resistant to disaster. It is this kind of family which offers its members the most support in taking up and keeping a job. It is this kind of family that *least* imprisons the individual within a particular role; that least deprives him of a constructive role; and that gives him the most opportunity to keep his place in the overall system of production and employment.

Bibliography

1. Bake (1940), in G. Friedmann and P. Naville *Traité de Sociologis du Travail,* Vol. 2, A. Colin, Paris, 1961, 299-324.
2. Bessaignet, P., Table ronde sur: *"les problèmes posés par les ressortissants des D.O.M. en France",* Paris, Institut des Hautes Etudes d'Amérique Latine, 2-4 Juin, 1969, (Comptes rendus á paraitrs).
3. Bourdieu, P., A. Darbel, J. P. Rivet and Cl. Seibel *Travail et Travailleure en Algérie,* Mouton & Co., Paris-La Hays, 1963.
4. Carrère, P., Etude sur le genre de vie des chômeurs, Nov. 1954-Janv. 1955, *Bull. Institut National d'Hygiène,* 10 (1955), 4, 883-920.
5. Chombart de Lauwe, P. H., *La Vie quotidienne des Familles Ouvrières,* Centre National de la Racherche Scientifique, Paris, 1956.
6. Dolto, F., Le Complexe d'Oedipe et la problématiqus humaine, *Pratique des Nots,* 3 (1968), 9.
7. Dumont, J. P., Les Jeunes sans emploi: vrais ou faux chômeurs?, *Le Monde,* 2-3-4 Avril 1969.
8. Islam, N., Les concepts et la mesure du chômage et du sous-emploi dans les économies en voie de développement, *Rev. internat. du Travail,* 89 (1964), 3, 34-51.
9. Ledrut, R., *Sociologie du Chômage,* Presses Universitaires de France, Paris, 1966.
10. Moscovici, S., *Reconversion Industrielle et Changements sociaux Un example: la Chapellerie dens l'Aude,* A. Colin, Paris, 1961.
11. Parmar, S., Chômage ou axil in, *Courrier de l'U.N.E.S.C.O.,* 22, Juillet, 32-34, 1969.
12. Roux, C., Cinquante sept pour cent des femmes désireraient travailler à temps partiel, *Le Monde,* 17 Avril, 1969.

13. Sarton, A., Pour une "thérapeutique" de l'emploi, *Psychol. francaise,* 10 (1965), 2, 164-170.
14. Servan-Schreiber, C., Quand le mari perd son travail, *Elle,* 28 Avril 1969, 1219.
15. Tausky, K. and E. Piedmont, The Meaning of work and unemployment: implications for mental health, *Internat. J. Soc. Psychiatry,* 14 (1967-1968), 1, 44-49.
16. Vexliard, A., Le Clochard. Les phases de la désocialisation, *Evol. psychiatrique,* 15 (1950), 4, 619-639.
17. Vexliard, A., Les Clochards. Le seuil de résistance à la desocialisation, *Evol. psychiatrique,* 16 (1951), 1, 133-150.
18. Vexliard, A., Le Clochard: un homme sans historie, *Evol. psychiatrique,* 17 (1952), 3, 507-527.
19. Williams, G., *Conseils pour les Groupes Spéciaux,* O.C.D.E., Paris, 1967.

Chronic Family Pathology

Editorial Comment

In this section, the contributors have attempted to deal with what Ackerman and his colleagues have referred to as chronic "interlocking pathology" as it exists within families. Once again, we see attempts to build theoretical bridges between the individual and group conceptions and the inner and outer aspects of personality. Ackerman, like the theorists in the dynamic section of this book, feels that it is important to base theory on observations made both from inside outward, as in the biological and psychoanalytic perspectives, as well as from the outside inward, that is, from the study of the family as a whole back to the individual member. Without this dual approach, the theoretical viewpoint in either case remains "incomplete, one-sided and selectively biased." Moreover, to obtain a more total picture, we need to examine "not only what the parent does to the child but also what the child does to the parent"; not only "how far the child is part of the family but how far the family is part of the child"; and we need to do all this across more than two generations and through wider environments. All this leads logically to the concept of family diagnosis and to the inclusion of the individual diagnosis within this system of the family diagnosis. In this context Ackerman offers the striking clinical observation that whereas some children in a family may represent its pathological aspect, other children are the stabilizing and healing powers and growth potential of the family.

Wolff's survey and bibliography are probably the fullest that we have in this area to date. She traces the influence of maternal and paternal pathology on the behavior of the children and finds it to be particularly pathogenic, especially in the case of maternal pathology and younger children. Paternal pathology appears more important in the genesis of adolescent delinquency in boys. However, she adds a necessary word of caution. Not all psychiatric disorders in children are reactions to parental pathology and there are many children with psychosis, organic brain disease, or constitutional variations of personality who have "perfectly normal parents." (If this "perfect normality" does indeed exist, it is often hidden under many secondary reactions to the children's behavior and what is primary and secondary then becomes increasingly difficult to distinguish.)

The remaining contributions to this section have all to do with the psychopathology of food intake, once again in the context of the family as regulator. Intrafamilial disturbances are rampant in such cases and may interfere radically with the smooth operation of the biological function. In addition, it may complicate the physiological working still further by an overload of distorted symbolism and conflictual fantasy. With regard to Bruch's work, we have the advantage of a commentary by Tolstrup who is one of the leading investigators in this field.

Dr. Selvini Palazzoli reviews for us the historical development of her own approach, illustrating to what a large extent the researcher is a child of his times so that his concepts and methods reflect the era in which he works. She has moved from the notion of a pathogenic mother-child relationship to the concept, as already stated by Ackerman, that the family is a total system of pathological interaction. It is interesting to compare her findings with those of Bruch because the data are obtained somewhat differently. Dr. Selvini Palazzoli makes systematic use of conjoint family interviews which she finds confirm and complete the observations that she made during her earlier phase of individual treatment. She has also found that the use of a co-therapist of the opposite sex is more effective in helping to break down the somewhat rigid family structures in the anorexic cases.

The child with a perverse appetite is different from the child with obesity or anorexia and the family characteristics are correspondingly different. The pica families are more akin to multiproblem families manifesting a high incidence of family instability and separation. The families, as a whole, are orally fixated so that both father and mother tend to suffer from obesity, alcoholism, and drug addiction. The authors feel that the circumstances may conduce to the development of addiction later on in the child. Since the therapeutic measures used are admittedly superficial, one cannot say that we get to know these families in any depth from reading this report, so that the area of inquiry remains relatively open for more intensive investigations. In the meantime, the two authors have done our field a great service by bringing an important and relatively overlooked symptom to our attention. If such explorations were common for the many symptoms that children manifest, we would be well on the way to developing a truly scientific system of child psychiatry based on the careful physical and psychological study of the individual and his family. It is the latter that was often overlooked in the past, but not by Freud who, as long ago as 1905, had this to say:

> We must pay as much attention in our case histories to the purely human and social circumstances of our patients as to the somatic data and the symptoms of the disorder. *Above all, our interest will be directed towards their family circumstances.*

Childhood Disorders and Interlocking Pathology in Family Relationships

NATHAN W. ACKERMAN, PEGGY PAPP,
AND PHOEBE PROSKY (U.S.A.)

Over a period of years [1-10] we have been trying to build a theoretical bridge between the traditional view of the psychiatrically disturbed child as individual and a broader conception of childhood disorder within the matrix of the psychosocial organization of the family unit. In this process of reorientation, three levels of analysis are involved: (1) the internal forces of child personality; (2) behavior influenced by one-to-one family relationships, such as the child-mother pair, child-father, or child-sibling; (3) behavior influenced by the child's integration into the whole family viewed as a behavior system and encompassing the interchange of family and community.

Up to now we have tended to formulate the determinants of child behavior in hierarchical series: heredity, embryonal factors, neurophysiological patterns, and the emerging stages of growth and development shaped by social process. In an earlier phase, there was a prime concern with inborn characteristics, with measurement of abilities, intellectual, neuromotor, and so on. Then came a shift of interest to the instinctual core of personality, to the organization of basic drives and needs related to successive stages of development; parallel with this came a concern with the child's response to mothering behavior. Still more recently, interest expanded to include the circular adaptive relations of child and family. Across time each sequential shift in emphasis and orientation brought a new kind of challenge and a greater appreciation of the complexities of social maturation.

To begin with, the approach was one-sided and oversimplified. Mainly, what are the biological roots of child behavior and what ingredients in the behavior of the mother, acting as an external influencing agent, exert a pathogenic effect on the child? Later, there came a broader interpretation of the problem, not only what parent does to child but also what child does to parent. At the present time there is a further broadening of the conceptual frame, an increasing concern with the circular relations and interchange of child and family across three generations, taking into account the circular processes of interpenetration and influence which occur at the interface of family and wider environment.

Thus far we have not been clear about the inner and outer aspects of child personality. We have not yet achieved a precise definition of the interplay and merging of biological and sociocultural forces in child development. We remain unsure as to how far the child is individual, how far the child is part of family, how far the family is part of the child. We do not yet have an adequate understanding of the border of the child's self and of the dynamics of interchange between self and the surrounding environment. Even to this day our conceptualization of such mechanisms as introjection and projection remains vague.

By tradition, the development of theory influenced by the biological and psychoanalytic perspectives moved from inside outward. Viewed in retrospect, this approach is incomplete, one-sided, and selectively biased. It needs to be balanced against observations made in the opposite direction, a conceptual movement from outside inward, from the dynamic study of the whole family back to the child or children.

What we learn about the nature of childhood disorders depends on how we learn it. Each procedure of study offers a special, though limited, set of potentials for understanding. No one of these methods is complete in itself. The position of the observer and his theoretical slant influence selectively both the findings and their interpretation. Each new method of investigation brings a different dimension, a change in perspective, and an altered conception of the nature of childhood disorders.

In this context the two conceptual approaches, from inside outward (i.e., from child to family) and from outside inward (i.e., from family to child or children) may be viewed as complementary procedures. The data derived from the two directions of study offer a reciprocal check on the validity of both findings and interpretations.

This point of view is exemplified in a comparison of study procedures twenty years ago and today. At the Child Development Center in New York, two decades ago, we studied a series of families moving conceptually, step-by-step, from an emotionally disturbed preschool child to the dynamics of his family group. To facilitate this purpose, we developed a scheme for organizing data leading to family diagnosis and a related outline for interpreting the mental health of child and family. At the Family Institute today we move conceptually from outside inward, from a psychosocial evaluation of the whole family back to its product, the set of children in the third generation. Toward this end, we have evolved an amended outline for family diagnosis.

For a better grasp of the implications of this theoretical development, it is useful to compare the two conceptual orientations in particular respects. This enables us to highlight differences in emphasis and perspective. Table 1 epitomizes these differences. In order to clarify the contrast of the two approaches, we now present several examples of family study, moving from child to family and from family to children.

Table 1 Two Conceptual Approaches to the Family

Points of Reference	From Child to Family	From Family to Children
Illness concept	One child is the "patient." The focus is on a single "breakdown."	The family is the "patient." "Breakdown" or illness encompasses the phenomenon of multiple disorders in the family group, their interlocking nature, and their emergence in series across time.

Table 1 Two Conceptual Approaches to the Family

Points of Reference	From Child to Family	From Family to Children
	The emphasis is on symptoms, on the overt clinical syndrome.	Thc emphasis is less on overt "illness" and more on interlocking vulnerability patterns among the family members.
	The emphasis is one-sidedly on the child's pathology.	The pathology of child is defined within the broader frame of total personality functioning.
	The pathogenic potential of family focuses on one child.	The pathogenic potential of the family is related to the emotional destiny of the entire set of children, viewed collectively as a subsystem of family. The joint identity, conflicts, fears, and defenses of parents and family are parcelled out in a special way among the entire brood of children. The stages of the family life cycle are correlated to the disturbances of each of the children in turn.
View of personality	The emphasis is on the child as individual.	The child is seen as an immature, incomplete being. The child is part of the family, family is part of the child.
Orientation to relationships	The emphasis is on one-to-one interaction. The child's behavior is related to mother as individual, to father as individual, etc.	The emphasis is on transaction. The child's behavior is related to the irreducible unit of family—the triad of mother, father, and child. Mothering, fathering, and "childing" are functions of the family as a behavior system, not just of individual personality.

Table 1 Two Conceptual Approaches to the Family

Points of Reference	From Child to Family	From Family to Children
View of causation	Causation is mainly linear, with an emphasis on direct, specific, and central elements of causation.	Causation is viewed as being multiple. It is circular, not linear. The contributing factors are both direct and indirect, specific and nonspecific, central and peripheral. They derive from conscious and unconscious experience and situational factors as well.
Development	The emotional development of the child is distorted by the pathogenic influence of each parent acting as external influencing agent.	The child's emotional development is shaped by the joint identity and complementarity of the marital and parental couple and the parent's relations with grandparents. The child's behavior is distorted by an imbalance and disharmony of family role relations. A critical warp of family functions precipitates symptoms in the child.
Coping	Coping with conflict is viewed mainly as an intrapsychic function of the child's personality.	Coping with conflict is a shared function, influenced by family interaction and the vicissitudes of family defense.
Healing	Healing is the resolution of intrapsychic conflict.	Healing is viewed as a shared process, a shift toward health in the complementarity of family relationships and in the interplay of individual and family defenses.
Temporal perspective	The emphasis is on past determinants, on the longitudinal vector.	The emphasis is on the "here and now," on the horizontal vector.

Table 1 Two Conceptual Approaches to the Family

Points of Reference	From Child to Family	From Family to Children
Level of conceptual analysis	Psychological.	Psychosocial.
Unit of examination	The behavior of the individual child.	The behavior of the child joined to his environment.
Unit of diagnosis	Individual personality of the child.	Child diagnosis within a system of family diagnosis.

From Child to Family

HENRY R

Problem in Light of Developmental History. Henry R., age 3½, was referred to the Child Development Center with complaints of total lack of speech and rituals around eating.

Henry was born 3 years after marriage; the birth was normal. He was nursed on demand and weaned himself at 8 months. Between 3 and 4 months, his father, a professional person, insisted he be given the yolk of a hard-boiled egg, on which he gagged. At 9 months, he gagged on coarse foods. His mother thought she was causing an eating problem, so she stopped the coarse foods and began feeding him chopped meat. He developed the habit of holding it in his mouth while he ate other foods. At 1 year, he began to eat solids, but became suspicious of new foods; he smelled and touched them before eating. He had never tasted candy, cake, or steak. As a baby he was never fed potatoes or other starches because his mother feared he would get fat. At the time of referral, he was drinking no milk and had developed food fads, such as at school he would eat only bananas. Eating has always been accompanied by rituals which he and his mother carry out; for example, when he eats Jello, he puts his hand on the glass and his mother says, "Henry, look out for the glass." When these rituals are omitted, he has tantrums, often severe and involving head-banging. His compulsions began at age 1½. His mother states that whenever he wanted anything she would point to it, name it, and explain what she was doing with it so he could learn from her. He began playing with his toys in the same order every day. Since 13 months of age, his favorite toy has been a tin can, which he carries at all times and at one time used in a dressing ritual. Henry's lack of closeness to other people was observed at 1 year, before which time he had been a "happy, friendly baby," except that he did not like to be held. He was suspicious of people and, by the time he was 2½, the family had "learned not to cuddle him." He was affectionate with and extremely dependent on his mother. He behaved as if he were unaware of others around him. He would stare at her as if trying to read her lips, and it became obvious that he had no need to talk because she anticipated all his wishes. She bound him to her by concentrated looking, and it seemed as if the child could continue to exist only through a return of the same concentration. Her speech, when directed at him, was stereotyped, ritualistic, and rhythmic. Henry's smile was constrained and he showed a monotony of mood.

Toilet training was accomplished easily between 1½ and 2½ years of age. Development of motor control was normal and there were no sleeping problems. Henry's performance on psychological tests was average, with some retardation related to his dependence on his mother. Defective hearing was ruled out. He was diagnosed as an obsessional neurotic—the same diagnosis as was given both his parents; the possibility of pre-schizophrenic morbidity was considered. Both parents were primarily concerned with Henry's speech difficulties, and felt he was otherwise a careful, gentle, intelligent child. They showed a striking lack of emotional contact and spontaneity with the child.

Family as a Group. The R's live in a fourth floor tenement apartment, where Henry has a small room which separates the parental bedroom from the living room. Mr. R says of his wife that she is the "loveliest, kindest person in the world," that their "marriage is wonderful," and that they were "made for each other." Mrs. R describes their sexual relations as "beautiful from the beginning." She says that her husband is very neat and cannot stand anything out of place; and that she was surprised to find someone neater than herself.

Mother. Mrs. R, age 26, was born in Atlantic City, the older of two children. Her father and mother owned a pharmacy. She described her family as "close and affectionate" and said she was "thrilled" with her home life as a child. Her parents were ideal and she felt as she grew up that she wanted to be like her mother and marry a man like her father. When she met her husband, she was surprised that she could love anyone as much as her parents.

Mrs. R, born during the first year of her parents' marriage, was premature and sickly. She was nursed, but the milk did not agree with her. She began refusing to eat; she was "starving, but they didn't know it." When she was force fed, she became constipated and was given enemas. At 5, she became an enormous eater. She wet her bed until she was nearly 5. Her brother was born when she was 6; they have always "admired" each other and been "very close."

Mrs. R did very well throughout school. Socially, her mother emphasized the value of "prudishness." Mrs. R, therefore, received no sex instruction and was told that a man and woman do not have to get together to make a baby. She was at first disgusted about sex and could not sit near her boyfriend in high school when she found out he had slept with a prostitute.

Psychological tests revealed that Mrs. R was emotionally immature and obsessive-compulsive; she was seen as "priggish" and complacent.

Father. Mr. R, age 25, is the older of two sons of a clothing cutter and his wife. His parents were strict, meticulous, and emphasized cleanliness. His father missed work only twice in his life—when he had heart attacks. His father had a short temper; his mother was a "sweet person" who tried to "soothe" his father.

Mr. R speaks in a precise, controlled manner and dresses with extreme neatness. Psychiatric evaluation described him as a severe obsessional with little emotional response, and with difficulty controlling his aggression.

Courtship and Early Marriage. Mr. and Mrs. R met in college; Mrs. R was not interested in him because they had "nothing in common." However, he wrote her a beautiful letter which she showed to her father, who asked her to reconsider, and she subsequently fell in love and married him. Mr. R's family was against so early a marriage, and they stopped his allowance, so Mr. and Mrs. R turned to her parents for support. They were separated for a year while he was at professional school, but he wrote every day. When Mrs. R found she was pregnant, she was "thrilled."

Treatment. In the beginning of his stay in the therapeutic nursery, Henry seemed to be in a world of his own. He showed no initiative and lost interest when external stimulus stopped. However, he was able to accept suggestions; his coordination was excellent. After a time, he began to pronounce words corresponding to pictures in books.

Mrs. R was seen individually only a few times; it was deemed wiser not to disturb her delicate pattern of integration. Mr. R was in a father's group.

MARVIN S.

Problem in Light of Developmental History. Marvin was referred at age 2, a sturdy child with a sad, dreamy expression. He showed specific fears and diffuse anxiety, an inability to separate from his mother, passive behavior with peers, inappropriate laughter and excessive talking—often bizarre—poor body coordination, a desire to be a girl, and feeding and toilet training difficulties. The Buhler test showed a retardation in body performance and manipulation of materials; a deficiency in capacity for identification; poor mother-child relations during his first year; and the possibility of organic defect and schizophrenia. His I.Q. was 110.

Marvin was a planned child, born 10 years after marriage. Delivery was normal. He was bottle fed because of his mother's fear of breast cancer, from which her own mother died. At 1 month he showed a fear of strangers. He was weaned at 15 months. He toilet trained himself at 18 months after an upset precipitated by his feces rolling out of his diaper onto the floor. He was slow to stand and stood only with help until he was 2. At 10 months he first showed anxiety when separated from his mother. He cried while urinating throughout his first year. At this time he underwent surgery for pinpoint meatus to open the urethral duct, for which he was hospitalized 2 days; this was followed by several painful dilation treatments and injections. After the operation he showed a concern with broken objects.

His mother seemed to relate to Marvin only through her anxiety. She handled him in a mechanical and restrained manner, lost her temper frequently, and experienced feelings of violence toward him.

She had little confidence in his abilities, and provoked his tears on separation by her own expressions of anxiety.

His father felt responsible for Marvin's difficulties. He was disappointed that Marvin was not immediately a mature person, was critical of him, and refused to help him answer questions. He resented any attention the child got and lost his temper frequently. Marvin reacted with fear of his father. His mother resented her husband's lack of involvement with the child; his father resented his wife's overinvolvement. Both parents feared aggression and suppressed it in Marvin.

Family as a Group. The S's lived in a cheap, 1-room apartment which appeared cramped and disorderly. Marvin slept in an alcove. Mr. S's mother and sister lived below. Mr. S was employed irregularly in menial restaurant jobs; Mrs. S had worked for several months as a bookkeeper, which she at first felt involved too much responsibility, but which she gradually began to enjoy.

The members of this family were depressed and not integrated in any way; Marvin seemed the most isolated and was expected to function independently. They appeared helpless and hopeless. Father seemed to dominate the group superficially but was basically passive; it was mother who provided the moving force. She threatened often to leave him, pushed him to work, and exploded at him, to which he reacted by leaving the house.

Mother. Mrs. S, age 35, Jewish, was the second of 4 children. Her mother died of cancer when Mrs. S was 8, and she was raised by her critical, domineering, paternal grandmother. Her father, a successful jeweler, remarried twice and had 7 children. Mrs. S was an obese, shy, insecure adolescent. She did well in high school, took business training, and held a series of jobs, among them selling tombstones, which she found depressing. While her husband was in the service and after her pregnancy, she suffered from asthma and heart attacks. Mrs. S presented as depressed and detached, but neatly dressed. She was diagnosed as psychoneurosis with phobic, compulsive, and conversion tendencies.

Father. Mr. S, age 41, Jewish, was born in Palestine, one of 4 children, one of whom was a polio victim and another of whom had two psychotic breakdowns with suicidal attempts. His mother was domineering and engendered in her children a strong sense of guilt, having heart attacks when opposed. His parents both worked and he was brought up by members of his extended family who lived in the house. At 16, he left home. He tried working in his father's corset business, but they did not get along. He subsequently worked irregularly in menial restaurant jobs. He felt that his army experience was the happiest time of his life. Mr. S was seen as unhappy about his life and status, continually anticipating tragedy. When he got depressed, he frequently left home for a couple of weeks at a time without notice.

Marital History. The S's were married after 2 years of courtship, although Mr. S did not want the responsibility of wife and children, and for the first year and a half after marriage they lived with his parents. Mrs. S felt protective toward him. Although Mr. S was not eager, they planned to have a child, who was conceived faster than they expected due to sexual ignorance; Mrs. S was pleased to be pregnant. Sex was good periodically. Marvin has been brought up in part by his paternal grandmother and aunt who live in the same building, both of whom frightened Marvin with demands for attention and were sadistic and critical with him.

Treatment. In his 2 years in the therapeutic nursery, during which time he also had individual therapy, Marvin did very well. He learned to separate from his mother and overcome many of his phobias; he improved his motor coordination and lost his female identification. His verbosity decreased and he developed good peer relationships. His mother was seen regularly in individual therapy. Although she did not seem capable of developing a close relationship, she gained some insight into Marvin's problems and learned to tolerate more aggression and be less anxious. His father eventually had some individual therapy but did not seem to benefit significantly.

Follow-Up (Marvin, aged 9½, 5 years later). There was a remarkable change in the emotional tone of this family since they were seen five years ago. Principally, they appeared much better integrated. Much of this had to do with a change in their behavior toward Marvin and a sizable change in Marvin himself. Marvin and his father had developed a good rapport and were spending much more time together. Both parents seemed to share a great deal of pride and pleasure in Marvin; they were no longer so anxious about him and related to him warmly. Marvin seemed to be a unifying and enlivening influence on the family. While they still occupied the same crowded apartment, it was more attractively decorated, and the aunt and grandmother had moved out of the building, which removed a strain from the family.

Marvin was doing well in school, had lots of friends, was poised, sociable, and friendly and no longer depressed or withdrawn; he seemed to have developed a capacity for independent, creative functioning. He still appeared tense at times, especially in school, and had some obsessive behaviors.

Mother and father felt their relationship was somewhat improved, especially because the father had become more involved in the family and no longer absented himself; however, they seemed resigned to their chronic marital situation and to finding their pleasure in Marvin. They remained isolated. Mother had developed many somatic symptoms and was quite preoccupied with these. Father was still having trouble holding a job and was dissatisfied with himself and his level of achievement. Both felt the need of further psychiatric help, but felt their family had benefited enormously from the help they had received.

From Family to Children

THE M FAMILY

The specter of death, mutilation, and suicide can be seen to haunt three generations of the M family. The main defense the family develops against the resultant anxiety is mutual rescue. The unique way in which these forces—death, mutilation, suicide, and rescue—originate in the grandparents, intermingle in the parents, and emerge in the grandchildren, is illustrated by the following family history.

The Maternal Side of the Family. The maternal grandmother was left motherless at 14 with six younger siblings to take care of on a poverty income. Two of the siblings died in her arms because of the family's inability to provide adequate medical care. The maternal grandmother blamed herself for the deaths. She developed a consuming, quasi-psychotic drive to save a child's life as a compensatory measure. Unable to have her own children, she adopted Mrs. M from the Salvation Army against her husband's wishes. By rescuing this unwanted child and giving it life, she hoped to find redemption.

She proceeded to rescue Mrs. M from every life situation. She waited on her hand and foot, made her decisions, did not allow her out of her sight, and protected her from the "monster" father who had not wanted her. Mrs. M was infantilized to a grotesque degree. Although not physically deformed she came to think of herself as a cripple, incapacitated by the symbiotic bond with her mother. Whenever she attempted to break this bond, her mother threatened suicide. She rushed into the kitchen and held a butcher knife to her throat. Mrs. M's growth, therefore, was ruthlessly stunted.

Her father displaced the hostility he felt towards his wife onto the daughter. He taunted her for her illegitimacy and predicted she would follow the wayward path of her mother. He committed suicide when she was 18. Mrs. M blamed herself for his death. She felt her very existence had killed her father. By the time of her marriage, Mrs. M was a confirmed emotional invalid, continuously seeking rescue.

The Paternal Side of the Family. The paternal side of the family consisted of two cold, rigid, puritanical grandparents of Pennsylvania Dutch stock. Thrift, duty, and self-discipline were the family values. The paternal grandfather was a tyrannical man who could brook no questioning of his authority. The family placed a high premium on conformity to church and community. When Mr. M was born with a withered, deformed hand, the family could not absorb the shock. They were ashamed of his deformity and taught him to hide his hand by keeping it in his pocket. Mr. M's fantasy was that he had been mutilated in his mother's womb because she did not want him. He sensed the family's secret wish to obliterate him and therefore believed that he must earn the right to live by servicing and salvaging others. This was his passport to existence.

Marital Union. When Mr. and Mrs. M met, they sensed each other's needs with an uncanny instinct. Mrs. M sent out the message "I cannot live without being saved." Mr. M sent out the counterpart, "I cannot live without saving." Mr. M hoped to repair his own feelings of mutilation by mending Mrs. M, and making himself indispensable. Mrs. M hoped to be made whole by putting her life in Mr. M's hands.

Their mutual attempts to compensate through marriage soon failed. Mrs. M discovered she resented her dependency on Mr. M; it made her even more helpless, inadequate, and inferior. She hated and feared him for the power he held over her. Her conviction that all men were monsters like her father was confirmed.

As Mrs. M was unable to express her hostility openly towards Mr. M, she became depressed, at times completely incapacitated. Mr. M would come home to find her still in bed, dishes in the sink, and no dinner. He was deflated over his failure to reform Mrs. M and felt erased by her withdrawal. In his absorption with saving her, he denied his own need to be saved. He labeled her the "sick one," blaming her for all their difficulties. The more rejected he felt the more viciously he attacked. The more viciously he attacked, the more depressed Mrs. M became. She turned to food, pills, and alcohol to save her. She gained 140 pounds in 18 months, became addicted to pep pills, went on drinking binges, and made several suicide attempts.

In desperation she sent out an SOS to her mother, who had been waiting in the wings for the chance to rush in and save her. A deadly enmity sprung up between Mr. M and the grandmother, as they vied for each other's job—who could save Mrs. M faster and better. Mrs. M capitalized on this by playing one against the other. The marriage became a round robin of three, each needing the other two. Mrs. M needed two mothers in case one failed. The grandmother needed Mr. M as the "monster" male, from whom she could rescue Mrs. M. Mr. M needed the grandmother to join him in a silent conspiracy to keep Mrs. M dependent and sick.

This "no exit" circle of the family tightened as each partner blocked the efforts of the other to escape. At various intervals Mrs. M would make a valiant attempt to extricate herself from her parasitic dependency on her mother and husband. She would stop drinking, go off the pills, diet, and register for courses to complete her education. These spurts of self-reliance were intolerable to both Mr. M and her mother. They were terrified Mrs. M would leave them if she ever managed to stand on her own two feet. One or the other would always subtly sabotage her efforts.

Mr. M turned to his work to rebuild his damaged ego. This threatened Mrs. M, so she sabotaged his studies by getting intoxicated and making exorbitant demands.

Child-Parent Relationship. It was into this environment that John, the first son was born—unexpected and unwanted. Mrs. M felt overwhelmed; she threw up her hands and cried for help. This gave Mr. M a second chance. Since his attempts to rescue Mrs. M had been thwarted, he could now rescue his son—from Mrs. M. He took over personally, saving the child from a dangerously incompetent mother. When he was away, the maternal grandmother took over. Mrs. M felt excluded, useless as a mother, and jealous of the attention diverted to the new baby. She broke down and was hospitalized for 3 months.

John never knew who his mother was. He had three – yet none. He was half-orphaned from birth. Because of his arrival at the most chaotic stage in the family life cycle, he was destined to wear the family crown of thorns. He became a silent, withdrawn, depressed child.

Since Mrs. M failed as a mother the first time, she decided she would try again. She never felt John belonged to her. It was as though she had given him up for adoption to her mother and husband, repeating her own life story. The next child was to be hers. Two years later she gave birth to another boy—her boy—Tommy; he even looked like her.

The birth of the two children served to polarize the split between the parents. Their failure to find solace in the marriage had intensified their feelings of loneliness and isolation. They now competed for the affection of the children.

Characteristically Mr. M tried to bind his sons to him by making himself indispensable to them. The price he exacted, however, was total obedience. To be disobeyed or questioned meant a loss of control and respect with resultant feelings of impotence. This made him the family tyrant—a view Mrs. M already held. She was quick to exploit it by seducing the children to her side and supporting their rebellion. The maternal grandmother was ever present to encourage the battle against the "monster" father.

Mrs. M retaliated by publicizing Mrs. M's every disability to the boys. He infected them with the idea that mother was incurably incompetent, could never be depended upon, and was out to destroy men. Mrs. M was more than accommodating, being frequently incapacitated by alcohol, drugs, or depression. At such times the boys felt betrayed and turned to Mr. M for sustenance. They trusted neither father nor mother.

When the boys were 9 and 11 a family crisis occurred which shifted the parental conflict into high gear. Mr. M lost his job as a research professor at a major university. The family moved to another city where Mr. M took a job in a smaller college. This was a severe blow to his self-esteem. It was also a traumatic experience for Mrs. M as she was forced to leave her psychiatrist, who had replaced her husband as her savior. She experienced the parting as a death and she never forgave her husband for the separation. As the bitterness and alienation between the parents increased, each chose a child as an ally in an effort to survive. Mr. M paired off with John, Mrs. M with Tommy. Each was jealous of the other's relationship with the chosen child and lumped child and partner together in a vicious scapegoating cycle. The children were torn between feelings of loyalty for one parent and extraordinary guilt for the other.

John adopted Mr. M's derogatory attitude toward Mrs. M, and often substituted for him in the family arguments. In so doing, he became the object of her stored-up hatred towards her father and Mr. M, fulfilling for the third time the maternal prophecy of the "monstrous male."

Conversely, Mrs. M, through her torrential outpouring of hostility towards John, fulfilled for him the paternal prophesy of the "mutilating female." She struck mortal blows at his masculinity. Like his father before him he was left feeling a crippled male.

Tommy was infantilized by Mrs. M which brought derision and ridicule upon him from John and Mr. M. Tommy associated maleness with ruthless tyranny and could not identify with it. The relationship between the two sons began to duplicate that of the parents, with John becoming overly aggressive and Tommy, through identification with the "female victim," becoming timid and effeminate.

In this civil war atmosphere with brother turned against brother, mother against son, and son against father, a bleak mood of despair and desolation prevailed.

John was the first to express the family despair in overt behavior. He failed in school, isolated himself from his peers, was chronically depressed, and saw the world as a "Vietnam." His suppressed rage would emerge periodically in acts of senseless violence—mutilating a rival's guitar, smashing windows and street lights, beating up a younger child. Finally, in order to cope with an overwhelming depression, he followed the path of his mother and turned to drugs, "it's the only time I feel warm and alive." His increasing use of narcotics veered toward the suicidal. Paradoxically it was his mother who came to his rescue—not his father. She rose up aghast when she saw her own self-destructiveness and agony emerging in her son. With evangelistic fervor she devoted herself to saving him. She aligned herself with the paternal defenses—discipline and self-control—and pulled with all her might. She persuaded John to join Synanon and accompanied him to the meetings. Mr. M on the other hand accepted his son's delinquent involvement fatalistically: "I've been waiting for it, now I have two cripples on my hands rather than one."

For several years John struggled with the crisscrossing introjects of his parents, "I have two people inside of me. One wants to give up and go to the dogs—quit school, live on drugs, and just be a bum. The other wants to do good things and serve other people."

He compromised by turning to a hippie religion—Hari Krishna. He controlled his self-destructive impulses through meditation and the sitar. He became a strict vegetarian and spent many hours reforming his former drug companions. At times he took over the role of father in the home, acting as Guru to mother and Tommy.

Tommy was able to handle his anxiety in a less destructive manner. He acted out the family themes with a menagerie of reptiles. Turning the home into a veritable natural history museum, he bred them, fed them, nursed them, watched them die, dissected them, and bred them again. The family themes had come full circle.

A FAMILY CLAN

Mr. B and Mrs. F, a brother and sister in their middle forties, came to our clinic with their families at about the same time. The oldest child in both families was showing delinquent behavior. Steve, the 15-year-old son in the brother's family, was given to violent temper outbursts in which he physically assaulted various members of the family, broke furniture, shouted obscenities, and vowed he would kill his parents. In the middle of family arguments he would throw open the window and yell "Help! Murder! Police! I'm retarded!"

Judy, the 18-year-old daughter in the sister's family, had quit school, refused to work, stayed out all night, and was addicted to amphetamines. She had violent fights with her mother in which she threatened to kill her.

The second child in both families was the "good one." Steve's 13-year-old brother, George, was the saving grace of the family—an A student, an usher in the church, industrious, dependable, and obedient. Judy's younger sister, Carol, was also virtuous—the family rudder—hard-working, prudent, and self-sacrificing.

In the process of treating these families, we discovered the older children were acting out against an entire family clan. Their threat to kill was in self-defense against the psychic killing in the families. The second children were protecting themselves by conforming to the clan's aims and values.

The clan consisted of seven families, all related, living within two blocks of one another—two sets of grandparents, a widowed grandmother, their four children, and twelve grandchildren.

This was a symbiotic clan, dominated by two powerful females—the widowed grandmother on the one side, and the eldest sister on the other side. They controlled all family functions for the entire group—child rearing, work, recreation, marital decisions, housekeeping, education, economics, and so on. The widowed grandmother had real estate holdings and intimidated the family through economics; she had a bad heart and threatened to have a heart attack whenever she was opposed.

Males were relegated to an inconsequential position on the periphery of the family. This was a tradition dating back many generations. Being extremely dependent and immature, they accepted their position and gave little support to their wives and children. Husbands, fathers, and sons were a study in impotence and rage—alternating between depression and violence.

The older generations were victims of immigration and the depression of the 1930s. Preoccupied with their life and death struggle for subsistence, they had had little time or energy to devote to the children. Family members were left with a profound sense of loneliness and apprehension. They compensated for this through a desperate clinging to each other, to their children, to possessions, to the old and the familiar. "We don't want to go without again." Tremendous emphasis was placed on money, status, and education as a defense against a recurring monetary and emotional poverty. Each grandchild was expected to excel; to win honor and prestige for the family; to wipe out past humiliation and failure. Born into this rigid format they were controlled, confined, and molded to fulfill clan ambitions.

Dominance and submission were crucial patterns in the clan system. Both of the mothers of the acting-out children were dominated by another member of the family, Mrs. F. by her mother, Mrs. B. by her older sister. Mrs. F. shared a duplex with her mother, a strong-willed, acid-tongued woman, who gained central control of the family and ruled with an iron hand. Since Mrs. F was her bulwark against loneliness, she had little inclination to share her with Mr. F. The couple was forced to elope and lived with the grandmother's daily insinuation that they should divorce. Mrs. F's main job in life was to juggle husband and mother in an effort to placate both. However, her mother always took precedence over Mr. F. She altered any decision which did not meet with her mother's approval. The family clan supported this "devoted daughter role" and reprimanded Mrs. F if she upset their mother. After several futile attempts to claim his wife for his own, Mr. F withdrew to the sidelines where he remained a silent observer—except for occasional violent temper outbursts due to sexual frustration. (To submit to a man would be a betrayal of grandma's dictum that sex was humiliating). Mr. F directed these outbursts toward the children, afraid to brave the women. Grandmother and mother were collusive in exaggerating the children's fear of the father's violence by admonishing "don't tell your father, no telling what he might do." This served to increase the distance between father and family.

Mrs. B lived with her older sister, Gladys, who had virtually raised her while their mother worked to support the family. Gladys was a vociferous, overpowering woman, who served as high priestess for the clan. Few major decisions were made without first consulting her. Both Mr. and Mrs. B resented her control, but both were afraid to pit themselves against it. This would mean challenging the entire clan system. Mr. B's contention that his wife belonged more to Gladys than to him was a constant source of conflict between them.

Both Mrs. F and Mrs. B were filled with chronic rage toward their mother and sister, yet felt separation would mean mutual death. They controlled their anger through compulsive talking, "I'd kill someone if I couldn't talk." Their families were subjected to an incessant, repetitive, maddening barrage of verbiage.

Steve, the first grandson, was expected to recoup the lost pride of two generations of males—that of his brain-damaged, semi-invalid grandfather, who had worked on useless inventions in a back room all his life, and that of his father who, in attempting to atone for his grandfather's failure, had heaped more failure on himself. Although he had been working on inventions for 15 years, he had patented nothing and remained a $150-a-week clerk. Mr. B looked to Steve to succeed where he and his father had failed.

From the first day Steve entered school, a massive pressure was exerted on him to achieve. Any evidence to the contrary raised the anxiety level of the family beyond their control. Steve was nagged and beaten unmercifully. In self-defense he decided not to learn at all. He truanted from school, locked the teacher in the bathroom and became the class clown, preventing anyone else from learning.

He was quick to sense and exploit the clan's Achilles heel—humiliation. He discovered the only time anyone was really emotionally involved with him was when he was disgracing the family. He therefore grew long hair, wore dirty clothes, used foul language in the neighborhood, and smoked cigarettes in front of the church on Sundays.

The parents' rage was so enormous it rendered them impotent. Mr. B still nursing the wounds of an unsavory father, now had an unsavory son. Both parents were held responsible for Steve's behavior by the clan, which plagued, criticized, advised, admonished, and threatened. The parents were afraid to tangle with Steve for fear they might kill him. On one occasion when the father was forced to strike him in self-defense, he broke down and sobbed, "I'm a murderer!"

When he was 15, Steve was hospitalized briefly for a severe anxiety attack. He ran to his parents' bedroom in the middle of the night, overcome with a nameless terror, repeatedly screaming "I love you mother, I love you daddy!" This was a frantic attempt to stave off the threatening patricide and infanticide. During a subsequent attack he shouted "call an ambulance! I'm going to have a baby"—a vivid testimony to the reversed sex roles in the family and his identification with the "dominant sex."

Judy's delinquent acting out, like Steve's, was an indictment of the entire clan system, which had subjected them to invalid-parenting. Judy deeply resented the grandmother's intrusion into the life of the home and blamed her parents for not protecting the family. She saw her mother as an agent of her grandmother, carrying out her orders, following her decisions, never free to establish a love bond with her. She was afraid of her father's violence, but saw him as a weakling, intimidated by women. Her adolescent development aroused separation anxiety and sexual fears in mother and grandmother causing them to tighten their control on her. They became frantically critical and domineering. Judy reacted by becoming derelict. She quit school, smoked pot, dressed like a tramp, and hung around on street corners. Her fantasies of killing her mother depressed her and she became addicted to amphetamines. Her father passively condoned her delinquency, remembering with pleasure his "wild oats days," before the dreariness of marriage.

Judy incorporated the maternal sexual phobia by turning her boyfriends into "brothers." Although she would sleep in their apartments, the relationships remained asexual. She was known as the neighborhood "big sister."

Within a year the underlying pathology in the "good siblings" emerged. Steve's brother, George, buckled under the family pressure, more excessive now due to Steve's defection. He had an anxiety attack in school before an exam, became hysterical, and had to be removed by his parents. He became surly and withdrawn, could not concentrate on his studies, and began to imitate his brother whom he had always secretly envied for his courage to disobey his parents.

Judy's sister Carol showed signs of depression and became preoccupied with death. She was afraid to go to bed for fear she would die in her sleep. She was plagued with fears of killing everybody in the world. She saw herself as a non-person, robbed of her individuality by her family. Each time she had attempted to assert herself, she was shouted down by her mother's "not you too. I'll kill myself or go crazy if I have two bad children." It was Carol's life or her mother's. She abdicated the "good sister" role and began her own rebellion.

SOME SPECIAL PROBLEMS

The path of development of this broader conceptual frame for the understanding of childhood disorder is fraught with hardships and complications. The unsolved problems are many. We formulate some of these as follows.

1. *The definition of the unit of family.* For the purpose of examining the adaptive relations of child and family, how do we determine the border of the family unit? Whom does it include, whom does it exclude? Do we elect to restrict ourselves to the nuclear family? Do we embrace, where possible, three generations of family? Under what conditions do we encompass collateral relatives? Which ones? The decisions regarding these questions are arrived at

partly on a theoretical basis, partly through pragmatic exigency. As a matter of principle, we try to involve all those members who share the identity of family, its way of life, and the struggle with emotions caught in conflict. We reach out to embrace those factions within the family entity that compete for the power to determine what the family stands for, what it does for the members, and what they in turn do for the family. The determination of the size and composition of the family is affected, obviously, by our clinical judgments as to the relative importance of one or another part of the family in shaping the complementarity of family relationships and the balance of family functions. Factors of social class, ethnic, and cultural background also play a part. Finally, there are the realistic limits imposed by the problem of the sheer physical availability of various family members for participation in family study.

2. *The theoretical foundations of the concept of family diagnosis.* The theoretical framework that underlies the concept of family diagnosis is intrinically incomplete, tentative, and relativistic. In our experiences it has proved necessary again and again to amend the outlines of family diagnosis in a flexible manner to suit the nature and aims of particular kinds of study. According to the special focus of the study, and the specific kinds of information being sought, the criteria and emphases of family diagnosis shift so as to favor observations appropriate to the aims of the study. For example, the outline of family diagnosis is pitched one way if we are investigating the relations of family process in drug-using adolescents. The outline is slanted a different way if we are focusing on the contagion of specific psychopathic tendencies across three generations. There is still another slant if we are concerned with the prevention of psychosis in the third generation offspring of vulnerable families.

On another level, the relative maturity of the nuclear unit, the stage of the family's life cycle at the point of clinical entry, its socioeconomic and cultural status also influence the specific design and application of the outline of family diagnosis.

3. *The inclusion of child diagnosis within a system of family diagnosis.* The challenge of placing child diagnosis within the dynamic context of family diagnosis, however complex and formidable, must nonetheless be faced. A more precise correlation of child and family requires the following:
   a. Criteria for the psychosocial structure and mental health functioning of the family group.
   b. Elucidation of the stages of development of the family.
   c. Classification of family types according to their mental health potential.
   d. A theory of child personality specifying the stages of development in terms of biosocial integration with the family group.
   e. A system of evaluating deviant units of child behavior within the context of total personality organization and adaptation to family roles.
   f. A classification of psychiatric disorders in children that can be joined to the principles of family diagnosis and family psychology.

4. *The evolution of a classification of family types.* This poses a task of huge proportions and yet it is important to work toward this goal. The sickness-inducing forces within the family need to be conceptualized within a broader frame of the healing and health-maintaining capacities of the family. Deviant behavior among members needs to be defined within the larger context of total adaptation to intra- and extra-familial roles. Toward this end we are in sore need of theoretical models of healthy adaptation for the family as a unit of living and for the special roles of mothering, fathering, and "childing."

It is within this larger conceptual orientation that we come to grips with the task of formulating the dynamic interplay of deviant behavior of the children and the constellation of interlocking pathology in family relationships.

5. *The theory of causation.* In rethinking the problems of causation of childhood disorders we must ask: How far does one or another conceptual orientation and investigative procedure light up selectively the multiple contributing forces. For example, is it so that the theoretical movement from child to family favors revelation of the predisposing and contributing factors of causation, while the opposite approach, from family to children highlights selectively the precipitating and reinforcing factors?

In conclusion, let us spell out the manner in which the parallel and complementary application of the two conceptual approaches facilitates our understanding of the dynamic relations of family and children.

1. The psychiatry of children expands to include a larger concern with the psychiatry of the family unit.
2. The theoretical orientation shifts from the traditional tendency to treat family as the extension of the child to a view of children as the product and extension of family. In child psychiatry and child therapy it seemed, for too long a time, that the tail was wagging the dog. Our perspective was upside down. The child held a central position, the family was relegated to a place of peripheral importance. Now, in contrast, we endeavor to define the disturbance of the child within the frame of the psychosocial pathology of the family unit. We join child diagnosis to family diagnosis.
3. The emphasis shifts from the deviancy of the single child viewed as "the patient" to the pathology of the whole set of children as a collectivity, a subsystem of the family phenomenon. The pathogenic potential of parents and family is divided up in a special way among all the children. The vicissitudes of such processes are affected by family change across time and by the interrelation of family and child at a particular stage of the family's life cycle. Each child in turn absorbs and reflects particular

aspects of the pathogenic contagion of the family. This is readily illustrated in those families where one child develops in an over-aggressive way, whereas another turns timid and submissive. One child internalizes his conflict experience and evolves a neurotic picture, whereas another externalizes his conflict and acts out. Or, for example, the pathogenic potential of the family unit is so transmitted that one child develops a psychosis, another a depression or a psychosomatic breakdown, and a third turns delinquent. The dynamic processes underlying such events are still obscure. Several mechanisms seem relevant, however. One is the extent to which, at a given stage of the family's life cycle, a particular child is locked into the living place of the family or is able to escape to the outside. Another relevant set of forces has to do with the dynamic role of scapegoating and the determination of vulnerability to breakdown. When in the history of family, how, and with what effects is a given child scapegoated? A related problem is the manner in which the family roles of persecutor, victim, and rescuer or healer are organized within the emotional life and role design of the family. Is it so, for example, that at a given stage, one child epitomizes predominantly the emotional warp of the family, another the stabilizing and healing powers, and a third the growth potential of the family?

Finally, of overriding significance is the shift in orientation to a broader conception of the phenomenon of breakdown or mental illness. We no longer think exclusively of the one member of the family as the sick or collapsed one, but tend rather to expand our image of mental illness as a cluster of interlocking vulnerabilities among the family members, within which, across time, the manifestations of clinical breakdown emerge in series, now afflicting one member, now another.

Bibliography

1. Ackerman, N. W., *The Psychodynamics of Family Life*, Basic Books, New York, 1958
2. "Adolescent Problems: A Symptom of Family Disorder", *Family Process*, Vol. 1, No. 2, Sept., 1962.

3. "Family Diagnosis: An Approach to the Pre-School Child", (with R. Sobel), The American Journal of Orthopsychiatry, Vol. XX, No. 4, October, 1950.
4. Hoch, P. and I. Lubin, "Psychiatric Disorders in Children – Diagnosis and Etiology in Our Time", in *Current Problems in Psychiatric Diagnosis*, Grune & Stratton, 1953.
5. Hoch and Lubin, eds. "Child and Family Psychopathy: Problems of Correlation", in *Psychopathology of Childhood,* Grune & Stratton, 1955.
6. "Interpersonal Disturbances in the Family: Some Unsolved Problems in Psychotherapy", *Psychiatry,* Vol. 17, No. 4, November, 1954.
7. "Prejudicial Scapegoating and Neutralizing Trends in the Family Group", *International Journal of Social Psychiatry,* Congress Issue, 1964.
8. "The Principles of Shared Responsibility for Child Rearing", *The International Journal of Social Psychiatry,* Vol. 2, No. 4, April, 1957.
9. Rado and Daniels, eds., "Interlocking Pathology in Family Relationships", in *Changing Conceptions of Psychoanalytic Medicine,* Grune & Stratton, 1956.
10. "Reciprocal Antagonism in Siblings", *Bulletin of the Menninger Clinic,* Vol. 11, No. 1, January, 1938.

Behavior and Pathology of Parents of Disturbed Children

Sula Wolff (U. K.)

Twenty five years ago Baldwin, Kalhorn and Breese, in their classical paper "Patterns of Parent Behavior," expressed the view that two factors are necessary to understand parents' child-rearing methods: the emotional attitude of the parents to the child, and their intellectual philosophy of child care [4]. Parent behavior was carefully observed and rated and a syndrome analysis revealed three dimensions. The first, Democracy versus Autocracy, reflected a general philosophy of child care; the second and third, Acceptance versus Rejection and Indulgence versus Nonchalance, were measures of the parents' emotional attitudes towards their children. Both were clearly related to the intelligence, education, and social background of the parents. The least well educated farming families were the most rejecting, nonchalant and autocratic; the culturally most sophisticated group, consisting mainly of college teachers, were predominantly accepting, democratic, and also nonindulgent. Excessively authoritarian parents tended to have passive children while democratic child-rearing methods produced socially outgoing and domineering children. The families studied were normal families, not seeking psychiatric care, and the children were not identified as problem children.

Nevertheless, the assumption was made that certain types of parent behavior, especially autocracy and rejection, assessed as being most prevalent in unskilled working class families, are detrimental to children, even if the parents themselves are otherwise well adjusted. This led the authors to suggest that courses in child care should be included in the curricula for high school students.

Child psychiatrists frequently face the dilemma as to whether their role is to treat children and parents who are ill or to teach them; whether it is their job to take care of the sick or to modify attitudes and inculcate skills. Child psychiatrists express this ambiguity about their role in the frequent avoidance of diagnostic labels for the parents they assess and even for the children they treat; and the term "treatment" for the interactions between social workers and their clients is often evaded not only by the parents but by the social workers themselves.

The knowledge that, except for a minority of clearly defined diseases (childhood autism for example, or obsessional neurosis), disturbed children display behavior disorders not at all uncommon in the population at large [57], perpetuates this ambiguity, and the voluminous literature on the relationship between parental attitudes and child behavior has not clarified the position.

Parental Attitudes

A major contribution of the Fels Institute Studies has been the development of reliable methods of rating parental behavior and attitudes on the basis of interviews with parents [4].

Short cuts using self-administered questionnaires have been widely explored but their results have been disappointing. Intercorrelations of items on such tests have tended to yield the same dimensions of authoritarianism-permissiveness and acceptance-rejection as have items derived from interview data. In addition, the relationship between test scores of the parents and children's behavior has often been tenuous.

As long ago as 1942, Brown found no correlation between maternal attitudes expressed on a questionnaire and children's emotional adjustment according to a children's personality inventory and teacher ratings [14].

In a recent review of what was perhaps the most widely used parent attitude questionnaire (the P.A.R.I.), it is pointed out that the test reflects the parents' education rather than more specific features of their relationship to their children, and that the correlations between the test and the children's behavior hold good only in middle-class families [7]. Certainly high scores on "bad" attitudes, such as authoritarian control and rejection, did not necessarily reflect pathogenic child-rearing attitudes.

Ryle, in a study of families in a London general practice, found no correlation at all between inventory assessments of parental attitudes of domination and acceptance, and assessments made by a social worker on the basis of interviews [54]. The inventory was known to reflect social class variations and was thought to show up differences in social desirability sets rather than differences in parental behavior.

West, in a study of pre-delinquent conduct disorders in boys also found minimal correlations between Psychiatric Social Worker ratings of parents and their responses on an attitude questionnaire [62]. Moreover, only insignificant correlations were found between mothers' scores for authoritarianism and under-concern, and teacher ratings of conduct disorders in the boys. P.S.W. ratings of parental attitudes based on interviews, however, correlated highly with the important variables of school conduct and performance in the children.

Refinements in interview assessment of parental attitudes were developed by Sears and his colleagues in their studies of maternal and child behavior in families belonging to different social classes [56].

Peterson, Becker, and their co-workers in Iowa assessed parental attitudes on the basis of the Sears structured interview [45, 46, 8, 9], using ratings derived both from the Sears scales and from Roff's factor analysis of the Fels behavior ratings [50]. Their researches into the relationship between parent attitudes and children's behavior disorders appear to have been more fruitful than previous such attempts [25]. In part this may be due to their incorporating the items constituting Roff's factor of general family maladjustment into their scales of child-rearing behavior.

In the Iowa studies a small group of Child Guidance Clinic attenders were compared with kindergarten and school children, not always well matched, and in some studies teacher ratings of behavior problems in larger samples of normal middle-class children were compared with ratings of parent behavior.

The relationships between parent behavior and children's disturbances varied somewhat in the different groups of families studied. The main conclusions were that fathers and mothers resembled each other in degree of hostility, restrictiveness, and sex anxiety; that the attitudes of fathers were at least as important as those of mothers in the genesis of maladjustment in children; and that, in line with Sears' findings [56], hostility and physical punishment on the part of parents were related to aggressive behavior in their children. However, no clear relationships were found between types of parental behavior and types of maladjustment in children.

The assumption is implicit in many investigations that correlations between parental attitudes and childhood behavior disorders in normal populations are necessarily relevant to the understanding of disturbed children who appear at a clinic [25]. The absence of significant correlations in normal populations, in which the proportion of seriously disturbed children is, of course, small [53], may not mean that such correlations will not be found in a group of disturbed children. David Levy proposed the hypothesis many years ago that situational determinants, such as infidelity of a husband or deformity or illness of a child, can change maternal behavior, making a "constitutionally" overprotective mother pathologically overprotective or a rejecting mother excessively rejecting. The constitutional determinants in the mother, Levy holds, become the situational determinants for her children [40].

Certainly comparisons between disturbed and nondisturbed populations of children have shown more convincing differences in the occurrence of adverse events and circumstances than of adverse parental child-rearing behavior, particularly since the good methods of rating such behavior depend on the interview, with all the possibilities of observer bias and halo effects that this can introduce [45a]. In studies of normal populations, social class bias may color the interviewer's ratings. In comparative studies of psychiatrically disturbed and normal children, the interviewers' knowledge of the child's pathology is likely to bias the assessment of the parents and vice versa [62].

Evaluations of attitudes can hardly be made without value judgments and this is of course recognized by the subjects of parental attitude enquiries: the parents. West found that non-response to a parental attitude questionnaire correlated as highly with disturbance in the child as did unfavorable questionnaire responses [62].

Adverse events and circumstances including parental illness can be defined more accurately than attitudes, and even the assessment of parental personality disorder is likely to be more valid and reliable. In any case even if certain child-rearing attitudes were found to be directly related to children's psychiatric disturbances, this is a matter more for the educator than the psychiatrist. Parents do not come to have their attitudes altered. While some may want their feelings towards their child to change, and are troubled by finding themselves reacting to their child in ways they do not themselves approve of, most of them expect relief from their own anxieties and improvement in their children to be brought about without having to relinquish their basic philosophy and cherished beliefs about child care. The distinction is important between emotional attitudes and beliefs in child-care methods held with conviction and those attitudes and reactions to their children of which the parents themselves disapprove. Attitudes held with conviction are likely to reflect the sociocultural background of parents, while patterns of responses about which parents themselves are ambivalent are likely to be pointers to parental pathology.

One study of parental attitudes must be mentioned separately because it tells us more about the views disturbed children have of their parents than about parental behavior as such [1]. Highly significant differences were found in the role perceptions of their parents between adolescent delinquent boys in a remand home and a group of matched controls. Delinquent boys perceived their mothers as more affectionate than their fathers and also as their main protectors. At the same time they thought their fathers ought to love them as much as their mothers loved them.

Adverse Family Circumstances and Events

While children attending child guidance clinics generally resemble children in the community with respect to socioeconomic circumstances, children identified as disturbed by coercive agencies come from socially deprived sections of society. Stein and Susser found this to be true for mentally defective children [58]; McCulloch and his co-workers, investigating teenagers seen by psychiatrists in Edinburgh, showed that children who were referred to hospital psychiatric departments usually by general practitioners, came from middle-class areas of the city, while teenagers seen in other settings, mainly in approved schools or in a general hospital after a suicide attempt, came from socially disorganized areas of the city [43]. A similar, although less marked difference, has been found between children referred to a psychiatric clinic by family doctors and by educational psychologists [47].

Delinquency is the preserve of the coercive agencies, and the social disadvantages of delinquent children are well documented [16, 26, 22, 49]. West, in a recent study of 9-year-old boys in a crowded urban district of London, found that social handicap (poor income, poor housing, large family, and dependence on social agencies) was the most important single factor discriminating between children with conduct disorders and those without [62]. This factor was also highly associated with instability of the mother, marital disharmony, lax parental attitudes to child care, and low intelligence in the boys. West points out that this does not argue for a direct causal link between the external handicap of social adversity and conduct disorders, but may well mean that parents with personality defects sink to the lowest level and hence suffer from poor housing, low income, and large unplanned families. Robins, in her book *Deviant Children Grown Up* [49], discounts the pathogenic influences of social class factors. She attributes the correlations of juvenile delinquency with low socioeconomic status and poor work records of fathers, and of delinquency in childhood with low social status in adult life entirely to the effects of parental personality disorder on child rearing and of early childhood experiences on later personality. This is a salutary reaction to the view that ameliorating poverty and overcrowding will of itself enable families to function better. Nevertheless, a more plausible theory is that parental personality and social adversity are factors which mutually reinforce each other.

Social handicap is characteristic of delinquent child populations. Family disruption has been shown repeatedly to be much commoner in psychiatrically disturbed children than in populations of nondisturbed children. Rutter showed that death of a parent, especially in the third and fourth years of life, is commoner in children who subsequently come to a child psychiatrist than in children in the community [51]. Adoption too is more often found in clinic populations [11, 34]. Illegitimacy, divorce, and separation of parents and also separation of the child from his parents for any reason are all highly correlated with children's psychiatric disorders [6, 26, 17, 12, 44, 51, 27, 65]. They are found in children with reactive disturbances and are more commonly associated with conduct than with neurotic disorders [10, 60]. While residential nursery care too is associated with subsequent emotional disorder in the child [12, 64], mother going out to work is not [65, 41, 62, 44, 22]. Working mothers on the whole have smaller families than mothers who stay at home, and their greater competence and better adjustment seem to outweigh any adverse effects their absence from the home may have on the children.

Family disruption is not an accident of nature to which all families are equally prone. Evidence is accumulating that, at least in the relatively wealthy and healthy regions of the Western world, family disruption like social adversity may be more important as an index of sickness or personality disorder in the parents than as a primary cause for psychiatric disturbances in children. Parents subject to illness and parents with personality disorders provide an environment for their children in which adverse events are not isolated episodes in an otherwise tranquil existence but follow each other, and in which many social disadvantages occur at the same time. Even such an apparently ordinary childhood stress as admission to a residential nursery during the mother's confinement, tends to occur in families in which the children have had more previous separation experiences and the parents are socially, although not geographically, more isolated from relatives and friends than in families who make private arrangements for their children at this time [55].

Concomitant Illness in the Family

The clustering of physical and psychiatric illness in individuals has been established by Hinkle and his associates [31]. Twenty-five percent of individuals in each of a number of widely differing populations studied experienced 50 percent of all episodes of illness during a 20-year period of young adult life. Those individuals with the highest rates of illness perceived their total environment to be most unsatisfactory, and this was independent of sex, of age, and of sociocultural background. Physical and psychiatric illnesses cluster not only in individuals but in families [20, 28]. Social problems in one member of a family are associated more often than expected with social problems in another member of the same family, and the incidence of illness and of social problems in families are related [33].

Children's psychiatric disturbances have been repeatedly related to illness, both physical and psychiatric, in the parents.[1] Bremer, in his wartime study of a small community in northern Norway [13], found the mental health of the parents to be the dominant factor in the environment of "difficult children," irrespective of their social conditions. In Hare and Shaw's household survey of an urban population, behavior disorders and general practitioner consultation rates for children were related both to neurosis and to a number of other indices of ill health in either parent [28]. Buck, in a sample of subscribers to a Canadian Health Insurance Scheme, found the frequency of emotional and physical illness and of accidents in children to correlate with psychoneurosis of the mother but not the father [15]. Brandon, too, found more psychiatric and physical illness among mothers but not fathers of children identified as disturbed by Health Visitors than among parents of nondisturbed controls [12].

The first study in which the health of parents was examined intensively in children with clearly defined psychiatric disorders attending a psychiatric clinic and in nonreferred controls, was Rutter's study reported in his book "Children of Sick Parents" [51]. He compared groups of children with reactive disorders referred to the Maudsley Hospital, with matched control groups of children attending pediatric and dental clinics, and also with a group of Maudsley Hospital children suffering from mental deficiency, epilepsy, and organic illness. He found that chronic and recurrent physical illness was twice as common among parents of the disturbed children as it was among the controls. Psychiatric disorder among parents was found to be three times as common in the disturbed group. Parental psychiatric disorder was most pathogenic for children when it took the form of personality disorder, when it affected both parents, and when the psychiatric symptoms of the parent involved the child. In Rutter's study, broad indices of parental psychiatric disorder were used and the data consisted of clinical case records and of brief interviews with parents of control children.

[1] See "The Mutative Impact of Serious Mental and Physical Illness in the Parent on Family Life," by E. J. Anthony, in this volume.

In Edinburgh a more detailed examination of illness and personality disorders among parents of primary school children with reactive behavior disorders was made [65]. The mothers of 100 consecutive new referrals to a psychiatric clinic, excluding children with brain damage, low intelligence, and psychosis, and excluding also children not living with mother figures, were interviewed intensively. A hundred mothers of control children from the same school classes, individually matched for sex, age, and occupation of father, were also seen.

Each mother was subjected to a standard, focused interview lasting about 3 hours. One part of the interview concerned the parents' own childhood experiences, their work and marital adjustment, and their illnesses. The names of all hospitals attended were noted and, as far as possible, the mothers' reports were checked against hospital records. Information about fathers was given by the mothers, except in a few cases. At the end of each interview, all information relating to the parents, but none about the children, was transcribed in the form of a life history, quoting the mother's own words whenever possible. On the basis of this history a number of ratings were made.

Since all interviews were done by one psychiatrist who knew which were clinic classes and which controls, some check for bias was necessary. The life histories were read by an independent psychologist who eliminated all psychiatric diagnostic labels and all value judgments unsupported by factual statements. An independent psychiatrist then read and rated the life histories of 25 consecutive clinic cases and of 25 controls without knowing which was which. Ratings of psychiatric illness and personality disorder were based on agreed definitions; ratings of social adjustment were based on anchor definitions. Agreements between the two raters were high. This procedure did not, of course, eliminate observer bias entirely, but it did provide some indications as to which were the more and which the less reliable indices.

Clinic mothers, but not fathers, were found to have had significantly more hospital admissions in the child's lifetime than mothers of control children. Mothers of clinic children had had significantly more medical attention for psychological disorders than mothers in the control group. Of the control mothers, 24 reported minor symptoms for which they had not consulted their doctor, while only 8 clinic mothers were uncomplaining sufferers. The difference was not however entirely attributable to the high consultation rates of clinic mothers: 24 had received hospital treatment for psychological illnesses, compared with only 6 in the control group. There had been 6 suicide attempts among clinic mothers and 3 among the controls. Fathers of the two groups of children did not differ in the amount of medical care they had received for psychological disorders.

Ratings of psychiatric illness were made only for mothers, because most fathers had not been personally interviewed. There was a significant difference in the incidence of psychoneurosis and psychosis in the two groups of mothers. The incidence of psychosomatic illnesses was the same.

Fifty-eight clinic mothers reported themselves as definitely suffering from "nerves" compared with 25 in the control group. Personality disorder was rated separately from psychiatric illness and was found to differentiate very highly indeed between mothers of clinic children and mothers of controls. The difference between the fathers was also significant but less great. Thirty-four clinic mothers had a "definite personality disorder," including 23 with hysterical personalities, compared with 15 (5 hysterics) among the controls. In addition 17 clinic mothers were sociopathic, compared with 3 among the controls. The only category of personality disorder which differentiated between the two groups of fathers was sociopathy and this occurred in 21 clinic fathers and 7 controls.

Four measures of social adjustment were used for mothers and one for fathers. There was no difference in the work adjustment of either parents and clinic mothers did not go out to work more than mothers of control children. The two groups of mothers managed the interview with equal competence. However, the care of the home was assessed as worse among the clinic mothers, and marital adjustment was very much poorer in this group.

One attitude scale was used: the Fould's Hostility Scale [24]. This differentiated significantly between the mothers but the difference was small.

Product-moment correlations between six indices of psychiatric disorder in the mothers of clinic children were calculated. The six indices were: psychiatric illness, treatment for psychological conditions, "nerves," hostility scores, personality disorder, and marital adjustment. Correlations above .30 were found between psychiatric illness and psychiatric treatment. Personality disorder, marital adjustment, and hostility all correlated with each other but not with psychiatric illness or treatment. "Nerves" correlated with all the indices except marital adjustment.

Because of Wardle's suggestion that broken homes were common not only in children attending child guidance clinics but also in their parents [69], mothers were questioned in detail about major family disruptions in their own and the fathers' childhood. The significant differences found between the two groups, and these were all small, were confined to separations of the mother from her parents lasting 6 months or more and occurring under the age of 5; serious childhool illnesses in which psychological factors played a part in the case of mothers; and an excess of psychiatric illness and psychopathy among the paternal grandparents.

The main findings of this study were first that mothers of children attending a psychiatric clinic make more use of medical services than mothers of nonreferred children and that they have more physical and psychiatric illnesses. Second, over one-half of the clinic mothers have clinically recognizable personality disorders (hysterical personality and sociopathy) compared with only one-fifth among the controls. Third, fathers of clinic children did not have an excess of illness and only severe personality disorder of the father (sociopathy) differentiated between the clinic and control groups. The children studied were of primary school age (mean age 8.3 years; range 5.3 to 12.5 years), comparable to the 9-year-old boys studied by West, who also found maternal but not paternal pathology to differentiate between disturbed and nondisturbed children [62].

This would not, of course, conflict with the findings that psychiatric disorders in older children, especially delinquency in boys, are related to absence or pathology of the father [27, 1]. Jonsson, in particular, found that both fathers and mothers of delinquent boys in Sweden had an excess of physical and mental illness [37].

The fact that psychiatric illness of the mother but not of the father is related to childhood behavior disorders in young children supports the assumption that the causal link is environmental rather than genetic. This conclusion was also reached by Cowie, who investigated the incidence of neurotic traits among the offspring of all ages, of psychotics and of patients with obsessive–compulsive reactions. Psychosis in the mother was more highly associated with disturbance in the child than psychosis in the father [19].

Psychiatrically disturbed mothers can be assumed to provide poorer maternal care than mothers who are not disturbed. The findings that both physical and psychiatric illness of the mother are related to behavior disorders in the child may merely reflect the commonly observed, but not yet explained, concurrence of organic and emotional illness. However, an additional interpretation must be considered. When a mother is admitted to hospital, children as a rule are cared for by people outside the immediate family, often outside their own homes [21]. Even maternal illness and personality disorder not leading to actual separations between mother and child commonly disrupt family life to a far greater extent than incapacity of the father. Pond, for example, has shown that neurosis in women but not in men is associated with poor marital adjustment [48], and the Edinburgh study demonstrates that this too is associated with psychological disturbances in children. Disabilities of the father, which are in any case rarer in this age group of parents, can be tolerated without disruptive effects on the children, so long as the family income is maintained from sources such as insurance benefits, and so long as his disorder falls short of sociopathy as manifested for example by alcoholism, violent behavior, or crime.

In their more recent investigations of the interaction between psychiatric disorders in parents and children, Rutter and his colleagues are studying the children of families in which one parent has been newly referred to a psychiatric service [52, 53]. The rates of childhood psychiatric disorders are higher than in families without a sick parent but, except for personality disorder, the diagnosis of the parents (most of them suffered from psychoneurosis or depression) was not related to the risk of behavior disorders developing in the children.

Rutter finds closer correlations between parental behavior than between parental diagnosis and childhood disturbance in this group of families. Nevertheless, one or other of the parents studied had been identified as ill or as suffering from a personality disorder.

Parental Characteristics and Childhood Disorders

There is some, as yet inconclusive, evidence for a genetic link between certain personality characteristics of parents and autism and schizoid personality in childhood. Lotter, in a population survey of autistic children, found their parents to be of higher socioeconomic status and more intelligent than parents of nonautistic children [42]. This suggests that the qualities of high intelligence, obsessionality, and emotional coldness that Kanner described in the parents of autistic children [39], may not have been due to referral bias, as was at one time thought, but may be pointers to a genetic link between schizoid traits in parents and autism in children.

In support of this, it was found that in a series of schizoid children there was often a parent or close relative with schizoid personality traits [63], and as long ago as 1946, Jenkins noted that children with schizoid traits had better educated parents of higher socioeconomic status than other child guidance clinic attenders.

Rutter has recently drawn attention to the fact that adverse environmental factors do not affect boys and girls equally [52]. All types of psychiatric illness affecting a parent lead to an excess of behavior disorders at school in girls but not in boys, while parental personality disorder and marital discord are specifically associated with antisocial disorders in boys. Rutter argues that genetic factors may in part be responsible for such sex differences.[2]

In an interesting study, admittedly based on a restricted population of adopted children, Weinstein found that the adjustment of boys was influenced to a greater degree by variations in neighborhood and home environment than the adjustment of girls. For example, a poor social environment and parental dissatisfaction with the child's school progress led to poorer educational attainments in boys than in girls; boys' but not girls' popularity among their peers depended on their parents' positive conception of their child's disposition. Like Kagan and Moss [38], Weinstein believes that the reasons for this difference lie in the fact that boys, like girls, are mainly reared by women, so that unlike girls, they have less access, especially in their early years, to satisfactory role models [61]. This may well be one of the crucial causes for the preponderance of boys among psychiatrically disturbed children.

That different influences affect children at different ages have been demonstrated recently by Stein and his colleagues, who examined the social and psychopathological causes for enuresis. They found that while physical maturation sets lower limits on the timetable which social forces can impose on the acquisition of sphincter con-

[2] See "Sex Differences in Response to Family Stress," by M. Rutter, in this volume.

trol, social class factors distinguished young enuretic children from children who had acquired toilet control, while maternal inadequacy and family disorganization characterized those children in whom enuresis persisted to a later age [59].

A great deal of work is available relating types of reactive disorders in children to types of home background. Specific neurotic syndromes have been linked to specific neurotic personality traits in mothers. Anthony, for example, found neurotic discontinuous soilers to have obsessional and coercive mothers [2], and that children with sleep disorders often had anxious mothers with irrational sexual fears [3]. Parents of school phobic children were more prone to psychoneurosis, according to Hersov, than parents of truanters [30].

When broader populations of psychiatrically disturbed children are studied, however, the associations between characteristics of parents and type of disorder in the children are less clear. Hewitt and Jenkins, in their classical study, related three behavioral syndromes to four situational patterns, defined in terms of family circumstances as well as parental attitudes [31]. Unsocialized aggression correlated with maternal rejection; socialized delinquency with parental neglect and family delinquency; overinhibited behavior with either family repression or chronic physical disability or illness in the child or his mother. A replication of this work, admittedly based on a much more homogeneous sample of children, failed to substantiate these findings [23].

Bennett could discover no association between neurotic disorders in the child and illness in the child or his parents [10]. In her study, illness was equally common in the families of neurotic and delinquent children. In fact only one of Hewitt and Jenkins' associations has been repeatedly confirmed: that between delinquency (but not aggressive behavior) and family disruption [5, 35, 10, 60, 18, 64].

Conclusions

Parental attitudes, especially as measured on pencil and paper tests, reflect culture rather than pathogenic child-rearing methods. Social disadvantages and family disruption, however, are major causes for reactive psychiatric disorders in children. Both are strongly associated with physical and psychiatric illness and with personality disorders in parents. While pathology of the mother is particularly implicated in the causation of behavior disorders in young children of both sexes, paternal illness and personality disorder may be more important in the genesis of adolescent delinquency in boys. When childhood psychiatric disorders are brought about by adverse circumstances and events, or by adverse parental behavior, the child psychiatrist needs to be alert to pathology in the parents which may require treatment in its own right.

This is not a plea for involving all parents of psychiatrically ill children in psychotherapy. Many psychiatric disorders in children are not reactions to parental pathology at all. In some cases the link between a parent's personality disorder and the child's disturbance is likely to be genetic, but there are also many children with psychosis, organic brain disease, or constitutional variations of personality who have perfectly normal parents. Furthermore, emotional reactions to serious or recurrent physical illness affecting the child himself can occur in children of healthy parents, and occasionally disasters befall a family and precipitate psychological illness in individuals previously well adjusted. In any case, psychoterapy is not equally successful for all psychiatric conditions, and personality disorders, especially sociopathy (most important from the point of view of the children), are notoriously difficult to treat.

Because the prevalence of personality disorders is high among parents of children attending psychiatric clinics, they provide an ideal population for research into these conditions, and evaluative studies of different treatment methods are long overdue. Social reformers, political planners, educators, social workers, and all doctors looking after parents and children have enormous opportunities for improving the environment of children and for preventing childhood emotional disorders. The greatest challenge facing psychiatrists, however, lies in the discovery of really effective treatment techniques for young adults with personality disorders.

Bibliography

1. Andry, R. G., *Delinquency and Parental Pathology*, Methuen, London, 1960
2. Anthony, E. J., An experimental approach to the psychopathology of childhood: Encopresis, *Brit. J. Med. Psychol.*, 30 (1957), 146.
3. Anthony, E. J., An experimental approach to the psychopathology of childhood: Sleep disturbances, *Brit. J. Med. Psychol.*, 33 (1959), 19.

4. Baldwin, A. L., J. Kalhorn and F. H. Breese, Patterns of parent behavior, *Psychol. Monog.*, 58 (1945), 1.
5. Bannister, H. and M. Ravden, The problem child and his environment, *Brit. J. Psychol.*, 34 (1944), 60.
6. Bannister, H. and M. Ravden, The environment and the child, *Brit. J. Psychol.*, 35 (1945), 82.
7. Becker, W. C., and R. S. Krug, The parent attitude research instrument – a research review, *Child Develpm.*, 36 (1965), 329.
8. Becker, W. C., D. R. Peterson, L. A. Hellmer, D. J. Shoemaker and H. C. Quay, Factors in parental behavior and personality as related to problem behavior in children, *J. Consult. Psychol.*, 23 (1959), 107.
9. Becker, W. C., D. R. Peterson, Z. Luria, D. J. Shoemaker and L. A. Hellmer, Relations of factors derived from parent-interview ratings to behavior problems of five-year-olds, *Child Develpm.*, 33 (1962), 509.
10. Bennett, I., *Delinquent and Neurotic Children*, Tavistock Publications, London, 1960.
11. Borgatta, E. F. and D. Fanshel, *Behavioral Characteristics of Children Known to Psychiatric Out-Patient Clinics*, Child Welfare League of America, 1965.
12. Brandon, S. *An Epidemiological Study of Maladjustment in Childhood*, M.D. Thesis, University of Durham, Durham, N. C., 1960.
13. Bremer, J. A Social psychiatric investigation of a small community in northern Norway, *Acta psychiat. neurol. Scand.*, supplement no. 62, 1951.
14. Brown, F. An experimental study of parental attitudes and their effect upon child adjustment, *Amer. J. Orthopsychiat.*, 12 (1942), 224.
15. Buck, C. W. and K. B. Laughton, Family patterns of illness: the effect of psychoneurosis in the parent upon illness in the child, *Acta psychiat. neurol. Scand.*, 34 (1959), 165.
16. Burt, C. *The Young Delinquent*, fourth ed. revised, Lawrence Verry, Inc., Mystic, Conn., 1925.
17. Burt, C. and M. Howard, The nature and causes of maladjustment among children of school age, *Brit. J. Psychol. (Statistical Section)*, 5 (1952), 39.
18. Collins, L. F., A. E. Maxwell and K. Cameron, A factor analysis of some child psychiatric clinic data. *J. Ment. Sci.*, 108 (1962), 274.
19. Cowie, V., The incidence of neurosis in the children of psychotics, *Acta. psychiat. Scand.*, 37 (1961), 37.
20. Downes, J. and K. Simon, Characteristics of psychoneurotic patients and their families as revealed in a general morbidity study, *Milbank Mem. Fund Quart.*, 32 (1954), 42.
21. Ekdahl, M. C., E. P. Rice and W. M. Schmidt, Children of parents hospitalized for mental illness, *Amer. J. public Health*, 52 (1962), 428.
22. Ferguson, T., *The Young Delinquent in his Social Setting*, Oxford University Press, London, 1952.
23. Field, E., *A Validation Study of Hewitt and Jenkins' Hypothesis*, Home Office Research Unit Report No. 10, H.M.S.O., 1967.
24. Foulds, G.A., *Personality and Personal Illness*, Tavistock Publications, London, 1965.
25. Glidewell, J. C., *Parental Attitudes and Child Behavior*, Thomas, Springfield, 1960.
26. Glueck, S. and E., *Unravelling Juvenile Delinquency*, The Commonwealth Fund, New York, 1950.

27. Gregory, I., Anterospective data following childhood loss of parent: 1. Delinquency and High School Drop-out, *Arch. Gen. Psychiat.*, 13 (1965), 99.

28. Hare, E. H. and G. K. Shaw, A study in family health: (2) a comparison of the health of fathers, mothers and children, *Brit. J. Psychiat.*, 111 (1965), 467.

29. Von Harnack, G.A., *Nervöse Verhattungsstörungen beim Schulkind*, Georg Thieme, Stuttgart, 1958.

30. Hersov, L. E., Persistent nonattendance at school, *J. Child Psychol. Psychiat.*, 1 (1961), 130.

31. Hewitt, L. E. and R. L. Jenkins, *Fundamental Patterns of Maladjustment*, Michigan Child Guidance Institute, Illinois, 1946.

32. Hinkle, L. E., Ecological investigations of the relationship between illness, life experiences and the social environment, *Annals Int. Med.*, 49 (1958), 1373.

33. Hrubec, Z., The Association of Health and social welfare problems in individuals and their families, *Milbank Mem. Fund Quart.* 37 (1959), 251.

34. Humphrey, M. E. and C. Ounsted, Adoptive Families referred for psychiatric advice: 1. The children, *Brit. J. Psychiat.*, 109 (1963), 599.

35. Jenkins, R. L. and S. Glickman, Common syndromes in child psychiatry: 1. Deviant behavior, *Amer. J. Orthopsychiat.*, 16 (1946), 244.

36. Jenkins, R. L. and S. Glickman, Common syndromes in child psychiatry: II. the Schizoid child, *Amer. J. Orthopsychiat.*, 16 (1946), 255.

37. Jonsson, G., Delinquent boys, their parents and grandparents, *Acta psychiat. Scand.*, Supplement no. 195, 1967.

38. Kagan, J. and H. A. Moss, The Stability of passive and dependent behavior from childhood through adulthood, *Child. Develpm.*, 31 (1960), 577.

39. Kanner, L., To what extent is Early Infantile Autism determined by constitutional inadequacies?, *Research Publications of the Association for Research into Nervous and Mental Diseases*, 33 (1954), 378.

40. Levy, D. M., Psychosomatic studies of some aspects of maternal behavior, in C. Kluckhohn and H. A. Murray, Eds., *Personality in Nature, Society and Culture*, Jonathan Cape, London, 1949.

41. Leys, D. G., B. Sammarco, C. O. Carter, P. A. Currie, H. Caunce, C. M. Maxwell and P. N. Swift, Mothers at work, *Brit. J. prev. soc. Med.*, 17 (1963), 145.

42. Lotter, V., Epidemiology of Autistic conditions in young children: 2. *Social Psychiatry*, 1 (1966), 163.

43. McCulloch, J. W., A. S. Henderson and A. E. Philip, Psychiatric Illness in Edinburgh teenagers, *Scot. Med. J.*, 11 (1966), 277.

44. Mitchell, S., *Study of the Mental Health of School Children in an English County*, Ph.D. Thesis, University of London, 1965.

45a. Oleinick, M., Bahn, A., Eisenberg, L. and Lilienfielz, A., Early socialization experiences and intrafamiliar environments, *Arch. Gen. Psychiat.* 15 (1966), 344.

45. Peterson, D. R., W. C. Becker, L. A. Hellmer, D. J. Shoemaker and H. C. Quay, Parental attitudes and child adjustment, *Child Develpm.*, 30 (1959), 120.

46. Peterson, D. R., W. C. Becker, D. J. Shoemaker, Z. Luria and L. A. Hellmer, Child behavior problems and parental attitudes, *Child Develpm.*, 32 (1961), 151.

47. Petriciani, J. C. and S. Wolff, Characteristics of referrals by school psychologists and general practitioners to a child psychiatric clinic, *Brit. J. Educ. Psychol.*, 38 (1968), 1.
48. Pond, D. A., A. Ryle and M. Hamilton, Marriage and neurosis in a working-class population, *Brit. J. Psychiat.*, 109 (1963), 592.
49. Robins, L. N., *Deviant Children Grown Up*, Williams and Wilkins, Baltimore, 1966.
50. Roff, M., A Factorial study of the Fels parent behavior scales, *Child Develpm.*, 20 (1949), 29.
51. Rutter, M., *Children of Sick Parents*, Oxford University Press, London, 1966.
52. Rutter, M., Discussion of Dr. Lee Robins paper "Follow-up studies of behavior disorders in children," *W.P.A. – R.M.P.A. Symposium of Psychiatric Epidemiology*, University of Aberdeen, 1969.
53. Rutter, M., P. Graham, D. Quinton, O. Rowlands and C. Tupling, The effects of the children of parental mental illness, work discussed at a *Conference on Current research in Great Britain on the early development of Behavior*, University of Sussex, 1969.
54. Ryle, A., *Neurosis in the Ordinary Family*, Tavistock Publications, London, 1967.
55. Schaffer, H. R. and E. B., *Child Care and the Family*, G. Bell and Sons, London, 1968.
56. Sears, R. R., E. E. Maccoby and H. Levin, *Patterns of Child Rearing*, Row, Peterson and Co., Illinois and New York, 1957.
57. Shepherd, M., A. N. Oppenheim and S. Mitchell, Childhood behavior disorders and the child guidance clinic: an epidemiological study, *J. Child Psychol. Psychiat.*, 7 (1966), 39.
58. Stein, Z. and M. Susser, The Families of Dull Children: Identifying family types and sub-cultures, *J. Ment. Sci.*, 106 (1960), 1296.
59. Stein, Z. A. and M. Susser, The social dimensions of a symptom, *Soc. Sci. and Med.*, 1 (1967), 183.
60. Wardle, C. J., Two generations of broken homes in the genesis of conduct and behavior disorders in childhood, *Brit. Med. J.*, ii (1961), 349.
61. Weinstein, E. A. and P. N. Geisel, An analysis of sex differences in adjustment, *Child Develpm.*, 31 (1960), 721.
62. West, D. J., *Present Conduct and Future Delinquency*, Heineman, London, 1969.
63. Wolff, S., *Children under Stress*, Allen Lane, Penguin Press, London, 1969.
64. Wolff, S., Clustering of behaviour disorders and environmental variables in primary school children referred to a psychiatric department, to be published (1969).
65. Wolff, S. and W. P. Acton, Characteristics of parents of disturbed children, *Brit. J. Psychiat.*, 114 (1968), 593.

Family Background in Eating Disorders

Hilde Bruch (U. S. A.)

It has always been known that eating habits, one's likes or dislikes, are determined to a large extent by what one has eaten as a child, and that there are great cultural differences, that what one society considers edible or even gourmet food may be considered inedible or repulsive by another. There is also general agreement that the amounts eaten are influenced by early experiences; families who set a rich table and enjoy food will be heavy and produce large children who are plump and happy.

Close personal contact with fat children reveals, however, that they are not just overweight and jolly, as has been popularly assumed, but that they suffer from serious disturbances in their behavior and personality [4]. Both the abnormal food habits and disturbed personality development are related to disturbing experiences within the family. This chapter deals with the question of what goes on in a family that raises a child that is conspicuously deviant in appearance as well as in behavior from the cultural expectation. The considerations will limit themselves to those children who eat abnormal amounts of food resulting in either obesity or cachexia (*anorexia nervosa*).

Childhood Obesity

The first systematic study of families was undertaken 30 years ago in a group of obese children who had come to the attention of the Department of Pediatrics of the Columbia Presbyterian Medical Center in New York. These children had been referred in the expectation of correcting an endocrine or other strictly organic defect. Contrary to the then current concepts, it was recognized that the abnormal body configuration, the overeating, inactivity, and awkward or seclusive behavior were not due to some endocrine dysfunction [5]. The hovering, anxious behavior of the mothers and their resistance against changing any aspect of a child's life, in particular the excessive eating, suggested the possibility of some disturbance in the psychological climate of these families [6].

The psychiatric literature of that time did not contain any family studies that might have served as model or offered a basis for comparison. What little there was came from child guidance clinics and seemed to limit itself to applying descriptive labels, such as "overprotective," "hostile," or "rejecting," to certain features of maternal behavior which were considered the causal explanation of a child's difficulties. References to the fathers' role were conspicuous by their absence. In our study efforts were made to get detailed information on the background and attitudes of both parents through repeated interviews and at least one visit to the home. Fathers were included but they were found to be reluctant to give information; some objected against any personal question as violating the sanctity of the home. It also appeared that they did not participate actively in the life of their families. The mothers, on the other hand, were eager to talk about themselves and used the interviews to express endless complaints and to reveal their unfulfilled aspirations. The mothers had suffered in their childhood from poverty, hunger, and insecurity, and felt that they had been thrown upon their own resources too early. Many of these parents were immigrants from poverty-stricken areas of Europe or were children of immigrants. The mothers had reacted to their experiences with self-pity and resentment and were overinvolved with their children. The differences in temperament between the parents was apparent in their marital relationships where disharmony expressed itself in open fighting or mutual contempt which many of these mothers expressed without restraint. An overall picture was gained which suggested that many fathers were weak and unaggressive with little drive and ambition, and that the mothers were dominant in the life of these families.

The families were conspicuous by their small size. Seventy percent of the children were only children or the youngest. There were many admitted abortions and more than 50 percent of the children had been "unwanted." The sex of the boys had frequently been a disappointment to the mothers who had hoped for a girl for companionship. Open dissatisfaction with the sex of a girl was expressed less frequently.

The observations were published in a lengthy report in *Psychosomatic Medicine* as "The Family Frame of Obese Children," in April 1940 [7]. The individual histories were published in detail to depict the wide range of individual manifestation of this composite picture of the family frame of a fat child. It was felt that the fundamental rejection which many mothers felt toward their children was overcompensated by overprotective measures and excessive feeding, and that, in a home environment without emotional security, food had been endowed with an exaggerated importance and was charged with a high emotional value substituting for love, security, and satisfaction. In all instances giving and receiving of food represented an important bond in the relationship between parent and child, and the parents would refuse to upset this precarious balance by withholding food when a diet was recommended. Muscular activity and social contacts, on the other hand, had been associated with concepts of danger and separation. It was felt that these circumstances made the simultaneous occurrence of excessive food intake and avoidance of activities comprehensible. They were considered less an expression of disturbances in weight-regulating mechanisms but rather that of poor social adjustment and delayed emotional maturation. The obesity was rarely a matter of concern to the parents in contrast to their exaggerated anxiety over other physical disorders, particularly fear of sexual maldevelopment. In a young child fatness was often valued as reflecting greater comfort than the parents had enjoyed.

The title "Family Frame" had been chosen to indicate that this part of the study represented an approach to the problem from the angle of the parents but needed to be supplemented by a study of the children's reaction to this traumatic climate. It was also recognized that social and cultural factors needed to be considered. Examined in retrospect it is apparent that many aspects of these families were not specific for obesity but reflected difficulties of immigrant families of lower-class status during the Depression years. The continuous reevaluation of the findings, in particular the incorporation of experiences with fat children and adolescents of middle- and upper-class background, leads to the conclusion that it is *not enough to give the family history in biographical or anecdotal detail, but there is need to formulate the essential aspects of the family transactions as generalized, even abstract concepts* which then may serve as the basis for comparison from family to family, and would apply to different social and cultural settings [8]. The same change in orientation can be recognized in the extensive studies of families of schizophrenics which flourished during the fifties and sixties [22, 26]. It was also recognized that in the study of psychosomatic disorders, such as obesity and *anorexia nervosa,* it is essential to surmount the age-old dichotomy of contrasting "external" and "internal" factors, of "biologic" and "psychologic" forces, but to view them as a feedback system in continuous interaction [9].

I shall present my material here under such generalized concepts. An early generalization was the recognition that fat children had been expected to compensate one or the other parent, usually the mother, for disappointments in their own life and had been raised as a precious posession to whom the very best care was given. The outcome were children who were essentially passive, lacking in individuality. In patients of upper-class background, the parents had not suffered from material deprivation but many mothers felt just as strongly that they were unfulfilled in their own lives and in their marriages, and they, too, kept the fat child in close emotional bondage.

The importance of differentiating between accidental features and the more abstract underlying aspects is vividly illustrated by a study that five Danish investigators conducted as a control to the observations reported in the Family Frame [11]. They did not work as a group but each approached the study independently on different groups of fat children. Their findings, made during the fifties in Denmark, differ from each other as much, if not more, as from my observations made during the late thirties in New York City. In a way their studies reveal more about different ways of investigators than about obesity. Only one, Lise Ostergaard, a psychologist, recognized that disturbances might manifest themselves differently in a different cultural setting [23]. By concentrating on dynamic configurations she was able to observe comparable psychological injuries. Three of the investigators found various manifestations of psychological disturbances and contrasted them to the New York picture [20, 21, 25]. Quaade limited his observations to school children whose weight was outside the standard deviation, with only very few children having a weight excess comparable to that of obese children observed in clinic settings [24]. He compared isolated aspects of the composite New York picture to isolated traits in Danish families but failed to make comparable observations. Needless to say, there were no children of first- or second-generation immigrants in Denmark.

Anorexia Nervosa

Psychological studies of *childhood obesity* are of comparatively recent origin. In *anorexia nervosa,* a "morbid mental state" had been recognized as characteristic since its description 100 years ago [18]. Yet there are few studies of the family background of these young patients. When mentioned at all, the emphasis is on the power struggle about food between mother and child *after* the condition has become manifest. In the few studies with focus on the pre-illness picture, observations are reported as generalized statements. Groen and Feldman-Toledano, for instance, speak of the "severe love deprivation" from which these children had suffered, and that the parents, too, seem to live in a loveless relationship, in marriages without satisfaction to either of them [17]. At the same time, the parents are obsessively concerned with exemplary education and the right way of behavior. Asperger describes abnormal family situations in which the mothers are unable to provide the necessary warmth and security because they themselves are neurotic personalities [1]. The mother's anxiety spreads itself in particular to all vegetative functioning. The fathers are described as soft, inactive, and unable to take a stand against their wives. Asperger does not feel that these traits prove the exogenous origin of the illness; to him they are manifestations of a constitutional psychopathy which is handed down from mother to child. Underlying the enormous negativism and stubbornness of these patients he recognizes a *"Befehlsautomatie"* which constitutes a relationship to schizophrenia. Blitzer, Rollins, and Blackwell, in a study of "Children Who Starve Themselves," speak of a "family neurosis," expressed in the parents' abnormal attitudes and concepts of eating and food, with several mothers obsessively concerned with weight [3]. Yet only about half of their patients had a history of early feeding difficulty; and even there the pediatricians had not felt the child was underweight but had considered the mothers to be overanxious.

Developmental Impediments in Obesity and Anorexia Nervosa

In order to come to an understanding of the not uncommon association of developmental obesity and *anorexia nervosa* with schizophrenia, it is necessary to define the forces that interfere with a child growing into a distinct individual with needs and impulses clearly differentiated from those of his parents, and with his learning how to organize his behavior and reactions in such a way that he can face the complexities of adult life [2, 12, 13]. In discussing eating and its psychological implications, one simple basic fact cannot be overlooked, namely, that feeding in the human infant *always* demands the cooperation of another person. The continuous ongoing interaction between infant and food giver is accompanied by emotional-affectional experiences which surround eating and food intake throughout life. This aspect has found ample attention in the clinical and psychoanalytic literature, and the early family studies were conducted under this orientation.

Such continuous interaction also has a bearing on the development of accurate perception and conceptualization of hunger as a discriminate sensation, a fact that has been comparatively neglected. Physiologists had drawn attention to this fact. Hebb, in particular, pointed out that even in an animal as low as the rat a certain amount of learning is necessary for "hunger" and "satiation" to be experienced discriminately [19]. In the clinical and psychoanalytic study of obesity and *anorexia nervosa* it could be recognized that underlying the many symbolic meanings of excessive eating or food refusal, there was a perceptual and conceptual confusion. The question of *why* food is used in an abnormal way needs to be supplemented by the question of *how* a body function as fundamental as food intake has been transformed in such a way that it can be misused for the pseudo-solution of an endless variety of nonnutritional problems. A common deficit in the background of these children was recognized, namely, absence or paucity of appropriate responses from the environment to cues indicating child-initiated expressions of his needs. These mothers would feed their children when they felt it was the correct time or when they themselves felt hungry, or for other reasons not corresponding to the child's need. In obesity many mothers had responded to any expression of discomfort on the part of the child by giving food, disregarding the child's real need. This would result in what has been described as overindulgent feeding. Others would overrigidly adhere to a prescribed schedule. The apparent contradiction in some of the older reports that children grow fat when their mothers are "overprotective," but also when they are "rejecting," can be resolved by rating the maternal behavior as "inappropriate."

Rarely, if ever, is the feeding situation the only one in which such inappropriate transactions take place [10]. The very fact that food is substituted for appeasement of nonnutritional needs will result in other forms of expression remaining undeveloped. The more impervious a mother, failing to give appropriate responses in many areas, the more extensive the deficits in the child who has been deprived of the opportunity to organize reliable tools for self-expression and orientation in the world around him. He fails to acquire the ability to express his needs in a way that they can find appropriate responses and fulfillment from others, and he will also be apt to misinterpret cues and messages coming from other people.

The outer constellation of the family will vary widely, from recognizable gross disturbances, with conflicts and openly expressed dissatisfaction, to seemingly well-functioning conventional family life. In families in whom a child grows fat during childhood the disturbances are more likely to be in the open. In contrast, families in whom a child develops *anorexia nervosa,* or where the obesity becomes manifest only at the time of puberty, function with the facade of normalcy.

Reconstruction of the early development of nearly 60 patients with *anorexia nervosa* revealed, as a composite picture, that they had been well cared-for children to whom many advantages and privileges of modern living had been offered. They had also been exposed to many stimulating influences, in education, in the arts, in athletics, and the like. Yet, on closer study, it was recognized that encouragement or reinforcement of self-expression had been deficient, and thus reliance on their own inner resources, ideas, or autonomous decisions had remained undeveloped. Pleasing compliance had become their way of life, which, however, when progressive development demanded more than conforming obedience turned into indiscriminate negativism, which was the most apparent psychological symptom after the illness had developed [14, 15].

The parents emphasized the normality of their family life, with repeated statements that "nothing was wrong," sometimes with frantic stress on "happiness," directly denying the desperate illness of one member. Often they emphasized the superiority of the now sick child over his siblings. The mothers had often been women of achievement, or career women frustrated in their aspirations, who had been conscientious in their concepts of motherhood. They were subservient to their husbands in many details, and yet did not truly respect them. The fathers, despite social and financial success which was often considerable, felt in some sense "second best." They were enormously preoccupied with outer appearances, in the physical sense of the word, admiring fitness and beauty, and expecting proper behavior and measurable achievements from their children. This description applies probably to many "success-oriented," upper-middle-class families. These traits appear more pronounced in an *anorexia* family. The great majority of anorexic patients come from upper-class or upper-middle-class families, with only very few of lower-class background.

The parents' denial of all difficulties in the present, except for their frantic concern with the weight loss, might suggest that earlier problems are not remembered, an expression of the same denial. Usually there is an excellent school record which supports the history of seemingly normal functioning.

Case History[1]

The seeming normality of the overt family constellation is one more puzzle in the understanding of *anorexia nervosa* where a well-cared-for and well-functioning child suddenly becomes desperately sick. I shall use as illustration Eric's history which fits this model of a nearly supernormal family where, in spite of devoted and conscientious care, his basic needs had been disregarded.

Eric had become sick when he was 12 years old. After summer camp he felt he was "too plump" with a weight of 91 pounds (height 56 inches). His parents had moved from a city apartment to a suburban home while he was away. Eric was unhappy in the unfamiliar

[1] This patient was observed at the New York State Psychiatric Institute in New York City.

neighborhood and new school and feared being ridiculed for his fatness, and that he would not be able to make new friends. He found himself wanting to run and exercise uncontrollably, and often he did this surreptitiously. When this was not effective in making him thin, he followed a diet his mother had used during the preceding year (and on which she had lost 20 pounds), but then ate less and less. There were occasional eating binges followed by self-induced vomiting. His weight dropped from 91 pounds in September 1952 to 57 pounds in May 1953. After he had refused any food at all for several days he was admitted to the Babies Hospital for feeding and evaluation. He was extremely negativistic and succeeded in getting himself discharged after 3 weeks, having gained only 4 pounds.

From then on he was nearly continuously in medical and psychiatric treatment. There were several hospital admissions, as life-saving measures and for study of his endocrine status. It was felt that pubertal and growth retardation were secondary to the severe malnutrition. He was alert and active throughout this period and graduated from high school (boarding school) when 17, weighing nearly 70 pounds. After that difficulties increased. There was so much tension and fighting that staying in his parents' home was impossible. When living alone he would completely neglect himself and not eat at all. He was admitted to the New York State Psychiatric Institute in March 1959, aged 18-1/2, with a weight of 49 pounds and a height of 59 inches. There were no signs of pubertal development and the bone age was only 13 years. He responded well, in spite of his initial negativistic attitude, to a treatment approach that had been developed to correct the deficits that had resulted from the distorting early transactional patterns. This treatment approach has been reported in detail elsewhere [16].

I shall here attempt to show how the essential patterns of the family interaction were reconstructed out of the enormous amount of often contradictory information. This was done through regular individual conferences with Eric [psychotherapy], occasional conferences with his parents, and several joint conferences which permitted observation of the ongoing relationship and of the changes as they occurred. This was supplemented by information from records of his earlier hospital admissions, and from reports by his previous psychiatrists. The first one had been in contact with the family during the first 4 years of the illness.

In descriptive terms this was a typical American family. The parents had grown up during the Depression years and their economic and social success was due to their own accomplishment. They took pride in their children and in their home. During the early years of the marriage, the mother continued to work because she enjoyed it and her economic contribution was needed. The family maintained good relationships with their background families and were particularly close to the family of the mother's sister who lived close by. The move to a home in the suburbs fulfilled their need for more space, was a sign of their success, but it involved loosening of important bonds.

At the time of admission the relationship between the mother and her anorexic son was so hostile and bristling that they had not talked to each other alone for nearly 2 years. The mother was frantic and unable to give objective information. In angry outbursts she would speak of her son as: "He is our supreme disappointment." Whatever details she remembered were of a negative nature, that he had always been difficult, "a problem." She was equally outspoken in her disappointment with psychiatry, that it had "nothing to offer," and that previous psychiatrists had made her feel that she had "failed." For years she has been preoccupied with the question of "Where have I gone wrong?" She felt it was unjust that only she was blamed for her son's illness, that her husband's emphasis on correctness and appearances had as much to do with his difficulties as her overconcern. Her glaring hostility was difficult to reconcile with information coming from the father, that until his illness Eric had been exceptionally close to his mother, that they had always been proud parents, that Eric had been an unusually competent child, healthy, well-built, outstanding in athletics, and interested and successful in his studies.

In spite of her defeated attitude the mother, too, stressed that they had provided an exceptionally good home. She had been somewhat of an expert in her neighborhood for other mothers when they had problems with their children. In a conference in 1961, 9 years after the onset of Eric's illness and after endless sleepless nights of soul-searching self-questioning, she would still emphasize: "We did things better than other families; there really was nothing wrong."

From every detail we could learn she had been a conscientious mother. Eric was her first child and she was determined to know as much about motherhood as there was to know. She was energetic and considered herself an independent career woman, but she acted, paradoxically, in a most conventional way. She went back to work when Eric was only 3 months old with the explanation: "That was the thing to do at that time; you had your baby and you went back to work."

Eric developed well, was tall for his age, and well nourished. After the *anorexia* and after repeated inquiries into his early eating habits, the mother gave a picture of his having "always" been difficult to feed. Without his serious illness the report would probably have been that he did alright, though somewhat fussy and demanding. An example of his being a willful child, who needed to be "forced," was an episode when he was 2 months old when he would not take solid food (banana). The mother's explanation was that "it was the thing to do at that time." One gained the impression that she was more concerned with being perfect and doing the correct thing than with observing and satisfying the child. She handled his refusal by not giving any other feeding until he would take what she gave him. This was characteristic of her handling of the food situation, and of other disagreements between them. She felt her approach was successful until she became concerned about his saying "No" so often, when he was 8-1/2 years old. At that time she wrote to a social worker asking whether this was a problem to be taken seriously. Until then she had felt confident about what she was doing. To quote from the letter: "I am sure I have made mistakes, but I don't think they were glaring ones which I see some parents making, to which I am very sensitive." She spoke of herself as "lying awake at night and worrying about it." His changed behavior was a complete puzzle to her.

> Lately there is one word in my boy's vocabulary which takes precedence over all others; that word is No. Whether it is putting on a raincoat in a downpour, having a bath, changing his pants on Sunday, or visiting his grandmother, no matter what the request, he seems to rebel. He can make it a major tragedy, if he has to wear a tie and makes it a point to object to anything we say or want him to do.

She gave the general background as:

> The child has almost everything a child can ask. We are a devoted family. My husband is wonderfully patient with the children, and on Sundays is always doing something with them. Playing ball with them, reading to them, playing indoor games, taking them places.

She described her husband as "sterner" than herself and felt that "as a consequence the child favors me" adding, "we always gave him love and affection, and I think we even leaned over backwards."

What was remembered about this episode was Eric's saying "No" all the time, and the question of discipline. The letter contained also information which, in retrospect, appears even more important, namely that he was "very tense and perhaps nervous" and

> . . . he does seem unhappy and will say, "I hate my name" or "I hate my face," or "I hate myself." We try to praise him in the things he does well, and he will still remark: "I don't play baseball well." Actually, he excels in baseball, we think.

Whatever the difficulties, Eric continued to function well in school, became even more absorbed in athletics, and was not too troublesome at home. His parents had high hopes for his career because he appeared to be an unusually bright boy and they showed great interest in his academic success. Later he blamed his mother for having expected extraordinary things from him. He reported, in a conference, rather defiantly, that she had wanted him to be the biggest mountain climber in the world: "When I don't do that my mother won't be satisfied." Of course, his mother had never expressed such ambition for him. It reflects his interpretation of an overall attitude, his feeling that too much was expected of him. He never blamed his father for having wanted the impossible from him, but there are implications that his father, too, saw in this boy the fulfillment of his hopes.

Throughout the long illness the father had been supportive and uncomplaining in his attitude toward his son. It appears that as the mother's despair mounted, father and son became closer. Until then they had had one great interest in common, namely, athletics. The father spoke of his pleasure in taking pictures of his children playing in the park, in particular in recording Eric's excellence in baseball. He summarized his attitude as, "I can only say that his interests were my interests," adding, "Even though we had all the trouble and sleepless nights, we also had had a happy period of having our children." During the first conference with the parents, when Eric was still desperately sick, the mother was unrestrained in expressing her resentment and disappointment in Eric as well as in the physicians who throughout his life had failed to give her correct advice. The father suddenly began to lecture on the joys of parenthood: "Even with all the troubles we have had, I would say that a person who has no children could just as well not have lived." Whenever a friend or acquaintance becomes a father he will congratulate him with this specific sentence: "Now you begin to live." This statement is repeated in every interview and conference so that one cannot escape the feeling that it has a profound meaning for him. Though successful, there is a certain blandness about him which suggests a detachment about his own life. The expectation that "my child will do my living for me" in its literal implication may have aroused in his son a fear of adulthood, a feeling that too much was expected of him, when his accomplishments were meant to give value to his father's life.

Even before he became manifestly ill, Eric had been enormously concerned with his manliness, with being fit and strong. Sports were his most intense interest, the one he shared with his father. Playing ball was not a source of enjoyment to him but a continuous proving ground where he felt he had to demonstrate that he was manly enough. One reason for his upset about moving to a new neighborhood was his fear that he could no longer excel in baseball. A new practical situation complicated matters. In his old school he had been in an advanced section of his grade, with his own age group. In the new school he was placed into a higher grade with older children; he was rated "too small" for sport activities and so felt left out.

Another symptom seems to be related to Eric's concept of his father, namely, his enormous stinginess. When reviewing his development Eric felt that probably the very first sign of his illness was this extreme concern with money and fear of waste. He reported as example that he would write very small on a piece of paper, filling in every corner, and that he did not want to have extra sheets in his loose-leaf notebook. He wanted to be sure that nothing was wasted. He thought this had begun when he thought he noticed that his father was worried about money. He became confused by the contradiction that shortly thereafter they moved to the suburbs, from a small apartment to a large house. He took upon himself the obligation to make sure that there was something left to fall back on. His father had been generous but had always been against useless expenditures and was careful to receive his money's worth.

Another aspect of this frugality, his absolute refusal to have any personal possessions, clothes or anything else, beyond the barest minimum, was related to the overwhelming sense of obligation he felt toward his parents, or anyone who gave him a present. He explained his refusal to eat and excessive exercising as a compelling need to burn up anything that came from "them." This was expressed at a time when he had recognized that his problem was related to his reaction to both his parents.

In the beginning of treatment he was full of complaints against his mother, that she had dominated his life, had planned and arranged everything for him, whether he wanted it or not. He focused on the clothes that mother bought because she liked them, with repetitious complaints about one pair of knickers which he disliked and which made his skin itch, but which she made him wear just the same. He felt there was nothing he could do about it; he had to wear what she had bought whether he liked it or not. He did not remember difficulties with eating before he became sick. He had always enjoyed good food, and did so again after he gave up his punishing attitude toward his body. During his illness food had become the focus of their fighting. "When I did not eat, the roof fell in. It gave me an empty feeling, there was no chance to please her. All my experiences with mother were displeasure."

As the tension in the family eased up somewhat, a number of small episodes occurred which illustrated the disturbing elements in seemingly well-meant acts. After a brief vacation the mother brought Eric a present, a cigarette lighter – and he was furious. To him this was typical of their relationship. He did not smoke and the mother knew this. She said, "You can light cigarettes for other people – it looks so gallant." That had been the trouble with all her gifts; they were always something that she wanted him to do, never what he wanted. "I would rather have nothing. I can't accept this with thanks – I feel I have to use it and I cannot throw it away." Thus the well-meant gift became a source of irritation for him. But it helped in the unraveling of the many small episodes which he had experienced as mother superimposing her will on him with disregard of his wishes.

When he felt well enough to be transferred to the open service, he spoke to his mother on the phone and she was skeptical whether he could make it. He was terribly upset about this: "The old story. She does not give me credit; maybe she is scared that I will be coming home soon." He felt disturbed that *he could never please her,* that this had been the story of his life. Even in the things where he was doing well there was always this aura of uncertainty. Though a good student and excellent athlete, he had always been afraid of making errors. "Maybe too many demands were made on me. Everybody jumped on me when I goofed." There was always pressure to improve. It had always been taken for granted that he was good but he never got as much recognition as he needed in order to feel secure.

He enjoyed being on the open ward and began to take part in activities. "No one is on your back. You are not responsible except to yourself. For the first time I am free. *I own my body.* I am not supervised any more by nurses or my mother." A few weeks later, on a visit home, he felt for the first time "happy" in his relation with his parents though they were not particularly demonstrative. He was just satisfied being with them. "For the first time Mother was *warm.* She brought me back to the hospital. She didn't need to do so. It showed she cared." He was also aware that he could accept her care now because he felt more independent. "I am closer to being well than before – I can do a lot for myself." He also noticed that his mother was less nervous; she had told him about her inability to sleep when she was worried about him and had said: "When you get better, I get better." Now he felt guilty for having caused them so much worry.

He now permitted adequate physical examinations. He needed extensive dental work and expressed guilt for having ruined his own body. He knew that the decay of his teeth was related to his long-standing malnutrition. "There is a general feeling of decay and I am responsible for it." While his teeth were repaired, a soft diet was prescribed, and he resented it. "I had to do without it so long, now I want it (referring to good food). Now if I lose weight it makes me feel sick, that I am losing something that is mine, that I am all washed out if I don't gain."

The fundamental significance of his repeated references to his owning or not owning his body was not immediately recognized, though he appeared to be preoccupied with this question. Its importance came dramatically into the open when he spoke of himself as "his parents' property." This occurred approximately one year after he had come to the Institute. When planning to go home for a holiday he was unable to decide whether to travel by subway and bus, or to phone his father to meet him with his car, as the father had suggested. Eric ruminated about not having the right to impose any special demands on his parents. When asked how he would act if the situation were reversed, if he were to pick up his parents, he answered with feeling: "I would be honored, because they are my parents and I owe them something. *I am their property,* that's why I owe them willingness to do things for them."

When the word *property* was questioned, he at first wanted to dismiss it, that of course he was not their property. But then he enlarged on it in a long talk which reflected that he had given it a great deal of thought.

> Everything I have and own comes from them. I feel guilty that I have nothing to show for it; I keep taking and taking from them. At least if I could produce, then they could be proud; that would be something they would get from me. But all I do is take and take – that's why I say everything is theirs and I am theirs – only after I have shown that something good comes out of me, that I can make something out of myself, then I can feel that things are mine.

He went on to speculate whether there had been a change in his feelings about wanting to be himself as he grew older. Maybe it was alright to *take* things until he was 8 or 9. That's when he began to say *No* continuously as if to prove himself as an independent individual. He became also exceedingly concerned about his fitness and, after they moved to the new neighborhood, when he was 12, he was doing more and more exercise to be sure that his muscles would develop correctly, like needing to prove that he himself was "something."

During this discussion he clarified that he felt that every possession made him more and more a part of his parents, increasing his sense of obligation and responsibility, and reversely, his guilt at not fulfilling his obligation toward them.

During this weekend, when the family had a meal in a restaurant, he became quite indignant when he observed other children "misbehaving." He reported that in one family the baby sitter phoned that she could not handle the baby's crying, and that the mother had to go home. He was outraged:

> The baby does not have the right to upset the family like this; of course, the baby doesn't know, but still he doesn't have the right. Why should this newcomer break up the family? The baby upsets the family nest and whatever pleasures they have.

He recalled how he had been an inconsiderate child, quite apart from the paradox that his illness, his striving for independence, had disrupted the family life in a most traumatic way. When he was 8 or 9 they had planned a winter vacation in Florida. He was afraid of flying and, thus, the family went by train. Now he felt acutely guilty for having forced a long train ride on them just because he felt anxious. He recalled another episode when he had refused to go to summer camp, thus forcing his mother to spend the summer with her children in the country, instead of letting her have a vacation.

The social worker who was in contact with the parents noticed that they had changed during this winter, had become much more aware of Eric's problems, and were dedicated to helping him. Optimism and hope that improvement was possible had replaced the defeatist attitude of the whole family. Yet, when a joint conference with his parents was suggested, Eric protested. At first he refused to come, then he agreed to attend but he would not talk. He was obsessively concerned with hurting his parents by what he might say, or with causing them new worries by not talking, that it might indicate he was sick in a new way.

> I cannot talk in front of her. She will think I do not cooperate. If I say all these memories and feelings, then it hurts her. I picture the glances from her to father. They will be watching me like a hawk, my every word and movement. I will never have such a conference again – I had one once – and everything was an attack on me.

It was explained to the parents that Eric just wanted to listen, and they accepted it without feeling handicapped in reviewing their own attitudes. It was helpful for Eric to hear his parents talk about their efforts on his behalf. He even agreed with his father who felt that he had observed that Eric as a child never was as frank and open in expressing his feelings as his mother would have liked him to be: "He was never ready to tell us off or yell at us."

Therapeutic work focused increasingly on Eric's inability to make decisions or to trust the reliability of his own impulses and plans. He brought innumerable examples of how he always had tried to do things that would please his mother. It had been puzzling that such a bright young man showed so few intellectual interests. In preparation for college he wanted to start a reading program. It became painfully clear that he was unable to select a book because he was preoccupied with the question of whether to read "to please mother or to please myself." As far back as he remembered, mother had chosen books for him and he had read them; the idea of reading for his own enjoyment or enrichment had not occurred to him. The same obsessive wavering "for whom he was doing it" came into the open when the question of further education and professional choice was discussed. It took many detailed discussions before he could accept that the life ahead was his own, and not something he had to produce in order to satisfy his parents.

The subtle ways in which the parents stymied him through well-meaning planning on his behalf were revealed in a joint conference preceding his leaving the hospital, in an atmosphere of relief about his improvement and pleasant anticipation. The parents brought up the question whether it would be advisable to move to a new neighborhood in order to spare Eric the embarrassment about having been in a mental hospital. Eric did not know what he wanted. In the conference, the emphasis was on two points, that if there was embarrassment, would this be one of the difficulties of living Eric was able to face. It appeared that his parents had been in the habit of anticipating problems and thus indirectly expressed mistrust in Eric's ability to handle them. In addition, during the last 2 years, he had done something he could take pride in, namely, having worked himself out of such a serious illness. If there was shame, then that was an indication that he still felt influenced by what others thought, something for which he needed continued therapy.

It was of interest how the mother picked up this point of his not having sufficient pride in himself by expressing her own concerns. When visiting his home Eric had wanted to go to a movie. His mother suggested: "Why don't you ask a girl to go with you?", and he had answered angrily: "What girl is going to look at me?" The mother explained: "That was painful to me. He does not think enough of himself that a girl would want to go with him." This was examined as another example of the mother's superimposing what she felt he should be ready for. The last 8 years, the time of adolescence for other youngsters, had left him not yet prepared for dating and similar activities. This was one more situation of negative feedback which had been so disturbing for his development. The fact that the mother expressed her discontent with his not yet being ready did make it harder for him to face the problems of growing up at a rate different from that of other young people. In order to engage in dating behavior, he needed to be much further along in his puberty development and more comfortable with himself. He also needed experiences of relaxed friendships outside the hospital before he could take the next step.

It was pointed out in general terms that, in facing his psychological handicaps, whatever plan would come from his parents before he was ready would arouse his old reaction of "there she goes again," and thus might interfere with his developing at his own rate. Father and son responded to this remark by giving many details of mother's "overdoing things." "The first thing when he walks in, 'Buy a pair of pants,' or 'Buy this or that,' or 'You promised to get another one,' She has a faculty to repeat it over and over and one can only characterize it as 'nagging.' " The father felt encouraged that for the first time Eric could let off steam and tell his mother off. He had such an outburst during the conference: "If you want to move to a new house – then move. Do it because you don't like the neighborhood or for whatever reason, but don't blame it on me and make me feel guilty."

The parents' greater alertness to their tendency to superimpose their plans on Eric made it possible to formulate what to avoid and how to meet problems that lay ahead. Eric came to recognize, during this conference, more clearly than he had done until then, his oversensitivity to the slightest expression of anxiety on the part of his mother. He felt more prepared to let her be anxious without his becoming involved in his old negativistic way.

When Eric left the hospital he went to live in the family home, while attending college, and encountered fewer difficulties at home and in new social situations than had been anticipated. He continued to be in treatment with the same psychiatrist for another year. After that he kept in touch with him through occasional letters.

Comment

Contact with this family over a period of time revealed how misleading it would have been to draw conclusions about the pre-illness relationships from the angry and hostile interaction that had developed after the condition has existed for some time. It would have been equally unjustified to consider the manipulative, deceitful, and aggressive, negativistic behavior of the patient as characteristic for his pre-morbid behavior. There are few conditions that evoke such severe emotional reaction as voluntary food refusal. The coercive power of hunger strikes is well known. To mention just two examples: the fight of the suffragettes for the vote for women, and Gandhi's struggle for the independence of India. The mighty English Empire was forced to interrupt prison terms to avoid causing death or damage to their political prisoners.

The detailed evaluation showed that the mother's description was essentially correct, that they were a devoted family with love and affection for their children. As relationships improved, Eric spoke often of "the warmth is coming back." The faulty attitudes and interactions that had resulted in the serious deficits underlying the *anorexia nervosa* syndrome were rather subtle in nature, but all pervasive and continuous. They were more readily recognized when, with improvement, the secondary reactions had subsided. The father summarized it well during the last conference when he spoke of "overdoing things," of planning too much for their children, and expecting too much in return. This had been expressed in the mother's overrigid adherence to an already rigid pediatric program, in her being overhelpful in all areas of her son's development, planning and selecting every detail of what he should eat, wear, or do, and in the father's overproud interest in his son's athletic achievement. Not one isolated act or attitude could have been called traumatic or abnormal. It was the aggregate of these influences that resulted in the child's experiencing an overall feeling that whatever he felt was not considered, or what he did was not for himself, never sufficient to please his parents, and that he did not even have ownership of his own body. The parents' conviction of their correctness blinded them to all signals indicating the increasing doubts and frustration from which their son suffered.

With this failure in communication, even benevolent and appropriate acts on the part of the parents are apt to be misinterpreted by a child as overcontrol, disregard for or belittling of anything that comes from him. In this family, eating had not been a particular problem, though the mother had made sure that he ate what she offered when he was an infant. Whether or not her having been on a diet prior to their moving to the new home influenced his resorting to non-eating as the most expressive symptom is possible but by no means certain.

In other families, preoccupation with slenderness and dieting may have been a pervasive influence. Of particular interest are situations where information about the later patient had been available before he became sick. In the case of a socially prominent upper-class family, there had been a consultation about an older daughter who was markedly obese at age 18 when the later anorexic girl was only 12 years old. The mother asked for help because she resented the older girl's obesity but was aware that her concern was excessive. She spoke in glowing terms about her younger daughter who in every respect was an ideal child. Her teachers would refer to her as the "best-balanced" girl in school, and would rely on her warmth and friendliness when a new child had difficulties in making friends. After the *anorexia* developed, it could be recognized to what extent the anxious and often punitive concern with the older sister's obesity had influenced the younger girl's thinking and self-concept, convincing her that being fat was the most shameful and deplorable condition. The rapid weight increase during puberty horrified her and she felt the only way of deserving respect was by being thin, and she went on a starvation regime. This coincided with her beginning to realize that life was not just filling the mold into which her parents had poured her, but that it was expected that she should be "master of her fate."

In another case the mother was in psychoanalytic treatment, with another analyst to whom I owe this information, because she felt dissatisfied in her marriage and had become depressed. The mother was of foreign (Scandinavian) background, from an educated, upper-middle-class family. Her husband came from a well-known, upper-class family and she felt he was "superior" to her in taste and social poise. In her background there had been great interest in good food with much emphasis on variety, interesting tastes, and artistic presentation. When she began her analysis she felt her relationship to her daughter was the one great satisfaction of her life. The girl (14 years of age) had always been a happy child who had had no problems and was perfectly contented now, she felt. Though the child had governesses, she herself had supervised her feeding, making sure that she always received the right diet. This was the one area where she felt sure of her superior knowledge. She knew exactly what a child should eat, how the food should be fixed, and how it should be offered.

Shortly thereafter, after a brief period of plumpness, the daughter became anorexic. She gave a picture exactly the opposite of what her mother had described. She remembered her childhood as a constant state of misery and frustration, that she could *never* have *what she wanted,* that it always *had to be exactly what mother had planned.* To give just one example: she longed to eat a whole orange, but there it was every day – orange juice, because mother felt this was better. She knew that mother discussed with the pediatrician the exact amount she should eat to keep her from growing fat, and felt that every bite that went into her mouth was watched. This concern about fatness was reinforced by father's excessive concern with appearance. He was a very successful man (though not quite as outstanding as other members of his family), handsome, well-built, and not at all a candidate for becoming fat. However, he was eternally preoccupied with his weight, continuously talking about going on a diet. This was a wealthy home and there was always a lavish array of food on the table. The father showed his superiority by eating very little and making snide remarks about people who just ate away, enjoying all this food.

When the girl became too plump at puberty, she tried to outdo her father in showing aristocratic control. Being slim was what she felt she owed to her background. After she had lost a great deal of weight, she knew that she looked ghastly but her ideal remained: "I want to come to the point where I don't eat at all." Her whole life was dominated by the question: "Can one ever satisfy Father?" Mother had been exceedingly submissive to him without ever quite reaching up to his standards. An older brother was rated by the father as inept and ineffective though he was successful by ordinary standards. She herself did quite well in her studies but was haunted by the fear of being found out to be "stupid," or of "not working enough." After she had become anorexic she summarized her life experiences as: "I never deserved what they gave me." She felt she had proven in a great many ways that she was "worthless" and keeping her weight low was her only way of proving hereself as "deserving" and as "having dignity."

In other families conflicts and problems are more in the open and may tempt one to blame them for the eating disorder. Sometimes such a direct relationship exists. More often the child's disordered food intake, his feeling inadequate and undermined in his basic sense of competence and effectiveness, must be related to persistent, often seemingly insignificant, errors surrounding his early feeding experiences and inappropriate responses to his other needs. If obesity develops during childhood, the picture is complicated because even mild degrees of overweight arouse hostile and condemning reactions. One may see mothers who literally persecute their child for being fat, but who, at the same time, in their every word and action, make it impossible for the child to develop control over his food intake, find other ways of combating anxiety and tension, or experiment with new forms of self-expression.

For effective treatment it is essential to clarify the disturbed interactional patterns so that the child can develop controls from within and become capable of experiencing himself as self-directed and as owning his body. Whether this can best be accomplished through individual therapy, or through conjoint family therapy, depends on the total situation. When difficulties have existed over an extended period and faulty self-awareness dominates the picture, individual therapy is essential to help a child learn to differentiate between different needs, and to assist him in becoming capable to stand up to the existing problems, without using excessive intake or food refusal in this bizarre way.

Summary

1. Feeding in the human infant *always* demands the cooperation of another person. The continuous ongoing interactions between infant and food giver are accompanied by emotional experiences which surround food intake throughout life. This aspect has found ample attention in the clinical and psychoanalytic literature, and early family studies of obesity and *anorexia nervosa* were conducted under this orientation.

2. The transactional patterns during early feeding experiences also determine the accuracy of perception and conceptualization of hunger as a distinct and identifiable sensation.

3. Obese and anorexic patients often are inaccurate in identifying bodily states, in particular, in differentiating nutritional need from other bodily sensations or emotional tensions.

4. Absence or paucity of appropriate responses from the environment to cues indicating a child's expression of his needs was recognized as a common deficit in the background of obesity and *anorexia*.

5. The broader the range of such inappropriate responses, the more extensive the deficits in total functioning, with schizophrenic development a not-uncommon occurrence.

6. The transactional patterns within a family with an anorexic son are reconstructed, from psychotherapeutic sessions and family conferences, to illustrate the occurrence of serious disturbances under the facade of seemingly normal functioning.

Bibliography

1. Asperger, H., Zur Problematik der Pubertaetsmagersucht, *Schweiz, Med. Wschr.*, 92 (1963), 66–68.
2. Bateson, G., D. D. Jackson, J. Haley, and J. Weakland, Toward a theory of schizophrenia, *Behavioral Science,* 1 (1956), 251–264.
3. Blitzer, J. R., N. Rollins, and A. Blackwell, Children who starve themselves: Anorexia nervosa. *Psychosom. Med.*, 23 (1961), 368–383.
4. Bruch, H., Obesity in childhood and personality development. *Am. J. Orthopsychiat.*, 11 (1941), 467–474.
5. Bruch, H., Obesity in Childhood. I. Physical growth and development of obese children, *Am. J. Dis. Child.*, 58 (1939), 457–484.
6. Bruch, H., Obesity in Childhood. III. Physiologic and psychologic aspects of the food intake of obese children, *Am. J. Dis. Child.*, 59 (1940), 739–781.
7. Bruch, H. and G. Touraine, Obesity in Childhood. V. The family frame of obese children, *Psychosom. Med.*, 2 (1940), 141–206.
8. Bruch, H., Changing approaches to the study of the family. *Psychiatric Research Report 20,* American Psychiatric Association, 1966, p. 1–7.
9. Bruch, H., Transformation of oral impulses in eating disorders: A conceptual approach, *Psychiatric Quarterly,* 35 (1961), 458–481.
10. Bruch, H., Falsification of bodily needs and body concept in schizophrenia, *Arch. Gen. Psychiatry,* 6 (1962), 18–24.
11. Bruch, H., N. Juel-Nielsen, F. Quaade, L. Ostergaard, T. Iversen, and K. Tolstrup, Adipositas – panel discussion on the Theory of Hilde Bruch., *Acta Psych. et Neurol. Scand.* 33 (1957), 152–173.
12. Bruch, H., Developmental obesity and schizophrenia, *Psychiatry,* 21 (1958), 65–70.
13. Bruch, H., Eating disorders and schizophrenic development. Chapter in *Psychoneurosis & Schizophrenia*, Lippincott, Philadelphia, Pa., 1966, p. 113–124.
14. Bruch, H. Perceptual and conceptual disturbances in anorexia nervosa., *Psychosom. Med.,* 24 (1962), 187–194.
15. Bruch, H., Anorexia nervosa and its differential diagnosis., *J. Nerv. Ment. Dis.*, 141 (1965), 555–566.
16. Bruch, H., Psychotherapy in anorexia nervosa., *J. Nerv. Ment. Dis.*, (in print).
17. Groen, J. J. and Z. Feldman-Toledano, Educative treatment of patients and parents in anorexia nervosa, *Brit. J. Psychiat.*, 112 (1966), 671–681.
18. Gull, W. W., Anorexia nervosa (apepsia hysterica)., *Brit. Med. J.*, 2 (1873), 527.
19. Hebb, D. O., *Organization of Behavior.* John Wiley & Sons, New York, 1949.
20. Iversen, T., Psychogenic obesity in children. I., *Acta Paediat.*, 42 (1953), 8–19.
21. Nuel-Nielsen, N.: On psychogenic obesity in children. II., *Acta Paediat.*, 42 (1953) 130–146.
22. Lidz, T., S. Fleck, and A. R. Cornelison, *Schizophrenia and the Family,* International University Press, 1965, p. 477.
23. Ostergaard, L.: On psychogenic obesity in children. V., *Acta Paediat.*, 43 (1954), 507–521.

24. Quaade, F.: On psychogenic obesity in children. III., *Acta Paediat.*, 42 (1953), 191–205.
25. Tolstrup, K., On psychogenic obesity in childhood. IV., *Acta Paediat.*, 42 (1953), 289–304.
26. Wynne, L. and M. Singer, Thought disorders and family relations of schizophrenics, *Arch. Gen. Psych.*, 9 (1963), 191–206.

The Necessity for Differentiating Eating Disorders—Discussion of Hilde Bruch's Paper on the Family Background

KAI TOLSTRUP (DENMARK)

In her paper, Hilde Bruch examines the family background of two distinct eating disorders in childhood, psychogenic obesity and *anorexia nervosa.* Psychogenic obesity is the condition with which her name is identified. Her vivid and empathic descriptions of these children and their families are still very much worth reading, being classics in the history of pediatrics and child psychiatry.

Few papers have been published on this subject since her original papers 30 years ago. The Danish studies, to which she refers, were carried out 20 years ago and have not been succeeded by similar investigations. Although differing in their conclusions, the Danish authors were in agreement, that Bruch's descriptions to some extent could be reproduced in a Danish population, but it was not possible to formulate a general hypothesis on the psychogenesis of obesity from these materials. Several different types of family background and possible psychogenesis were found. Some of the Danish studies concluded that obesity was not a specific phenomenon, but that cultural, social, and somatic factors, to varying degrees in each child, determined the development of the presenting symptom. In my opinion these studies add useful knowledge to Bruch's work, and I find it useful to read, for instance, the extensive work by Quaade [3] as a supplement to the former's intensive studies.

The Copenhagen Experience

The child psychiatrist rarely sees truly gross cases of psychogenic obesity. During my 15 years in child psychiatry, I have seen fewer of these children than during a single year in a pediatric setting. These cases are therefore not only rare, but they are generally usually seen by the general practitioner and the pediatrician and extremely seldom by the child psychiatrist. The reason for this probably is the lack of motivation with respect to psychiatric examination and treatment in both the obese child and his mother.

During 10 years in a hospital department of child psychiatry (Rigshospitalet, Copenhagen), I have seen two or three outspoken cases of obesity among 2000 in- and outpatients, but between 30 and 40 patients in a state of fully developed *anorexia nervosa*. This would most likely be the experience in other clinics too: that in a child psychiatric setting *anorexia nervosa* will appear much more often than obesity. For that reason I shall restrict my discussion to the family background of *anorexia nervosa* evaluated in the light of my experience in a child psychiatric clinic. I have personally treated about 30 patients. The duration of the treatment was from a few months to 3 years, and in some of these cases the patients have been in need of some form of therapeutic contact for an even longer period.

SURFACE SIMILARITIES BETWEEN FAMILIES

On a superficial level the similarities between the families are striking. A nice and respectable appearance, secure and well-ordered social and economic conditions, a tolerant atmosphere in the home, and a very cooperative attitude towards therapy once the parents have accepted the unpleasant fact that the eating disorder cannot be coped with inside the family. It is moreover conspicuous how often the mother is the active and energetic person in the marriage, and that she looks less feminine and shows less empathy in relation to her child than a mother usually shows. From the same superficial view the father appears weak and not very masculine, but in possession of more tact and understanding for the sick child's needs and problems.

This frequently observed outer family frame is, however, by no means only seen in patients with *anorexia nervosa.* Children suffering from other types of neuroses (e.g., school phobia) live in a similar family pattern. Moreover, you will occasionally find other distinct family patterns in otherwise typical cases of *anorexia nervosa*, for instance, a family in which the father is very successful, with a masculine and expansive personality, whereas the mother is self-effacing and markedly feminine; or, in another case, you meet a mother, who shows much empathy, indulgence, and resignation towards a severely neurotic, aggressive, and impotent father.

DIFFERENCES IN DEPTH BETWEEN FAMILIES

This seemingly common characteristic of the family appearance fades away as the therapist becomes acquainted with the patient and the relatives. The conflicts, which at first are so strongly denied, now become obvious, but they differ from case to case. In some, the girl's strong, unreleased aggressiveness towards the mother dominates whilst in others, the rivalry with an admired elder brother, or the status as an elder sister having nearly motherly obligations towards younger siblings commands the conscious field of conflict in the patient. The few patients who are able and willing to be engaged in an open, verbalizing psychotherapeutic relationship, show conflicts of the same sort as found in other children and youngsters, conflicts which are not bound specifically to the syndrome of *anorexia nervosa*. A common core, made up of some central etiologic, pathogenetic factors, is only found among the characteristics of puberty crisis. By this I mean the intrapsychic struggle between the fear of and the desire for growing up, fulfilling the obligations connected with adulthood, and acquiring the corresponding rights. This common conflict of puberty becomes acutely and psychopathologically aggravated in the patients suffering from *anorexia nervosa*, but the underlying causes for the condition vary individually.

Is it surprising that the seemingly specific family structure disappears on closer examination? In my opinion it is not. Although I find it justified to consider *anorexia nervosa* a nosological entity because of the distinct symptoms and the urgency for treatment, there are still so many differences from case to case, that it would be reasonable to expect distinct differences in the family pattern too.

ESSENTIALS OF THE CLINICAL PROFILE

A precise clinical description of the patient suffering from it must include a differentiation as to (1) sex, (2) age, (3) personality structure, and (4) symptomatology. I shall briefly discuss these four items with regard to the family background.

As is well known, it is characteristic of this disease that girls outnumber boys—the relative frequency (female:male) being of the magnitude 10:1. Thus the very instructive case history given by Bruch is an exception. The psychogenic factors, for example, the body-image and the symbolism of the food and the eating, have a different meaning and significance for an adolescent girl than for an adolescent boy. Fantasies about conception and pregnancy, ideas of a heavy body as a sign of strength—those are areas where the imagination has a different background of reality for the two sexes. The final sexual identification depends on the dynamics of the family. In those conflicts, which determine the emotional constellation of the parents and bring psychopathology into the puberty crisis, girls must be different from boys.

The factor of age, too, influences the actual family structure. Although my conclusion in comparing the youngest with the oldest age group was that the oldest patient (26 years old) very much resembled the youngest (8 years old) in the manifestation of her illness, the age of the patient is not negligible in regard to family structure. A child just before or at the beginning of puberty provokes quite different expectations in her parents than a patient in late puberty or young adulthood. Similarly, the parents' opinion of, demands, and influence—and perhaps also dependence—on the daughter (son) differ in the course of that decade when the family has to adapt itself to the situation of a member changing from child to adult. In the case of the youngest patients, the onset of the disease may be precipitated by a particularly severe intrafamilial psychic conflict. On the other hand, the pre-pubertal child is so easily influenced and plastic that the therapeutic process aimed at developing independence goes more easily. For the older patient—that is, the youngster in fully developed puberty or young adulthood—the detachment from home is particularly painful and connected with special social implications, for instance, society expects a young woman or man to have a job and a flat of her own. Finally, the child and the fully sexually mature young woman obviously have different sexual problems. The young woman may painfully sense her parents' expectations that she should have a male partner. I have several times seen these patients trying to pacify the parents by establishing a "pseudo-love," so that they could demonstrate their "being like other young people."

The personality structure varies a good deal from patient to patient. As described by Theilgaard [1] and myself [2] it is practical to work with three (perhaps four) main types, according to the resemblance with (1) obsessive-compulsive neurosis (the core group); (2) hysterical neurosis; (3) psychotic borderline states; and possibly (4) endogenous depression. This classification according to personality type does not imply that you identify the cases with the psychopathological states that they resemble. We consider it practical for therapeutical reasons to make such a diagnostic subgrouping, still keeping the common diagnosis, *anorexia nervosa*, intact.

According to my experience, the hysterical type of patient shows particularly obvious infantile fixations manifesting themselves through more undisguised feelings of love towards her father and more easily observed aggressive feelings towards her mother than is the case with other personality types. The neurotic secondary gain is presented openly and dramatically in a way that involves the family very strongly, resulting in severe secondary family reactions and demanding special therapeutic measures. The intrafamilial conflicts of the obsessive-compulsive type (the "core-group") are not so easily disclosed because the patient entrenches herself behind a silent defiance, prepared for fight. The personality type bordering on psychosis is characterized by a severely injured sense of reality with regard to her own body and by a tendency to break through eating impulses with bulimic attacks. These "partially-psychotic" personality disturbances appear much too undisguised, thereby indicating very defective defense mechanisms. The patient suffers extremely, experiencing consciously and overtly the horror and disgust at the hunger which she cannot manage and the intense feelings of dislike for her own "fatness." This feeling borders on delusion. In the other types of personality the same phenomena are only suspected and much better covered up and kept in the unconscious by the ego defenses.

In my patient material there is a significant tendency towards a heredity of severe mental diseases in the families of the type of personality bordering on psychosis. In one such family, for instance, the mother was schizoid and the father harassed by depressions. One may say that these families in appearance, too, are of a different kind from the "typical" decent, respectable family.

In my experience the depressive type is so rarely seen that I am not able to talk confidently about any characteristic family structure.

Finally, it is necessary to differentiate *anorexia nervosa* according to symptomatology. By this I mean that the refusal to eat and the pathological ideas of the body dominate the clinical picture to different degrees. There may be great differences in the patient's subjective suffering connected with her compelling feelings of not allowing herself to eat. These feelings stretch from the daily, continual inner struggles between desire for eating and the fear of eating, sometimes combined with the problem of masochism. Yet, they all have one thing in common, a constant preoccupation with and conscious awareness of food, pondering over and fantasying about eating. In addition, the ideas and concepts of their own body vary greatly from patient to patient. This extends from the extreme of a contented *belle indifference* to the other extreme of painful fantasies of an ugly body combined with paranoid and hypochondriacal ideas. These delusions comprise not only the idea of fatness (in spite of extreme emaciation), but also include delusional ideas about isolated parts of the body. One of my patients stated that her main complaint was the ever-conscious thought of her hips being too fat—although she was well-proportioned and of a beautiful, feminine shape. This "partially-paranoid" idea was closely associated with severe, hypochondriac ideas of the bowel function and a constant preoccupation with constipation that in reality was negligible.

To some degree this symptomatological differentiation parallels, but is not identical with, the subgrouping into personality types. However, I have not found any correlation between symptomatological variations and distinct family constellations.

Some girls constitute a very special and very interesting group. They are of normal bodily appearance, suffering from violent bulimic attacks, to which, in great anxiety, they yield, followed by strong feelings of guilt relieved by self-induced vomiting. Between the outbursts of eating they voluntarily starve themselves. The result is that weight fluctuates only a little, and the appearance is therefore inconspicuous, neither fat nor thin. These girls are also constantly and consciously preoccupied with the struggle against their eating impulses, and the realistic menace of growing fat. I also had, among my patients, two girls, who were addicted to drugs and alcohol but such symptoms are, in general, uncharacteristic of cases with *anorexia nervosa.*

Conclusion

I want to emphasize that the characteristic eating disorders in childhood and adolescence, psychogenic obesity and *anorexia nervosa,* are not generally and unequivocally correlated with a distinct familial background. As far as obesity is concerned, some relatively rare markedly psychopathological cases are found in which the child and the mother are tightly and pathologically fixated on each other in a characteristic ambivalent way (Bruch's syndrome). The family of the patient suffering from *anorexia nervosa* often presents an outer constellation which, superficially viewed, seems characteristic, but this appearance does not comprise all cases of the condition and it may also be seen in children and adolescents suffering from other psychiatric disturbances. A deeper investigation of each case upsets this finding of an apparently uniform and common family pattern. It is also necessary to differentiate according to, among other things, sex, age, personality type, and symptomatology. When this is done, it becomes clear and understandable why one should not expect to find a family background which is specific for *anorexia nervosa.*

Bibiliography

1. Theilgaard, A. *Anorexia nervosa,* J.-E. Meyer and H. Feldmann, Eds., Stuttgart, 1965, pp. 122-128.
2. Tolstrup, K., *Anorexia nervosa,* J.-E. Meyer and H. Feldmann, Eds., Stuttgart, 1965, pp. 51-59.
3. Quaade, Fl., *Obese Children,* Copenhagen, 1955.

The Families of Patients with Anorexia Nervosa

Mara Selvini-Palazzoli (Italy)

The anorexic patients whom I have been studying for nearly twenty years (approximately 60 cases, 30 of which received intensive psychotherapy) are female subjects immediately before and during puberty (German-speaking authors refer to this condition as *Pubertätsmagersucht*[1]

Historical Perspective

My clinical experience with the families of these patients may be divided into two phases. In the first phase, I received information concerning the family both from the material obtained in the patient's individual psychotherapy and from direct contacts with relatives, almost exclusively the mothers. These contacts consisted of interviews which were held prior to therapy and which, in certain cases, were continued during therapy with the patient's consent.

[1] The three cases of undereating in males which I studied were cases of pseudo-anorexia. One was a monk who soon developed paranoid delusions: by fasting he thought he could redeem the corrupt members of his order. Another was dominated by hypochondriacal ideas of a schizophrenic type, centered on his digestive system. The third was the closest to true A.N., also because of the presence of neuromuscular hyperactivity. This patient, however, showed two atypical signs. In the first place, he explicitly declared he longed for food as if it were a "paradise lost," whereas true anorexics never admit this longing. In the second place, he liked to exhibit his fasting performance, unlike female anorexic patients who constantly claim they have eaten a great deal.

In the second phase, which started three years ago, I began to explore with direct and participant observation the type of family relationships and the overall way of functioning of these families.

THE FIRST PHASE: THE MOTHERS' PHASE

This first phase of my clinical experience was almost exclusively focused on the anorexic patient's relationship with the pathogenic mother, which coincided with a trend prevailing at the time in general psychiatric research [6].

THE SECOND PHASE: THE FAMILY OF THE ANOREXIC AS A TOTAL SYSTEM OF PATHOLOGICAL INTERACTION

There are now extensive and numerous studies of the pathological way of functioning of families presenting a member designated as a psychiatric patient, and of the various methods of psychotherapy which have been suggested. I began to take a thorough interest in these studies only a few years ago, in 1965.

Most of these studies, and maybe the most important, concerned families that presented a member designated as schizophrenic. I had been struck by what Haley [4] had written ever since 1959 about the evolution of psychiatric research in schizophrenia:

> A transition would seem to have taken place in the study of schizophrenia; from the early idea that the difficulty in these families was caused by the schizophrenic member, to the idea that they contained a pathogenic mother, to the discovery that the father was inadequate, to the current emphasis upon all three family members involved in a pathological system of interaction.

If this was the conclusion to which research on schizophrenia clearly seemed to lead, it was natural to try and apply it as a working hypothesis to another severe psychiatric disorder such as A.N. *(anorexia nervosa.)* From a methodological point of view, moreover, this seemed to me to offer an advantage. Schizophrenia is still a vague nosographic category, applied to patients belonging to subgroups that differ widely in type of thinking disorder, affect disturbance, and course [9]. A.N., if correctly diagnosed, could provide a more precise and uniform area of family research because of its almost monotonously typical clinical picture.

Maybe this is also the reason why more recent pioneer research has been systematically expanding from the families of schizophrenics to the families of patients belonging to a great variety of diagnostic categories. The findings enabled Framo, in agreement with Laing and many other clinical and experiemental workers, to state in 1966:

> From the standpoint of a transpersonal family concept, schizophrenia, *or any other type of mental illness* (italics mine), can be looked upon as the only logical adaptive response to a deranged, illogical family system.

The theoretical problem could thus be extended to the family of the anorexic patient. Could A.N. be the only possible means of psychic survival for a given subject in the context of a given type of family functioning? Could a family system typical for the development of A.N. be discovered? A definite answer to these problems, if any such answer is at all possible, will require further years of clinical and experimental research and above all of systematic longitudinal follow-ups.

At any rate, the mere fact of becoming aware of the existence of the problem led me to adopt the new work methods, which could enable me to become a direct and participant observer of the type of transpersonal system of collusion in the families I wished to study. Laing had made a shrewd remark which was too obvious to justify any further methodological doubts:

> If one wishes to know how a football team concert or disconcert their action in play, one does not think only or even primarily of approaching this problem by talking to the members individually. One watches the way they play together [5, p. 7].

The Research Approach

So far, for the purpose of clinical research and therapeutic verification, I have set up some new working situations.

a. One or more conjoint family sessions, at the same time explorative and therapeutic, which systematically precede the individual treatment of patients referred for psychotherapy.
b. Psychotherapeutic treatment of the parents of a patient undergoing individual psychotherapy with a colleague.
c. Intensive co-therapy treatment, together with a male colleague with whom I have been working for years, of the parents of a cured anorexic patient of mine. The parents asked for therapy 3 years after the daughter's recovery.

(This treatment, among other things, enabled me to make an illuminating comparison between the material obtained at the time of the individual psychotherapy of the daughter and that obtained from the parents.

d. Intensive co-therapy treatment, together with the same colleague, of a young couple in which the wife, a chronic anorexic since adolescence, had also become a severe dipsomaniac after marriage.

Every time a patient suffering from A.N. is referred to me, I invite all the members of the family, including the designated patient, to the first interview. Almost invariably, the parents start the interview with the following statement: "If only we didn't have this daughter who drives us crazy with her obstinate refusal to eat, we'd be a happy family." However, when sufficient experience and capacity for observation have been acquired, even a single session of this kind, if long enough, enables one to become aware of the atmosphere of conflict and psychological violence in which the patient is placed and to which she contributes. Sometimes it is even possible, from the very first session, to observe and make the participants observe certain highly significant ways of behavior and transaction. Quite often, already in the course of these family sessions, I succeed in sending the designated patient a therapeutic message, in which I somehow, also by non-verbal means, try to convey to her that I realize how unbearable, at times tragic, her situation is.

The systematic use of conjoint family interviews has provided me with some valuable direct clinical material confirming or completing the observations I had made during the earlier individual treatments. It has also given me a unique opportunity, previously unsuspected, to motivate certain negativistic patients who were inaccessible to individual treatment.

Some Psychodynamic Formulations

The type of family functioning which I have so far been able to ascertain may be outlined as follows.

a. A fixation of the mother on a latent homosexual level. The father has deep passive tendencies, which may be concealed by counterphobic mechanisms. He often has an obsessive character structure.

b. A sadomasochistic relationship between the parents. More commonly, the more apparent sadistic behavior is shown by the father. The mother, however, knows how to exert an underhand influence and succeeds in being highly castrating, even with apparently submissive and nonverbal attitudes.

c. The designated patient is subjected to the mother's needs and cut off from any relationship with the father, who, for his part, accepts and reinforces this isolation.

d. The system prevents the designated patient from differentiating herself from the mother and going through a valid Oedipal experience.

THE HUSBAND-WIFE RELATIONSHIP

Neither spouse has ever adequately freed himself from the ties with his family of origin. If, as Bowen says [2], it takes at least three generations to "produce" a schizophrenic, it also certainly takes more than one to produce an anorexic. The husband never "really" married the wife, but only an idealized mother image of an oral type: attentive, efficient, protective, devoid of any identity or needs of her own and totally identified with his own needs, values, and duty patterns. Therefore, every time he sees an aspect of his wife's personality that is at variance with his fantasies, he feels abandoned, misunderstood, and unfairly treated. Very soon, sadistic communications convey his aggressiveness due to the frustration of his deep fantasy needs.

The wife, for her part, because of the husband's needs, sees in him many hateful characteristics of her own mother. She has had, and often still has, a very close relationship with her mother, made up of slavery, guilt, and hostility. The mothers of these women were demanding, hypercritical, possessive, and apparently strong. They segregated their daughters in a sort of superego matriarchate, in which the husband was considered a mere accident, socially and economically inevitable. The mothers of anorexic patients have for years humbly served their own mothers, in different ways according to circumstances and social condition. They acted as confidantes, servants, or nurses, and their obligations prevented them from developing an existence of their own, with its own meanings.

Sperling [7], in a paper of his, has correctly laid great stress on the harmful influence of the grandmothers in the families of anorexic patients. As Schwidder rightly points out [cited in 7], even when these grandmothers were not actually present in the family, or had been dead for years, their domineering spirit and influence continued to prevail, as alive as ever. The maternal grandmother's role may sometimes be assumed by the paternal grandmother.

Therefore, marriage appears to the mothers of anorexics to be a sort of liberation, the achievement of social status, dignity, and independence. Clinging to their dream, they choose not to observe in their partner, during their engagement, the many signs that should warn them of a conflicting reality. There is a symmetrical omission on the part of the future husband. They get married with the best of intentions and with many secret expectations which they have never dared to express clearly. Very soon, only the good intentions remain.

As for their sexual life, none of these women, because of their history, has reached a genital level. They are all clearly fixated at a latent homosexual level. The husband's sexual demands, which are sometimes insistent because of his need to be reassured about his virility, make them feel they are only an instrument for physical satisfaction.

These women are unsatisfied or depressed. Not only do they not dare to verbalize any of their deep feelings, but they often refuse to become fully aware of them. Communication between the two spouses, both terrified of acknowledging the failure of their relationship, becomes progressively more restricted, allusive, and disappointing.

Burning subjects, such as personal feelings, secret expectations and desires, and the resentment caused by relationships with the families of origin, are avoided by tacit consent. But behind the facade of order at any cost, there is permanent underground tension which produces moodiness, sulking, and irritability. Occasional aimless bickering about secondary matters provides effective concealment of the real problem. Periodic phases of stubborn silence show that both have given up communication in despair. The family atmosphere becomes progressively heavy and ritualistic. Feeding rites play an important part. Feeding in these families is often a complicated and tiring undertaking for the mother, who considers it a sacred duty and a burden. Various members follow different diets of have food fads. Feeding is pedantically and aggressively emphasized, and meals take place without joy, in a tense and moody atmosphere.

THE MOTHER-DAUGHTER RELATIONSHIP

The unsatisfied and unhappy mother very soon reestablishes with her daughter, with a vengeance, the same relationship she had with her mother. The chosen daughter is unconsciously consecrated to the consolation of her mother. She cannot afford *not* to be good, compliant, sensible, quick to satisfy her mother's expectations, without fancies and problems of her own (if she dares to ventilate any, the mother promptly provides the solution with some sound advice). It is very rare to find in the childhood of the anorexic the normal manifestations of the oppositional phase. If there were any, they are found to have been systematically eliminated and doomed to repression. Also, the school history of the anorexic is very often that of a model pupil, obsessively trying to live up to parental expectations.

If there are other children in the family, interesting patterns may be observed. The male is generally more respected, at times even highly considered. In any case, he is less involved in the pathological needs of the parents. If there is another daughter in addition to the designated patient, the mother establishes an entirely different kind of relationship with her. It is extremely rare to encounter two real anorexic patients in the same family (at the most, a sister may occasionally "copy" the symptom for entirely different dynamic reasons). I have had the opportunity of studying only one such case, in which, however, the fourth-born daughter became anorexic at puberty several years after the death from anorexia of the eldest daughter. In this case, an absolutely typical family system was built up again around the fourth-born daughter after the death of the eldest daughter.

More commonly, after the "sacrifice" of the designated patient, the sister or sisters are allowed to develop in comparative freedom. In my experience, however, when the designated patient had a sister, I often observed a different situation: there was a mutually highly erotic relationship between the mother and the sister of the designated patient. This sister is often very beautiful. Based on the latent homosexual tendency, the relationship between the two women is stormy and exhausting, constantly disturbed by quarrels due to mutual provocation. Deep down, however, the mother is in love with the rebellious daughter, she admires and envies her, for the daughter does all those things which the mother never dared allow herself to do. This daughter also knows how to be seductive with her father, albeit in an inauthentic and manipulative manner, and thus succeeds in obtaining much from him. The designated patient, for her part, has highly ambivalent feelings towards her sister: she admires, envies, and detests her. But, since she is incapable of inflicting frustration on such a suffering mother, she does not dare to imitate the sister. On the contrary, she emphasizes her compliance towards the mother and her perfectionism, in an attempt to obtain the consideration which seems to be denied to her. Eventually, only in the "illness" will she find the means to express at the same time her despair, her protest, and her desire to communicate. In several of the families of anorexic patients which I have studied, the erotic and stormy relationship of the mother with the rebellious daughter is for years a burden on the whole family and does not even cease when the daughter gets married. Actually, however, this daughter's adjustment is also very uncertain. I had evidence of this in two cases: after the psychotherapeutic recovery of the anorexic sister, the so-called healthy sister developed manifest neurotic symptoms.

In the course of the conjoint psychotherapy of the parents of the cured anorexic patient, we were surprised to find that one daughter, the rebel, seemed somehow to have impersonated the mother's id, while the other daughter, the anorexic, seemed to have impersonated the superego. These two agencies were irreconcilable within the mother and seemed to have found in the two daughters their respective "embodiments."

The following extract from a recorded session with the above-mentioned couple shows a striking connection with the bodily destruction carried out by the anorexic daughter.

> Wife (to husband): What did you see in me, then? Why did you keep coming close to me (i.e., having sexual relations) if there was no intimacy between us?
>
> Husband: Human frailty!
>
> Wife: And am I supposed to be the object of your frailty? (turning to the woman therapist) Ah! Mrs. S., how often at night, in bed, I longed to destroy my body, to reduce it to nothing, in order that he shouldn't have it. . . .

The latent homosexuality of the mothers of anorexic patients has always become obvious in their relationship with me. They very soon become seductive towards me and unconsciously competitive with me and with the daughter undergoing psychotherapy, for not only do I take her away from them, but she, for her part, takes me, the mother figure, from them.

Thus, the unresolved tie with her own mother prevents the mother of the anorexic from having a real marital and maternal experience. She is a highly ambivalent parthenogenetic mother. Her obsessive concern with her children makes her husband feel excluded from any relationship with her and with them. Though she is distressed by the husband's coldness towards the children, she persists in making him share only in the bothers, worries, and small daily mishaps concerning them.

THE FATHER-DAUGHTER RELATIONSHIP

The father, who for his part is already ambivalent and jealous towards the children because of his own dependence on his wife, becomes still more confused and irritated by the double-bind situation in which his wife places him. As he is incapable of clarifying this situation and changing its rules, it increases his isolation.

As far as the designated patient is concerned, she is almost completely cut out from a relationship with her father by the exclusive tie with her mother. If the daughter attempts to approach the father, the mother immediately interferes, using a thousand and one rationalizations: the father is too busy, she has to look after everything, report to the father, explain, act as mediator between the two (just as the daughter effectively acts as mediator in the couple's silence). The tendency to prevent the daughter from having an authentic relationship with the father is obvious, both in the family transactions and in the course of individual psychotherapy. In the second year of treatment of a 15-year-old anorexic, an only daughter, when the girl started having some timid positive feelings towards her father, the mother suddenly felt the need to reveal a secret to her daughter: she was only alive thanks to the mother, for at the first signs of pregnancy the father had insisted that the wife should abort.

The father, on the other hand, obeys the secret rule and does not attempt to approach his daughter. If he happens to be left alone with her, he is embarrassed, moody, and irritated. She is a stranger to him, a riddle which becomes unfathomable as the symptom develops. I remember the case of one father, a colleague of mine. He came by order of his wife to speak to me about his 14-year-old daughter, already a severe anorexic, and to entrust her to me for treatment, and he did not succeed in telling me anything more than his wife had told him to report. He had no personal observation, no intimate recollection, no experience of his own to contribute. The girl was literally a stranger to him. This experience has recurred repeatedly with many fathers of anorexic patients, including some who came to the interview dutifully primed on anorexia, having read my writings or even drawn a long chronological report on the daughter's "case."

Conjoint Therapy with Co-therapists

In addition to the positive results already obtained in other cases, two observations led me to apply conjoint therapy in these cases, in association with a male co-therapist.

a. The difficulties I encountered when I tried to conduct therapy alone with a mother-daughter couple were hard to overcome on account of the competitiveness which soon developed towards myself.
b. In my opinion, it is hard for only one therapist to modify this type of rigid family homeostasis, organized in dyadic subsystems. Many deep situations and defenses may be revealed, and the homeostatic system may thus be broken up, if a couple of therapists of different sex is introduced into the family situation, acts as a comparatively adult and maturely cooperating couple, and *stirs up and works mainly on transference and counter-transference reactions.*

Our experience so far is very limited and is restricted to the two couples mentioned above. It allowed us to make one interesting observation, however, because it repeated itself in both cases in identical terms. Despite numerous clarifications and the man therapist's determined efforts to enter emotionally into the situation, he was systematically excluded from it for months on end. Both partners seemed to connive at this resistance and would turn exclusively to the woman therapist, who was seen as a powerful and redeeming maternal figure.

Eventually, taking advantage of some emotionally charged situation, the man therapist succeeded in effecting an approach and in making his presence felt. This produced in both spouses anxiety reactions and the appearance of various resistances, including acting out in the form of missing sessions or leaving earlier on vacation. Then the resistence gradually broke down. Husband and wife started expressing strong emotions towards the man therapist, at times positive ones (the longing for a strong, protecting, and good father figure), at other times intensely negative ones (because he did not seem to participate actively enough, or because of fear of being criticized and abandoned by him). *When strong affective relationships with the man therapist made their appearance, the "idyllic" relationship with me also underwent rapid change.* The wives were the first to find the courage to express aggressiveness towards me. The dipsomaniacal wife, however, actually needed to enter into a clearly hypomanic phase in order to find the courage to behave in an overtly seductive manner towards my co-therapist. But at this point, my actual presence, though transferentially distorted, became crucially important. She was testing above all my reaction to her undertaking. Would I allow her to compete with me, to take my partner away from me, to take my place in the relationship with him?

In both our cases, the decisive moment of change came when the man therapist was no longer excluded, namely when a third member entered into the relationship and strong differentiated and differentiating emotions towards the members of the therapeutic couple arose. In the specific case of the dipsomaniacal wife, she relinquished her symptom the very moment she succeeded, in the positive relationship with the man therapist, in experiencing her body no longer as the symbiotic body for the mother but as the erotic body for the father.

These findings, however, should be repeated in other similar cases and with other therapeutic couples in order to control as systematically as possible the variables dependent on the type of functioning of a given therapeutic couple in its impact on a given family system.

For the time being, we may cautiously limit ourselves to saying that our type of functioning as a therapeutic couple in its impact on the two above-mentioned couples, has given rise to the finding described above. This in itself is sufficient to give an idea of the boundless complexity with which the psychotherapy of the family is faced in theoretical terms.

The Family and the Anorexic Crisis

At this point, research is faced with crucial problems. How does the designated patient's anorexic crisis fit into the type of family functioning described so far? Why does this type of functioning correspond to an anorexic syndrome at puberty and not, for example, to an adolescent psychotic crisis?

Only to attempt to answer the first problem would imply the comparative description of the intrapsychic and interpersonal dynamics of the puberal anorexic crisis, which lies outside the scope of this paper.

As for the second problem, I may try to suggest an hypothesis, though further data need to be obtained from control studies. In the course of individual psychotherapy, as I have tried to show in earlier writings, it appears that the anorexic crisis is *an extreme defense against psychosis.* Although very rarely, some families of anorexic patients present another member diagnosed as schizophrenic. In two families which have recently arranged for psychotherapy and have not yet been thoroughly studied, the anorexic patient is in one case the sister of a male who became schizophrenic at the age of 18, in the other case the sister of two young male schizophrenics, one paranoid and the other hebephrenic. Moreover, in studying some severe overeating and undereating patients, I was able to ascertain, by means of the technique of Thaler Singer and Wynne [8], disturbances of thinking, experience, and communication of a schizophrenic type. It may thus be inferred that in the families presenting only an anorexic patient the communicative distortion and the pathological way of functioning do not reach the degree of psychoticism to be found in the families of schizophrenics. In the families which, in addition to the anorexic patient, also present schizophrenic siblings, though there are severe distortions in the family system, the defect in the primary relationship and the anorexic patient's psycho-emotive involvement in the pathological system do not reach the extreme degree to be found in the case of the schizophrenic sib. The designated patient may find it possible to organize a complex defensive strategy which allows her, among other things, to keep a hold, although a tiring and precarious one, on reality and social relationships. This hold, however, implies the cruel sacrifice of a fundamental relationship with primary reality, that with her own body, its needs, and its rights. The attempt to survive as a person may thus become so distorted and tragic as to bring about the death of the very person that was trying to emerge.

Acknowledgments

I am greatly indebted to my co-therapist, Dr. S. Rusconi, and to the other members of the team, Drs. G. Boscolo, G. Chistoni, and S. Ferraresi Taccani, for having taken part in the discussion of the sessions.

Bibliography

1. Boszormenyi-Nagy, I and J. L. Framo, *Intensive Family Therapy*, Hoeber, New York, 1965.
2. Bowen, M., The use of family therapy in clinical practice, *Comprehensive Psychiatry*, 7 (1966), 345.
3. a. Bruch, H.,Transformation of oral impulses in eating disorders, *Psychiatric Quarterly*, 35 (1961), 458.
   b. Bruch, H., Perceptual and conceptual disturbances in Anorexia Nervosa, *Psychosomatic Medicine*, 24 (1962), 187.
   c. Bruch, H., "The psychiatric differential diagnosis of Anorexia Nervosa," in J. E. Meyer, and H. Feldam, Eds., *Anorexia Nervosa*, Georg Thieme Verlag, Stuttgart, 1965.
4. Haley, J.,Family of the schizophrenic: a model system, *Journal of Nervous and Mental Disorders*, 129 (1959), 357.
5. Laing, R. D. and A. Esterson, *Sanity Madness and the Family*, Basic Books, New York, 1964.
6. a. Selvini Palazzoli, M., *L'Anoressia Mentale*, Feltrinelli, Milano, 1963.
   b. Selvini Palazzoli, M., "*Interpretation of Mental Anorexia,*" in J. E. Meyer, and and E. Feldman, Eds., *Anorexia Nervosa*, Georg Thieme Verlag, Stuttgart, 1965.
   c. Selvini Palazzoli, M., Contribution à la psychophatologie du vécu coporel, *Evolution Psychiatrique*, 1 (1967), 149.
   d. Selvini Palazzoli, M., Die Bildung des Körpers bewusstseins, Die Ernährung des Kindes als lernprozess, *Psychotherapy Psychosomatics*, 15, 293.
   e. Selvini Palazzoli, M., Die Bildung des Körpers bewusstseins. Beitrag einer neuen Auswertung des Rorschach tests zur Untersuchung von Stoerungen der Korperlichkeit, *Psychotherapy Psychosomatics* (in print).
7. Sperling, E., "Die ≪Magersucht-Familie≫ und ihre Behandlung," in J. E. Meyer, and H. Feldman, Eds., *Anorexia Nervosa*, Georg Thieme Verlag, Stuttgart, 1965.
8. Thaler Singer, M., and L. C. Wynne, Principles of scoring communication defects and deviances in parents of schizophrenics. Rorschach and T.A.T. scoring manuals, *Psychiatry*, 29 (1966), 260.

9. a. Wynne, L. C. and M. Thaler Singer, Thoughts disorders and family relations of schizophrenics, *Archives of general Psychiatry*, 9 (1963), 191-9.
   b. Wynne, L. C. and M. Thaler Singer, *Archives of general Psychiatry*, 12 (1965), 187.

Address of the author: Mara P. Selvini, M. D. Director, "Centro per lo Studio della Famiglia", Via Keplero, 10 -20124, Milano, Italy

The Child with Pica and His Family

FRANCES K. MILLICAN AND REGINALD S. LOURIE (U. S. A.)

Introduction

The term pica, which has been broadly used to describe the craving for unnatural substances, the ingestion of substances unfit for food, or as a depraved appetite, has its origin in the Latin word for the scavenger bird, magpie. Our study of this problem at the Children's Hospital of the District of Columbia (Washington), United States, began with a need to find out why young children ate the substances which produced lead poisoning. Soon, children with pica which had not resulted in lead poisoning were included. These children persistently ate many different substances, included laundry starch, plaster, paint, paper, wood, crayons, cigarette ashes and butts, and frequently sought them in preference to food or sweets. Explorations of these patterns of ingestion led to consideration of the problem of accidental poisonings in preschool children. The presence of pica in many such cases made them appear less "accidental" than had been previously assumed, and revealed them to be a part of the pattern of pica in many children. Iron deficiency anemia has also been found to be an accompaniment of pica [2, 10] and led to our study of the relationship between certain nutrients and pica. These findings provided an indication for child health workers to include questions

*This study was supported by Public Health Service Grants M-1445 R MH, RG-5923R1, and the follow-up study by RO1 MH 15443.

about pica in the routine health care of all young children, and to consider all children with pica as possible lead-poisoning cases.

Pica was found to be widespread, no respecter of social class, an indicator of the existence of distortions in the mother-child relationship, and a manifestation of the use of oral activity as a solution to problems in close relationships. Previous studies of the psychologic aspects of pica include those of Kanner [8], Van der Sar and Waszink [23], Mellins and Jenkins [16, 17], and Wortis, et al. [25]. This report on children with pica not only presents our findings but describes the successive stages of the research as it developed.

The Research

Children normally explore their environment by mouthing, and occasionally even ingesting something, beginning about 5 months of age [5]. It is necessary to distinguish such normal oral activity from that which by its intensity or prolongation indicates that psychopathology in the form of an oral fixation or regression is present. We, therefore, arbitrarily defined a pica case as that of a child 18 months or older who had persistently ingested nonfood substances for at least 3 months immediately prior to the study. Only 9 of the children studied were over 6 years of age, the oldest being 14 years.

The research team consisted of a psychiatrist, a psychologist, a pediatrician, a social worker, and a nurse. There were two separate studies by the research team: (1) psychiatric and (2) nutritional. In the psychiatric study there were 154 children (125 Negro and 29 white) of whom 95 were children with pica and 59 were control cases (27 normal and 32 psychiatric controls). In the nutritional study all the children were Negro including 54 children with pica and 28 normal control children.

The basic diagnostic study consisted of history from the parents, psychological testing of the child, psychiatric playroom interview with the child, and Rorschach evaluation of 115 mothers. Seventeen children with pica and their parents were also seen in psychotherapy, thus providing better and more detailed understanding of these cases. The data was augmented in the course of the nutritional study through information gathered in home visits, socio-environmental survey, psychological testing of the children, and observations of mother-child interaction through a one-way viewing screen.

In order to meet the pressing medical and social needs of the pica children and their families, a Pica and Lead-Poisoning Clinic was established at Children's Hospital in 1957. The clinic has also furnished us additional data through the hundreds of children who have been seen there since then. Most of the pica children from the two research projects were followed in the clinic for several years after the initial evaluation. It was also found that the characteristic evidence of reluctance to participate previously manifested in many broken appointments in the department of psychiatry, was not as evident in the medical clinic setting, and we were thus able to reach more of the children who needed help. Here too, however, the families most in need of help often found it difficult to avail themselves of the clinic's services and "reaching out" was found to be necessary.

ILLUSTRATIVE CASES

The following cases of children with pica illustrate the types and varieties of problems encountered in them and their families.

CASE 1

Andy, the first child studied, was hospitalized with lead poisoning at the age of 3 years. He was referred to the psychiatry department a year later after two more hospitalizations related to lead poisoning. His craving for and ingestion of nonfood substances had continued since his first hospitalization. As is almost always the case in children, his pica produced lead poisoning because he chewed on substances painted with lead-containing paint. For him these included furniture, window sills, doors, and old wall plaster. Andy's pica had started at 27 months, soon after he left the grandmother who had cared for him since he was 2 months old and had returned to his parents, whom he had not seen meanwhile. For a long time after his return he was described as quite passive. Handling frustration was difficult for him. His mother was neglectful and he had difficulty in expressing his aggression toward her. Hyperactivity, lack of ability to control aggression and impulses in general, and distractibility suggested that he had suffered organic brain damage from the lead poisoning. Subsequently he developed convulsive seizures. During psychotherapy, separation problems were resolved, and he gave up his pica, although he occasionally used it as an aggressive threat, telling his mother that he would eat paint again if she did not meet his demands.

CASE 2

Ann was a 2-year, 7-month-old Negro girl who was admitted to the hospital in convulsions due to lead encephalopathy. In spite of immediate therapy for the lead poisoning, she was unable to hold her head erect, to see or hear. One month later there was some return of vision; motor development returned to the 15-month level, but in all other areas she functioned at the 9-month level. Her vocalization consisted of babbling. She put everything in her mouth. The parents gave a history which was somewhat vague as to time sequences, and were quite unaware of what had been happening in her everyday life. She was still receiving formula from the bottle at the time she was hospitalized. A pacifier had been used from 6 to 12 months. She had been toilet trained prior to hospitalization and said some words beginning at about 1 year. Nothing in the history indicated organic brain damage prior to the lead poisoning.

Ann's illness had occurred in the aftermath of a move by the family from a small Southern town to Washington, D.C. The father moved before the rest of the family and the child was separated from him for about 6 months, beginning at about 14 months of age. The mother had been depressed over the move because she had been reluctant to leave her home and felt exceedingly lonely, frightened, and overwhelmed by the new situation in which she was cut off from the usual support of her family and friends. For a number of months she spoke to no adults except her husband. She was resentful toward him, feeling that he did not give her adequate support for household expenditures; but she was unable to discuss this with him. Ann had always preferred her father and, in addition to the separation from him, at the time of the move she saw little of him in the new environment because he was employed at two jobs. Ingestion of peeling paint and plaster started after the move to Washington, although she had begun mouthing objects when she was about 9 months old, and had ingested some pebbles and other small objects including crayons, toys, and sticks when she started walking at 1 year.

The mother had great difficulty in relating to Ann and dealing with the realities of the child's illness. It seemed that not only had the child suffered the separation from the father, but also her mother had withdrawn from involvement due to her own depression. Our impression of the mother's personality from our study and work with her in the clinic and from the Rorschach testing was that of a somewhat schizoid, depressed, anxious woman who was only partially available for her mothering responsibilities. She seemed unable to accept the reality of the danger from pica. Even after extensive work with the staff of the pica clinic on the problem of the child's continuing pica, the mother blandly stated that she did not know what substances contained lead. In addition to her apparent unawareness, there was a strong cultural acceptance of pica in her family. She herself previously had a mild degree of pica. Later, in the mothers' group, when discussing pica she said very defensively, "All children eat dirt," citing her third child as an example. Her fostering of oral activity in her children was illustrated by continuing her children on the bottle with only perfunctory attempts at weaning. The patient had been given a minimum of solid food up until the time of hospitalization.

During the long follow-up of this child, it became evident that the organic brain damage which she had suffered limited what we could do toward her improvement. There was a partial return of hearing but no return of speech, and toilet training was accomplished with difficulty several years later. Her severe organic brain damage and retardation appeared to be the factors which made it impossible to stop pica. She was hyperactive and her uncontrolled aggressiveness included biting people. Plans were begun for eventual institutionalization when home management was no longer possible.

CASE 3

James, a 22-month-old Negro boy, was hospitalized along with his two older brothers because they had together ingested a bottle of aspirin tablets. Both the older boys had a history of pica and James, in addition, had blood lead levels indicative of asymptomatic lead poisoning, for which he was treated.

The parents had separated about 2 months prior to James' hospitalization. When the mother was interviewed, we learned that she had received shock treatment for schizophrenia following the birth of the baby sister. and subsequent tubal ligation, 5 months previously. The mother was quite depressed and was hallucinating at the time of the study. She was unable to care for the children, slept most of the time, neglected to feed them, and allowed the patient to play unattended in the street. During the course of the study the mother had to be hospitalized for mental illness and chronic alcoholism. The father assumed responsibility for the children, hired a housekeeper, and invited the grandmother to live with the family. James formed an extremely close attachment to her. The medical social worker with the Visiting Nurse Association helped the family with planning for the care of the children.

History revealed that both parents had eaten dirt themselves as children. Several unsuccessful attempts had been made to wean James from the bottle. He was able to form a relationship with the clinic staff. He was quite active in his play, displaying considerable evidence of oral concerns. He continued with some mouthing of objects but no ingestion. There was no evidence of Organic brain damage.

Subsequent to cessation of pica, James had nightmares, enuresis, soiling, and nail-biting and was obviously a very unhappy little boy. There were several shifts in mother substitutes in the family and later James required additional child guidance treatment because of behavior problems. We also learned that the sister subsequently developed pica, having been introduced to it by James. James himself had earlier been introduced to the habit by his next older sibling.

CASE 4

Billy was 4 years, 3 months old when he was referred by a physician because he spoke poorly and seemed to have emotional difficulties. He was the older of two sons of a 24-year-old Negro mother who had been separated from Billy's father since he was 2 years old. Both parents had some education beyond high school. They had been married two months after Billy's birth. The family lived with the great-grandparents who resented having to share the responsibility of caring for the children. Actually the mother had had very little to do with Billy's care from the beginning, since she had rejected her maternal role from his birth and did not like to hold him for feeding. However, she was the one who had to rock him to sleep until he was 1 year old. At 6 months of age, when he still had no teeth, he was fed table food.

Billy showed considerable upset about his brother's birth when he was 1 year, 9 months old and would steal the baby's bottles and drink them. At 3 years, Billy began nail-biting, and 10 months later he began to have pica which consisted of eating pencils, crayons, and chewing on the desk. He was afraid of the dark and could not sleep until his mother sat beside him. Even at age 4, he was expected to do household chores. At the time of the evaluation, he was found to have an I.Q. of 125. He showed a frantic desire to relate to adults in the hope of getting his dependency needs met. He showed considerable anxiety about aggression. The mother openly rejected him and identified him with his father. She competed with him for having her own needs met. On one occasion in the waiting room she took the child's candy bar away from him and ate it. It was reported that he in turn would often steal his mother's beer to drink. On one occasion the mother told Billy's therapist in the child's presence that she would be delighted to give the child to the therapist. His unmet infantile needs seemed to be represented by infantile speech, pica, and sleep disturbances. After psychotherapy Billy's pica stopped. It returned, however, for two periods later: at the age of 5 when the termination of therapy coincided with his beginning school; and again a year later at age 6 when he returned to stay with his mother after spending the summer with his grandmother.

Factors Responsible for Pica

Pica has been known since ancient times and occurs on every continent [1, 2, 11]. In the United States pica is common in the urban slums, in the southeastern states, and in some Indian tribes. In this study we were concerned with pica in a population most of whom lived in the economically deprived sections of the city and most of whom were Negro. The sampling was not random; we studied those children who were referred to us and whose families were willing to participate. Some of the multi-problem families were so disturbed that they were unable to follow through on referral, even with active support from us.

The results of the research have led us to conclude that a combination of factors underlies the selection of pica as a symptom, with these various factors contributing to a different extent in each child. Some of the factors are from the child's constitutional makeup and others occur in the course of development in relation to interaction with his family and his environment [12-14, 19-21], including problems involving availability of the mothering functions.

CONSTITUTIONAL FACTORS

Children with the types of marked organic brain damage or mental retardation which made controls difficult seemed more prone to the development of pica, and in these children the symptom was very difficult to modify. Kanner [8] and Wortis [25] have also reported upon the association between pica and organic brain damage and retardation.

Constitutionally, children differ in the degree of intensity of normal oral drives and also in their willingness to relinquish oral activities. An extra amount of help may be necessary from parents both of the damaged child and of the normal child with a high degree of oral activity in order to help the child relinquish these activities and move on to the next phase of development. The combination of a high level of oral interest, prolonged hand-to-mouth activity, and unavailability of someone to supply controls from the outside, set the stage for the next step, ingestion.

CULTURAL AND ECONOMIC FACTORS

From early in these studies more children with pica from Negro low-income families were being referred to us than from the white or upper-income population. In order to determine whether this ratio

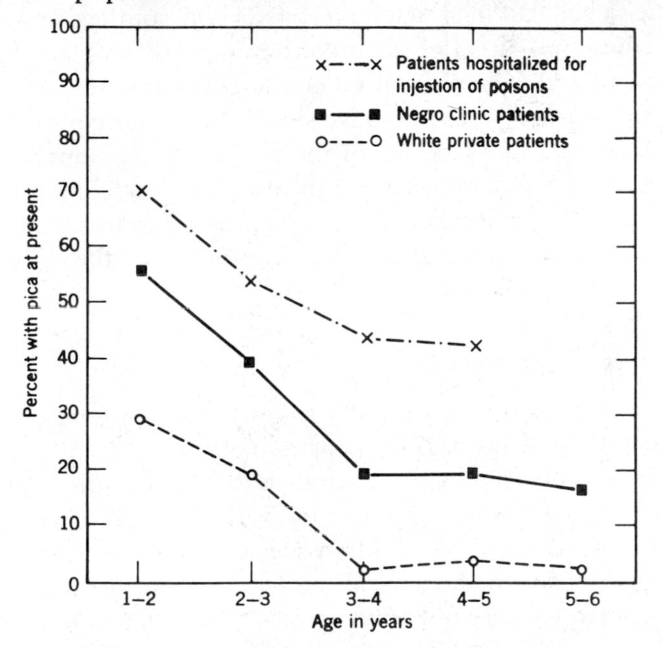

Figure 1 The prevalence of pica.

was representative or merely a function of our sources of referral, a survey of the prevalence of pica was undertaken (see Figure 1) [20]. Three segments of the population known to Children's Hospital were surveyed: Group I, children from low-income families; Group II, children from middle- and upper-income families; Group III, all children hospitalized for the ingestion of poisons over a specified 11-month period. The children surveyed were from 1 to 6 years of age. Of the 486 children in Group I, 32 percent ingested nonedible substances, whereas only 10 percent of the 294 children in Group II did so. Of the 79 children in Group III, 55 percent had pica, indicating the close association between pica and accidental poisoning. The prevalence of pica dropped sharply in both groups after the age of 3 years, but was still higher among the Negro children at all age levels. The difference between the occurrence of pica in the Negro low-income group and in the white middle-income group was statistically significant. Small samples suggested that children in the white low-income group and the Negro middle-income group had pica to a degree comparable to that occurring in the Negro low-income population.

For the Negro children studied, cultural factors were particularly important. The families to which this segment of the research population belonged had migrated largely from the southeastern United States, where the eating of earth containing clay, and laundry starch is a frequent and widely accepted custom. The mothers of the children with pica were found to have significantly more pica themselves as adults than did the mothers of the two control groups without pica. Sixty-three percent of the children with pica had mothers who also had pica. Some mothers taught their children to eat such substances as laundry starch or dirt, but in other cases the child simply identified with his mother's pica [12].

NUTRITIONAL FACTORS

It has been suggested repeatedly that pica is an attempt to supply some essential missing nutrient, particularly iron [2, 10]. It is probably true that pica has been resorted to throughout the centuries to assuage hunger pains when food is unavailable [1, 2, 11]. It was observed that a few of the children seen in the pica clinic were grossly malnourished and a number of them were anemic; therefore, it was decided to carry out a nutritional study at Children's Hospital of D.C. to determine the influence of nutritional deficiencies in the etiology of pica.

Results of this nutritional study showed children with pica to be normal by anthropometric evaluation and on clinical examination when they were compared with control children. They did tend, however, to have had less adequate diets, showed lower levels of ascorbic acid in the plasma, have slightly lower hemoglobin concentrations, have more reported respiratory illnesses, and have more recorded days of hospitalization than the control children without pica. In spite of these findings two double-blind experiments failed to show that iron given intramuscularly or that a multi-vitamin and mineral preparation given daily were any more effective than were placebos in eliminating or modifying the habit of pica. From these studies we could not conclude that pica was caused by a deficiency of any of the nutrients which we studied. It would seem, though, that poor economic conditions and inadequacies in child care are factors both in the etiology of the symptom of pica and of inadequate nutrition of the child [6, 7]. The reverse, however, can be true as has been shown in two reports where the prolonged eating of large amounts of dirt has produced anemia and even death [4, 18].

PSYCHIATRIC FACTORS

The major diagnoses of the children with pica are given in Table 1. Only the primary diagnosis for each child is tabulated for the total group of 95 children, but for all children over the age of 5 years both primary and secondary diagnoses are recorded. In the older age groups it will be noted that these children had the most severe psychopathology, as would be expected.

Although the psychiatric diagnoses varied, certain behavioral characteristics were significantly present in the pica children. They had a high degree of other oral activities including mouthing of inedible objects in addition to ingesting them, thumb-sucking, nail-biting, and feeding problems. They were, as a group, somewhat retarded in their use of speech, and some even withheld speech.

Pica children had some characteristics in common with those reported by the McCords in a longitudinal study of children who later became alcoholics [15]. They showed conflicts about their dependency needs and also conflicts around the handling of aggressive feelings, with considerable negativism. As would be expected, the pica children exhibited various other symptoms: rocking, head-banging, hair-pulling (and sometimes eating). In older children there were fears, nightmares, enuresis, temper tantrums, uncontrolled aggression, fire-setting, stuttering, oral-genital sexual play, compulsive masturbation, and phobias.

Twelve of the 95 children in the pica and lead-poisoning group had severe or moderate organic brain damage which was not due to lead poisoning and preceded the pica. Eleven more children had suggestive evidence of brain damage which was not the result of lead poisoning. The children over 3 years of age with pica showed the most severe psychopathology. In these cases pica seemed to occur more frequently in children whose weak or defective ego functioning was due to organic brain damage or schizophrenic disorders. Neuroses and personality disorders, especially impulse control difficulties, also occurred in this group. As with the older children in general, the 17

Table 1 Diagnoses of Children with Pica

	Major Diagnosis, Total Group (*N* = 95)	All Diagnoses		
		6 Years and Over (*N* = 9)	5 Years (*N* = 8)	4 Years (*N* = 13)
None	2			
Brain damage	14			
Severe		2	4	5
Suggestive		3	3	1
Mental deficiency	1			
Severe		2	3	2
Mild		4	1	1
Psychosis	9	3	2	3
Psychophysiological	0			
Neurosis	8	2		2
Personality disorder	28		6	6
Schizoid		3		
Other		1		
Transient personality disorder	33			

white children in the study also had more severe difficulties. For the younger Negro children their mothers' cultural acceptance of pica was of major etiological significance. In these cases the children very frequently identified with their own mothers' pica and there was less internalization of a prohibiting superego in regard to pica in the child's immature ego. Where this occurred, the basic psychopathology was not usually as severe as among the white children or the older Negro children.

PSYCHODYNAMIC FACTORS

As is obvious from the case reports, separations from one or both parents or emotional difficulties in the mother which made her unavailable for nurturing the young child were found in many (47 percent) cases. Although the patients studied were largely from the marginal income Negro population where there is a high incidence of family instability, separations of a major order were still more frequent in the pica group of children than in the normal control group. That these patterns are not characteristic of this Negro group alone is evident from the reports of Pavenstedt, et al., in *The Drifters* [22], which describes the functioning of 3 multi-problem families, only 3 of whom were Negro. The clearly delineated psychosocial characteristics of the nursery-school-aged children in these families and the family psychodynamics have marked similarities to the largely Negro population of our study.

The incidence of pica (63 percent) in the mothers of the pica children was significantly higher than in either of the control groups. Mothers who had pica themselves also showed evidence of other forms of oral fixation: obesity, alcoholism, and drug addictions. Alcoholism and drug addiction were also found among the fathers of the pica children. The psychiatric diagnoses most frequently found among the mothers of the children with pica were passive-aggressive personality disorders and neurotic depressions. The mothers who were psychotic, alcoholic, depressive, or with personality disorders of passive-aggressive, schizoid, or paranoid types were particularly unavailable to nurture the child's dependency needs.

One of the most important factors in the choice of pica as a symptom was the mother's encouragement of oral satisfaction as a substitute for a satisfactory personal relationship when dealing with the child's anxiety. One mother described this: "Whenever he fusses I give him about an ounce of milk in a bottle." The mothers seemed unable or uninterested, frequently, in exploring the children's feelings or responding to them but rather shunted the child to oral satisfaction as a way of dealing with anxiety. Encouragement of oral activity also occurred in the form of late weaning (i.e. after 2 years) or vacillating weaning, or by the use of pacifiers well beyond infancy. Pica was seen most frequently where there was excessive gratification of the oral drive; excessive frustration was found in some cases, however.

The Therapeutic Approach

The first approach to treatment was through the pica clinic. The staff consisted of pediatrician, social worker, nurse, and psychiatrist or psychologist. Medical aspects included follow-up of cases of lead poisoning to prevent repetition, and early detection or prevention of lead poisoning for other children with pica. In an effort to prevent neurologic sequelae, children with pica were screened for toxic blood lead levels. Anemia was treated, if present.

An educational approach was employed with the mothers, since most of the children were quite young. Since lead paint and crumbling ploster were frequently found in the older homes of the inner city, where many of the patients lived, the mothers were particularly warned about the dangers of paint ingestion. They were told which substances contained lead and of the danger that the child with pica, in particular, might ingest other poisons such as medicine and household cleaners. They were encouraged to discontinue excessive oral satisfactions in older children by weaning them from the bottle. It was recommended that children be firmly directed away from pica, and that the mother at the same time, if possible, also devote some time to the child. Although we recognized the difficulties, both conscious and unconscious, that might prevent a mother from carrying through on such a recommendation, many mothers were able to change their handling. Counselling was also offered about developmental and behavioral problems.

The role of the social caseworker was extremely important in helping the family with the problems that were interfering with their care of the child. Social casework dealt with critical financial problems, marital problems, and relocation into more adequate housing. Families were guided toward further help from other community resources. In many cases, when family stresses were reduced, and the mothers had some of their own dependency needs met, they were able in turn to provide better nurture for their children. Many younger children were still flexible enough in personality structure that their pica disappeared.

This more superficial supportive and educational approach was effective in the large majority of cases. When it seemed indicated by the persistence of the symptom of pica, or the presence of other symptoms, a complete diagnostic psychiatric evaluation was performed. The children with more fixed or severe psychopathology, principally the older children, usually required psychotherapy.

Follow-up and Outcome

In the psychodynamics of many of the cases, pica had many of the qualities of an addiction. There was a distorted instinctual satisfaction which was impulsively engaged in as a defense against the loss of security [3]. This led us to postulate that these children who had turned to an oral craving to solve a relationship problem might be addiction prone – and might return to orality as a solution to problems in later life [9]. Fortunately in June 1969, we were able to begin a follow-up study of the children from the original study whose ages now range from 12 to 24. This study has just begun, and it is too early to draw any conclusions as to our hypotheses at this stage.

Early information suggests that we are finding a wide spectrum of outcomes, with some children functioning quite well, and others having deteriorated. For a number of families there has been an improvement in family income and overall sufficiency. This may be partly a reflection of social changes in this country, and partly that the families have been able to use the assistance offered them. Some of the children are functioning well in school or on jobs, and three are enrolled in colleges. On the other hand, for some of the pica . children, the difficult experiences of their early years have continued. They have suffered further parental deprivations in the form of death, desertion, or hospitalization for mental illness. Information is being collected about the persistence of oral habit patterns that could lead to later, or true, addiction.

Summary

Pica is the persistent ingestion of substances not fit for food and is the cause of practically all cases of lead poisoning in children. It is also associated with "accidental poisonings" and was found to occur in 55 percent of such children hospitalized for other nonlead poisoning. It is important from the psychological point of view because it is evidence of an oral fixation or a regression. The psychiatric findings reported here were based upon the study of 95 children with pica and 69 children studied as normal or psychiatric control cases. The nutritional study comprised 54 children with pica and 28 normal control cases. The relevant factors operating in the etiology of a given case vary in their relative importance in each child. Those discussed are constitutional, cultural and environmental, nutritional, and emotional. Eight percent of the children studied had suffered moderate or severe organic brain damage prior to lead poisoning. These and other constituional differences in the strength of the child's oral drives and the child's endowment of ego apparatus account for a small proportion of differences in oral activities and thus in pica. The infant begins exploring the environment by mouthing and occasionally ingesting substances at about 5 months of age. For the next year, adequate mothering is needed to control ingestion. The attachment to inanimate objects begins early in this period and is the beginning of transitional phenomena as described by Winnicott [24]. A deficiency in the cathexis of the mother and a distortion of the normal progression to attachment to the symbolic transitional object may occur, with a fixation on the early libidinization of pica substances. Pica is often related to the loss of the mother and as such is related to depression. Severe persistent pica even before 18 months of age is suggestive of some degree of psychopathology.

Many of the Negro mothers of children with pica came from a cultural background in which pica is accepted, and 63 percent had pica themselves. If the mother thus accepts pica or consciously or unconsciously fosters the use of oral defenses against anxiety (by late or vacillating weaning or late use of a pacifier), the child is more likely to both identify with the mother's pica and her use of oral activity as a defense against anxiety and to continue to have pica. However, maternal fostering of oral activity of itself does not produce pica unless parental deprivation occurs concomitantly. Even within the low economic subculture where separations from parents and the use of many mother surrogates are commonplace, separations occurred much more frequently in the pica group than in the normal group. Emotional difficulties in the mothers, particularly personality disorders of the passive-aggressive type and neurotic-depressive patterns, interfered with their ability to respond to the children's needs and to help them to deal with their feelings. Often the child was shunted to oral satisfaction.

Personality studies of the mothers revealed passivity, narcissicism, poor control of impulses, manifest anxiety, and neurotic and depressive personality structures. Two mothers were psychotic. There were significantly more oral habits (alcoholism, drug addiction, and pica) among the parents of children with pica. White children and Negro children over the age of 3 years who still had pica had the most serious psychopathology. In children over 6 years of age, poor reality testing due to brain damage or psychosis in either the mother or child played a major role. In these children pica is a very difficult symptom to treat as is the basic pathology. Other psychiatric diagnoses of older children with pica included neuroses and personality disorders, both situational and fixed types.

Certain behavioral characteristics were significantly present throughout the cases. Children with pica had a high degree of other oral problems, including thumb-sucking and psychological feeding problems. As a whole, they were somewhat retarded in speech development and some withheld speech. They showed conflicts about dependency needs and about handling of aggressive feelings and exhibited considerable negativism.

That multiple factors contribute to the etiology of pica means that the treatment must be comprehensive, including medical, family social services, and psychiatric services.

Bibliography

1. Anell, B and S. Lagercrantz, *Geophagical Customs*, Upsalla, Sweden, Amquist and Wiksells Boktrycheri Ab, 1958.
2. Cooper, M., *Pica*, Charles C. Thomas, Springfield, Ill., 1957.
3. Fenichel, O., *The Psychoanalytic Theory of Neurosis*, Norton, New York, 1945, pp. 65-66, 375-386.

4. Gardner, J. E. and F. Tevetoglu, The roentgenographic diagnosis of geophagia (dirt-eating) in children, *J. Pediat.*, 51 (1957), 667.
5. Gesell, A. and C. S. Amatruda, *Developmental Diagnosis: Normal and Abnormal Child Development,* Paul B. Hoeber, New York, 1941.
6. Gutelius, M. F., F. K. Millican, E. M. Layman, G. J. Cohen, and C. C. Dublin, Nutritional studies of children with pica, *Pediatrics,* 29 (1962), 1012-23.
7. Gutelius, M. F., F. K. Millican, E. M. Layman, G. J. Cohen, and C. C. Dublin, Treatment of pica with a vitamin and mineral supplement, *Am. J. Clin. Nutr.,* 12 (1963), 388.
8. Kanner, L., *Child Psychiatry,* 3rd Ed., Charles C. Thomas, Springfield, Ill., 1957.
9. Knight, R. P., The psychodynamics of chronic alcoholism, *J. Nerv. Ment. Dis.,* 86 (1937), 538-548.
10. Lanzkowsky, P., Investigation into the aetiology and treatment of pica, *Arch. Dis. Child.,* 34 (1959), 140.
11. Laufer, B., *Geophagy,* Field Museum of Natural History, Anthropological Series, 18, No. 2, Chicago, Ill., 1930.
12. Layman, E. M., F. K. Millican, R. S. Lourie, and L. Y. Takahashi, Cultural influences and symptom choice: clay-eating customs in relation to the etiology of pica, *Psychol. Rec.,* 13 (1963), 249.
13. Lourie, R. S., E. M. Layman, F. K. Millican, B. Sokoloff, and L. Y. Takahashi, A study of the etiology of pica in young children, an early pattern of addiction. In *Problems of Addiction and Habituation,* Hoch and Zubin Eds, Grune and Stratton, New York, 1958.
14. Lourie, R. S., E. M. Layman, and F. K. Millican, Why children eat things that are not food, *Children,* 10 (1963), 143.
15. McCord, W. and J. McCord, *Origins of Alcoholism,* Stanford University Press, Standford, 1960.
16. Mellins, R. G., and C. D. Jenkins, Lead poisoning in children, *Arch. Neurol. Psychiat.,* 77 (1957), 70.
17. Mellins, R. G., and C. D. Jenkins, Epidemiological and psychological study of lead poisoning in children, *J. Amer. Med. Assn.,* 158 (1955), 15.
18. Mengel, C. E., et al. Geophagia with iron deficiency and hypokalemia-cachexia africana, *Amer. Med. Assn., Arch. Int. Med.,* 114 (1964), 470.
19. Millican, F. K., E. M. Layman, R. S. Lourie, and L. Y. Takahashi, Study of an oral fixation: pica, *Jour. Am. Acad. Child Psych.,* 7 (1968), 79.
20. Millican, F. K., E. M. Layman, R. S. Lourie, L. Y. Takahashi, and C. C. Dublin, The prevalence of ingestion and mouthing of non-edible substances by children, *Clin. Proc. Child. Hosp. D.C.,* 18 (1962), 207.
21. Millican, F. K., R. S. Lourie, and E. M. Layman, Emotional factors in the etiology and treatment of lead poisoning, *Amer. Med. Assn. J. Dis. Child.,* 91 (1956), 144.
22. Pavenstedt, E., Ed., *The Drifters,* Little, Brown & Co., Boston, 1967.
23. Van der Sar, A., and H. M. Waszink, Pica (report on a case), *Docum. Med. Geog. Trop.,* 4 (1952), 29.
24. Winnicott, D. W., Transitional objects and transitional phenomena, *Int. J. Psycho-Anal.,* 34 (1953), 89-97.
25. Wortis, H., R. Rue, C. Heimer, M. Braine, M. Redlo, and A. Freedman, Children who eat noxious substances, *J. Amer. Acad. Child Psychiat.,* 1 (1962), 536.

Family Variation and Mental Health

*Introductory Comment**

G. CONDOMINAS (FRANCE)

One of the fathers of modern ethnology, Marcel Mauss, in the course of a discussion which followed the communications of the psychologists, Pierre Janet and Jean Piaget, at the third international meeting on Synthesis in 1931, made the following comment on the second of the two speakers:

> Piaget, in my opinion, has not constructed a general psychology of childhood but a psychology of highly civilized children. It is necessary to consider other kinds of children coming from very different social and cultural enviroments [20, Volume 3, pp. 300].[1]

As a matter of fact, psychologists and psychiatrists have, for a long time, confined their interest uniquely to Western society, satisfied with extrapolating to other cultures the conclusions that they have drawn from observations made in this particular one; as a result, they have simply looked for elements of divergence from these Western standards among the so-called primitives, as manifested in dreams, myths, and certain aspects of ritual, notably the ritual of procession. One can recognize this attitude in the work of Freud [2, 4, 5].

*Translated by E. J. Anthony.

[1] This statement must be considered within the historical context of the year 1931 and in relation to the fact that it came not from a prepared text but from a spoken intervention, so that the terms, used by Mauss, such as "highly civilized children" and "very different environments" would be better understood today as "children of Western societies" (speaking technologically) "and cultures" (in the sociological sense) [19].

The ethnologists, in their turn, soon discovered explanatory possibilities in the casework of psychiatrists, observing analogies between certain types of behavior and reasoning of "primitives" and those suffering from mental disorders in their own Western society. The work of Levy-Bruhl furnished them with numerous illustration [11, 12]. Psychoanalysis, from its beginning, also exercized a very powerful influence on investigators in this area. The names of such pioneers as Malinowski, Roheim, and Mead, among others, bear witness to this, and it was from this point of departure that they developed interests in problems of education, psychology and psycho-pathology of children [13-17, 22-24, 26-28].[2]

What lies behind the development of these interests among ethnologists? Right from the beginning, as if in some way the study of the individual interferred with the understanding of the group, sociology experienced considerable difficulty in establishing itself as a separate discipline from psychology. A reading of the three volumes recently published by Mauss makes this abundantly clear [21].[3] Ethnology, in contrast, had, for the past two hundred years, focused its attention on non-Western societies, with emphasis on cultural differences, and had arrived more easily to the point of recognizing the structure and functioning of groups as such. In their case, it was the individual facets of behavior that came as a surprise. Some of this behavior did not correspond at all to that was considered normal in the Western societies from which they came. This raised the crucial question whether the norms of mental health were valid only for a particular setting or were universally applicable. Would the behavior of an individual that was diagnosed as pathological in a Western setting be regarded as such by members of his own group? It must be surely admitted that this is not the case. For example, the comparison of non-Western societies by Benedict demonstrated the existence of radically divergent norms each imposing its own "normal" patterns of behavior that differed completely in different archaic societies, so

[2] I have not mentioned in the bibliography the earliest books and articles or those only bordering on the present topic. I am also not directly acquainted with the work of Roheim published in Hungarian which I have nevertheless included in the reference [26].

[3] In his examination of the relationships between the two disciplines in 1924, Mauss, thanks to his erudition and unusual sensitivity, clearly saw the directions of research that was realized very much later. On this point, the preface by Levi-Strauss to *Sociology* and *Anthropology* should be consulted [20].

that a particular form of conduct could be considered an abnormal in one group and not only justified but recommended by another [1].

The gold mine of information that biographical inquiries and autobiographical accounts laid bare to ethnographers has been a factor in bringing them closer to psychologists and psychiatrists, from the point of view of both content and the mode of investigation in which interviewing played a major role. It was from this that the ethnologist's interest in certain aspects of psychoanalytic technique originated [2, 3, 9, 29]. One particular book that proved a landmark in the history of effective collaboration between ethnologist and psychiatrist was *The Individual and his Society* by the psychiatrist-psychoanalyst Kardiner, who collaborated with the ethnologist Linton [7]. This work was published in 1939 and along with a subsequent book by Kardiner on the concept of the "basic personality" [8] demonstrated to psychiatrists the necessity for making observations from the point of view of other cultures, having a different frame of reference regarding normality. It laid particular emphasis on the educational process, especially the type of infant care. Kardiner insisted on the consequences of these factors for the child's subsequent adjustment as an adult in his society.

The enormous work load on the level of everyday living forced on psychiatrists by the industrial and urban societies have not only tended to turn them away but also caused them to forget the seminal findings of Kardiner and his colleagues.

The work presented here has the special merit of reminding us of the exceptional richness the combined ethnological and clinical approach offers to the child psychiatrist and psychologist working in various cultures and more especially non-Western ones.

The Five Studies

These five studies do not pretend to cover the totality of problems that cultural differences give rise to in child psychiatry across the world. The sample is too restricted and, moreover, if ever there was a research area requiring a thorough and deeper approach it is that concerned with childhood and education. Nevertheless, these examples are sufficiently varied to demonstrate the specificity of certain traits or the interrelatedness of different characteristics and the practical consequences that ensue from this.

ECOLOGY OF CHILD REARING

After reading through the entire series, a preliminary thought presents itself. In relation to the Indian, Turkish, African, and Sudanese examples provided by Kahtri, Sumer, Collomb and Valantin, and Cederblad, Haggard's account of the isolated farm life on the mountainous regions of northern Norway seems categorically different. Ecology has enlarged (may one say to the point of exasperation) on the type of systematized relationships involving young children and adults that is met with frequently in the different environments of Western Europe. In the arctic world, on the farms of the northern mountains, the young mother, overwhelmed by her multiple tasks, is forced very early to abandon her baby to his own resources leaving him by himself at first in the parental bedroom and later in the kitchen. As a contrast, in the four other societies studied, one is struck by the nonisolation of the infant, socialization being constant. Characteristically, a sensual quasi-symbiotic dependency ties the infant to his mother for both nourishment and transport. She carries him continually on her back whether she be at home or out in the fields and even when she sleeps she keeps him pressed against her body. And the more she gives him the care he demands, the more does he manifest his imperative wishes.

Toilet training and weaning take different forms in the four societies. Weaning, especially, is a critical event, since it marks the rupture, more or less brutal according to the society, of the exclusive dependence on the mother. But even when this separation is brought about in the most precipitate fashion, the baby is by no means thrust into isolation. Depending on the type of care sponsored by each of the four societies, the separation is in part compensated for by the fact that the familial environment is more than the nuclear group; it is part of a much larger system which is the extended family, clan, or lineage. The infant is thus constantly in the milieu of "uncles" or "aunts" (to use our terminology) who are ready to take care of him.

MODERNIZATION, URBANIZATION, AND ACCULTURATION

Whatever the consequences of this kind of upbringing from a psychiatric point of view, the whole business becomes complicated by the intrusion of the modern world or, rather, the absorption by the modern world of all these societies. None of them, backward or isolated as they may be, are able to escape this process. This gigantic acculturation, which penetrates the entire surface of the globe to its remotest corners, starts slowly but gets increasingly accelerated. It is with this that these various authors are chiefly concerned; not so much with adequate medical aid or the development of techniques of mass communication (obviously of great importance for education) but rather with the fact of rapid urbanization that is responsible for the destruction of traditional social structures beginning, in the first place, with the family group and subsequently with other various groupings of individuals. The source of trauma for the adult originates in the struggle with the norms and techniques brought about by the new socio-economic conditions in the absence of any visible link to the previous way of life, and if the effect is as powerful for children as for adults, it is because the child's security is undermined by the fact that he is dependent on parents who are themselves maladjusted to their new environment.

It is clear from this that the crisis stemming from urbanization does not spare the isolated mountaineers of the north, the ancient nomadic Sudanese, or the Turkish peasant. But in the urban setting itself, the matter is somewhat different and viewed differently. Both adult and child see their social horizon enlarged and experience less misery, since the standard of living is relatively high. This is what drives the migrant to the city, for it offers him the social benefit of more or less regular contact with a circle of individuals who are other than members of his immediate family. One must not underestimate the material attractions of a life which is not only less arduous but offers many distractions. This is no less the case for the African as for the Turkish peasant; the latter finds that the life he leads in the transit camps of Istanbul and Ankara is more acceptable to him than what he had in the village from which he came. This urban migration has occurred in all places where the extended family group still continues to exist. Following migration, the life of the child is confined to his nuclear family, and even when the separation that follows weaning from the mother is rendered less brutal (as in India for example), he is no longer able to find, as in previous times within the larger family, surrogate mothers with which to replace her. Moreover, his mother goes out more often to work. It is, perhaps, in relation to the woman that modernism and particularly the urban revolution has brought about its most striking changes, especially in Turkey and in India where the woman was greatly debased. It cannot be denied, least of all in relation to this, that modernism has made some very positive contributions to the life of the family.

Conclusions

These interesting problems, as much theoretical as practical, made prominent by these five studies should hopefully encourage the child psychiatrist and psychologist to extend their investigations to a larger number of different social environments. The diversity of cultures, providing a variety of groupings and the many consequences on the level of pathology should make it possible, even if limited to the practical aspects alone, to better understand and treat more effectively the increasingly frequent and serious disturbances provoked by urbanization. The study of the psychiatric problems of childhood within the framework of urban living must certainly be carried out for every culture which means in every city; a city, in effect, constitutes a new culture in the process of formation. The study of a single urban variable is not enough, because there is nowhere in the Western world where one can, with any justification, claim that the new culture is in equilibrium or moving towards it. And yet, this is what one does imagine when confronted with the external monolithic appearance of a great metropolis like New York, Paris, or London. Everywhere, the conflicts and the mixtures between the cultures and the original subcultures of the migrants demand that we study not only the immediate effects but also use these as a starting point for other studies that will allow us to achieve a better understanding of the crises stemming from this type of urbanization. There is also a need to mention the relevance that this kind of research has for theory, within the frame of the diversification of a major variable in the development of the child, cultural variability.

Bibliography

1. Benedict, Ruth, *Patterns of Culture,* Houghton Mifflin Co., Boston, 1934.
2. Devereux, George, *Reality and Dream: The Psychotherapy of a Plains Indian,* Prefaces by Karl A. Menninger and Robert H. Lowie; psychological tests edited by Robert R. Holt. International Universities Press, New York, 1951.

3. Dollard, John, *Criteria for Life History, with Analyses of Six Notable Documents.* Published for the Institute of Human Relations by Yale University Press, New Haven, 1935; Reprinted, 1969, Peter Smith, New Haven.
4. Erikson, E. H., *Observations on the Yurok: Childhood and World Image.* University of California Publications in American Archaeology and Ethnology, 46, No. 10; Berkeley, 1943.
5. Freud, Sigmund, *Totem und Tabu.* French translation *Totem et Tabou,* Payot, Paris, 1929.
6. Janet, P., and J. Piaget, "L'individualité," *Centre international de synthesè. Troisième semaine internationale de synthèse,* 1931, pp. 51 sq., 118-120 sq. Alcan, Paris (Interventions de Marcel Mauss reproduites dans *Oeuvres* III, pp. 298-302, sous le titre "Debat sur les rapports entre la sociologie et la psychologie"), 1933.
7. Kardiner, Abram, in association with Ralph Linton, *The Individual and His Society.* Columbia University Press, New York, 1939.
8. Kardiner, Abram, with the collaboration of Ralph Linton, Cora Dubois, and James West, *The Psychological Frontiers of Society.* Columbia University Press, New York, 1945.
9. Klunckhohn, Clyde, "The Personal Document in Anthropological Science," in Louis Gottschalk, Clyde Klunckhohn, and Robert Angelli (eds.), *The Use of Personal Document in History, Anthropology and Sociology,* Social Science Research Council, New York, Bulletin 53, pp. 70-173, 1945.
10. Lévi-Strauss, Claude, "Introduction à l'oeuvre de Marcel Mauss," in Mauss, 1950, pp. IX-LII, 1950.
11. Lévy-Bruhl, Lucien, *Les Fonctions mentales dans les sociétés inférieures,* Alcan, Paris, 1911.
12. Lévy-Bruhl, Lucien, *La Mentalité primitive,* Alcan, Paris, 1922.
13. Malinowski, Bronislaw, *Argonauts of the Western Pacific.* An Account of Native Enterprise and Adventure in the Archipelagoes of Melanesian New Guinea. With a Preface by Sir James George Frazer. Routledge and Kegan Paul, London (Studies in Economics and Political Science, no. 65), 1922.
14. Malinowski, Bronislaw, "Psychoanalysis and Anthropology," *Psyche,* IV (April), 293-332 (reprinted in Malinowski, 1927), 1924.
15. Malinowski, Bronislaw, *Crime and Custom in Savage Society.* International library of Psychology, Philosophy and Scientific Method. Routledge and Kegan Paul, London, 1926.
16. Malinowski, Bronislaw,*Sex and Repression in Savage Society.* International library of Psychology, Philosophy and Scientific Method. Routledge and Kegan Paul, London, 1927.
17. Malinowski, Bronislaw, *The Sexual Life of Savages in North-Western Melanesia.* An Ethnographie Account of Courtship, Marriage and Family Life among the Natives of the Trobriand Islands, British New Guinea. With a Preface by Havelock Ellis. Routledge and Kegan Paul, London, 1929.
18. Mauss, Marcel, "Rapports réels et pratiques de la psychologie et de la sociologie," *Journal de Psychologie Normale et Pathologique,* XXI, pp. 892-922 (Reprinted in Mauss, 1950. pp. 281-310.), 1924.
19. Mauss, Marcel, cf. P. Janet and J. Piaget, 1933 and Mauss, 1969.

20. Mauss, Marcel, *Sociologie et Anthropologie*, precédé d'uné Introduction a l'oeuvre de Marcel Mauss par Claudé Levi-Strauss. Presses Universitaires de France, Paris (4e édit. augmentée en 1968), 1950.
21. Mauss, Marcel, *Oeuvres*. Présentation de Victor Karady. Paris. Les Editions de Minuit; Vol. I. *Les fonctions sociales du sacré*, 1968; Vol. II. *Représentations collectives et diversité des civilisations*, 1969; Vol. III. *Cohésion sociale et divisions de la Sociologie*, 1969 (includes Mauss 1931), 1968-1969.
22. Mead, Margaret, *Coming of Age in Samoa*, W. W. Morrow, New York, 1928.
23. Mead, Margaret, *Growing Up in New Guinea*, W. W. Morrow, New York, 1930.
24. Mead, Margaret, "An Investigation of the Thought of Primitive Children, with Special Reference to Animism," *Journal of the Royal Anthropological Institute*, Vol. 62 (1932), pp. 173-90.
25. Mead, Margaret, "Research on Primitive Children," in L. Carmichael (ed.), *Manual of Child Psychology*, John Wiley and Sons, New York, 1946.
26. Róheim, Géza, "L'ours et les jumeaux" (en hongrois), *Ethnographia*, Vol. 25 (1914), 93-97.
27. Róheim, Géza, *Australian Totemism*, Allen and Unwin, New York, 1925.
28. Róheim, Géza, *Psychoanalysis and Anthropology:* Culture, Personality, and the Unconscions. International Universities Press, New York. *(Psychanalyse et Anthropologie.* Culture- Personnalité - Inconscient Traduction francaise par Marie Moscovici; avant-propos et bibliographie des travaux de G. Róheim par Roger Dadoun. Gallimard, Paris, 1967. Collection "Connaissance de l'Inconscient"), 1950.
29. Talayesva, Don C., *Sun Chief. The Autobiography of a Hopi Indian*, edited by Leo W. Simmons. New Haven: Published for the Institute of Human Relations by Yale University Press. (*Soleil Hopi. L'autobiographie d'un Indien Hopi.* Textes rassemblés et preséntés par Léo-W. Simmons. Traduction de Genevieve Mayoux Préface de Claude Lévi-Strauss. Paris: Plon 1959. Collection "Terre Humaine"), 1942.

The Black African Family

H. COLLOMB AND S. VALANTIN (SENEGAL)

Introduction

To speak of *the* African family presupposes a homogeneous Black Africa (south of the Sahara) where all the institutions, cultures, and individuals are identical.

Africa is certainly not a monolithic i.e. institution where all men live, think, and feel in the same way, where all social systems and cultural values are identical. The human milieu is as diversified as the landscape and the physical environment.

Nevertheless, all those who have had the opportunity to study African populations, both inside Africa and outside the African continent, have been able to discern, beyond the diversities of languages, customs, and social heritage, a comprehensive cultural unity comparable to what we call Western European, Islamic, or Indian civilization. This unity, made up of the whole of the elements common to all societies within traditional Africa, is *"Africanity"*.

"An inventory of these common elements covers all the cultural domains: production techniques (e.g., the cultivation of burnt land), economy (e.g., team work on collective fields), politics (e.g., decisions based on unanimous rather than majority opinion), kinship (e.g., solidarity with their family line), family (e.g., plurality of wives), religion (e.g., veneration of ancestors), philosophy (e.g., the idea of the unity of a vital force underlying the multiplicity of living beings), the arts (e.g., the representation of man's mental image in an expressionist manner), etc...." [2] This enumeration gives only one series of examples.

For the subject which interests us here, we could add maternity customs (e.g., the carrying of babies on the mother's back), the place accorded to children, the passage rites from one phase of existence to another (e.g., ritual circumcision), and the organization of age categories.

The origin of this imposed unity is of little importance and is perhaps due to a physical environment which is hardly favorable to economic development and which has contributed to sparseness of population, to the historic isolation of the African continent, and to inter-ethnic mixing inside the continent. This leads us to speak in a general way of an African civilization, an African culture, the African family.

The unity of the African family depends on a traditional idea of the family. But this traditional organization is today subject to external pressures due to the rapidity of modern social changes. These disintegrating forces grow as the phenomena of Western acculturation, urbanization, and industrialization become more widespread. Some regions, groups of the population, and social classes are more affected than others by these processes which impose an evolution towards other kinds of family organization, and the resulting diversification is parallel to the degree of penetration by foreign models rather than to ethnic dissimilarities.

Our experience is essentially limited to Senegal. The literature concerning the African family is made up, above all, of descriptive ethnological, sociological, or anthropological monographs. Few physicians, psychiatrists, or psychologists have studied the dynamics of relationships inside the family. The ideas that we are going to try to delineate are based on close contact with the families of the mentally ill, on surveys, and on naturalistic observations of the families. We will borrow heavily from the work in process at the Center of Psychopathological Research at the University of Dakar [20, 19]. This will help us to extend our ideas to include Black Africa in general.

There is no general theory about the family which could serve as a reference and as an analytic instrument. The sociological definition is purely descriptive: it is either a conjugal group composed of parents and children (limited, nuclear, elementary family); or it is a primary group with structures differing according to matrimonial modes (extended family).

The meaning of the word "family" includes a system resulting from the behavior of society's individual members as well as an institutional subsystem. In family behavior, it is possible to separate a series of determinants (somatic, psychological, social, and cultural) in the same way that it is possible to analyze the integrative capacity of each member within his own status and his own roles. As an institution, the family is a part of another dynamic system with its prohibitions and rules of conduct which are laid down by the society as a whole with its economic and political imperatives, its process of growth and change. "To want to explain the family is to want to explain the conditions of man's existence and to ask the most fundamental questions about human existence" [10].

However, it is impossible for us to deal with this here. We will limit ourselves to some of the aspects of the African family, chosen because of their interest for the clinician. After a summary definition of physical and demographic frameworks as well as social and cultural ones, we will consider family life and intrafamily relationships, and finally the transformations of the family and their effects on mental health along with social changes.

Physical And Demographic Frameworks

THE PHYSICAL ENVIRONMENT

The physical environment has often been considered to be one of the basic elements in the structure of men and societies. Generally speaking, the physical environment in Africa is hostile to man. In this elementary fact lies an explanation for many human problems.

Schematically, intertropical Black Africa lies within a belt of 5000 kilometers, between two deserts – to the north the Sahara and to the south the Kalahari – which separate it from the temperate zones (North Africa and South Africa). However diversified the landscape may be (savanna, forest, or even mountain), it does possess common characteristics: immensity, sparseness of population, absence of "humanization," that is to say, of changes brought about by man.

The contrast between the small village, the usual form of settlement, and the vast expanse of the bush or the forest, is striking. The bush represents nonsocialized space, entered only with great precaution, where certain essential and basic activities are forbidden (for example, procreation). It is the locale of dangerous spirits, of evil encounters, of the asocial madman. Living space is arranged into three areas: the village, field, and bush; social and economic activity is limited to the first two. Beyond them lies a universe without limits, hostile and threatening.

Time is measured by seasonal rhythm, a dry season and a rainy season, which regulates activity (sowing, harvesting). In desert or forest areas, the seasons last longer: the continuous drought in the desert or the unceasing rainfall in the forest.

Although varied, the climate is characterized everywhere by intense heat, continuously high humidity, brutal variations between the dry and the humid season. Beside the fact that this climate hardly stimulates activity, it influences human pathology (adaptation to seasonal changes, the extent of diseases transmitted by insects).

In rural environments, the general hygienic conditions favor the spread of *diseases*. The African child is still today subject to serious endemic or epidemic diseases (malaria, measles, meningitis) which are difficult to cure, particularly since the lack of protein weakens his defenses and retards his development. However, Africa is not a continent suffering from malnutrition, in comparison with other areas of the world. Dietary deficiencies are far less widespread than is usually supposed, despite an extremely low average income: $80 (U.S.) per year per person [12].

Four-fifths of the inhabitants live in centers of less than 2000: the characteristic entity is the small village. The number of people living in *cities* is still low; but this urban population poses special problems. Life is easier than in the bush from which there is a continuous exodus. African cities are expanding with dizzying speed (a progression from 6 to 15%, compared to 2.5% for all of Black Africa). Within the last 100 years, Dakar has gone from 1600 to 500,000 inhabitants. This accelerated urbanization has had a profound repercussion on family organization.

DEMOGRAPHIC DATA

Demographic data, although only fragmentary and approximate, tally and make it possible to define, within a broad general outline, the populations of Black Africa.

Two hundred million inhabitants[1] are spread out over a vast expanse south of the Sahara, with a density of 8 persons per square

[1] Aside from the rare states where a white colony exists (Rhodesia, the Union of South Africa), the proportion of Europeans is very low, always less than 1%.

kilometer. Wide variations exist: 0.8 in Mauritania, 50 in Nigeria, 200 on the high plateaus of East Africa. This populaton is made up of some *300 ethnic groups* which until now have succeeded in remaining pure-bred. Every 200 or 300 kilometers the "race," the language, the customs change. Each country includes at least ten ethnic groups. In Tanzania (East Africa), there are more than 120 "tribes." This polymorphous aspect of the African population has not yet been explained; it does not contradict the idea of Africanity.

In spite of the great number of urban migrations, the still essentially rural population remains attached to the traditional ways of life. The usual pattern is as follows (just about the same for each state): a large city drains away 10 percent of the population; 10 percent are divided between cities of 10,000 to 50,000 inhabitants; the remaining 80 percent are in the villages. Nigeria and East Africa are an exception to the rule because of the density of their population.

The *sex ratio* (number of men for every 100 women) is on the order of 97, higher than in Europe. The *age pyramid* is characteristic of a young population. In the French-speaking African states as a whole, more than 50 percent of the people are under 20 years of age; 35 to 45 percent are under 15 years of age.

Polygamy is practiced in all animistic societies and is legal according to unwritten African law, which is often inspired by Islam. On the one hand, it is observed by a well-to-do minority and the traditional chiefs and on the other by the rural populations and the small wage-earners of the big cities. In Dakar, one man out of 6 is a polygamist; out of 100 polygamists, 83 have 2 wives, 14 have 3 and 3 have 4. The number of wives increases with age. Bachelorhood is the exception.[2] Men marry later than women, at 25 and 18 years of age, respectively. Divorce and repudiation are very frequent; in Dakar, 50-year-old women have, on an average, been married twice.

Throughout all of Africa, the *birth rate* is very high: 40 to 50 for 1000 inhabitants (France 18.5, U.S.A. and U.S.S.R. 25). The African woman has repeated pregnancies which begin soon after the marriage and occur on an average of every 3 years; the number of pregnancies varies between 8 and 12. The rate of reproduction is also very high; each woman gives birth to 3 daughters on an average. Sterility has

[2] In the cities, 4 percent of the women are unmarried.

not been properly estimated as yet; however, the ratio seems rather high (17 wives out of 100 to the north of Senegal). Gynecological ailments, and above all inbreeding, might be responsible for this.

The *mortality rate* is also very high: for French-speaking Africa, 19 to 35 per 1000, with an average of 27 (in France 10.8). Life expectancy is between 38 and 42 years of age (in France, 70 years); for those children who live to 6 years of age, life expectancy is likely to be 55 years. An *extremely high rate of infant mortality* is characteristic. Miscarriages are frequent and many infants are stillborn. Strictly speaking, infant mortality varies from 150 to 250 per 1000 with an average of 230 for French-speaking Africa (in France, 21 per 1000). This rate is lower in the cities where endemic-epidemic diseases are less serious and a higher level of medical assistance exists. There are two dangerous periods: the first 2 weeks of life (death almost immediately after birth due to malformation of the pelvis or premature birth), and towards the twelfth month when the infant succumbs to infections, parasitic diseases, the consequences of feeding errors (insufficiency or suppression of mother's milk). After the first year, the mortality rate remains high: 1 child out of 2 does not live longer than 5 years; half of the deaths registered in the cities are those of children under 5 years of age.

Migrations are very frequent, motivated by economic reasons, by the attraction of the big cities, or by some obscure tendency (the migrating instinct). The consequences vary a great deal. They depend on family cohesion, the receptiveness of the new environment, ethnic solidarity, the potential for adaptation and the state of the labor market. Quite often the city is not prepared to receive the migrant who comes to look for work to improve the lot of his family which is remaining behind in the village. In spite of this, the risks of maladjustment, of delinquency, or of drug addiction are still relatively small and mainly confined to adolescents.

The African population is even now characterized by a high birth and mortality rate. It is undergoing rapid growth and progressive aging. The physical environment continues to be brutal, despite the advances in sanitation.

Cultural And Social Frameworks

Most African societies are in a state of transition. The changes brought about, first by colonization then by modernization, have left their mark on the cultural and social frameworks according to the degree of penetration of foreign patterns, of economic evolution towards a monetary system, and of diversification of professional activities.

The African is traditionally a farmer and only incidentally a shepherd or fisherman. The technical differentiations are limited to several skilled specializations (blacksmiths, jewelers, woodworkers, leather workers, cloth weavers). The caste system still adheres to a very rigid stratification in many of the societies (nobles or chiefs, warriors, peasants, artisans, *griots*[3] or singers). The social unit is the family in the broad sense of the word (extended family), organized according to systems of kinship. The head of the family, determined by age, exercises final authority, administers the collective property, distributes its proceeds, and settles conflicts. Education is based on fidelity to tradition, which ensures group cohesion and maintains the group's adhesion to its family line. Religions and cosmogonies tie man to his ancestors and to the universe, and they lay the foundations for his intimate participation in the spiritual and physical world.

While these frameworks continue to organize existence, they are being weakened in the cities. There are two signs indicative of this latter tendency: the growth of the educational system and the increase in new job activities. About 30 to 40 percent of the children between 6 and 14 years of age are now attending school; in some countries the figure reaches 60 percent (Gabon) and even 80 percent (Congo-Brazzaville). The distribution of activity still falls short of that of the European countries[4]: the primary sector, the exploitation of resources (agriculture, fishing, mines), still occupies 80 percent of the men and 90 percent of the women who work; the secondary sector, transformation and transportation industries, 5 to 10 percent of the men and 1 to 3 percent of the women; the tertiary sector, services, 7 to 12 percent of the men and 2 to 5 percent of the women. However, new categories of workers, wage earners, employees, and government functionaries have appeared; and, above all, the idea of the individual salary and a monetary economy to replace the subsistence economy has been introduced.

[3] A *griot* is an itinerant musician often credited with supernatural powers.

[4] In France, the distribution is approximately one-third for each sector.

On all levels of economic and social life, interference by the State and by political institutions is growing, resulting in a modification of family structures. Power has not yet changed hands; the family still plays a great number of its roles, but evolution is effecting a gradual change from traditional economic and social units toward the modern State.

Imported religions (Islam, Christianity) also modify the family structure and transfer a part of its authority to religious chiefs (marabouts or priests). In some completely Islamized countries, the family model has evolved towards the Moslem type which gives greater authority to the husband and depends less on the family line and ancestors. In the Christianized societies, polygamy has diminished and God has replaced the family lineage as the point of reference.

In the series of structures which continue and overlap – the individual, the family, the society – the family is growing weaker, while the individual and society are growing stronger.

It would be difficult to form a synthesis and to present clearly defined types of families, although it is always possible, given a concrete situation, to uncover the different pressures that have modified the family structure and the play of intrafamily relationships. In an effort to show the foundations on which the African family continues to rest, despite the recent contributions of colonialism and imported religons, and those, more recent still, of modernity, we will analyze its traditions and dimensions while indicating the modifications they have undergone or are in the process of undergoing.

FILIATION AND LINEAGE

"Rights, privileges, obligations are all determined by kinship. Any individual must be either a real or a fictive kinsman, or a stranger to whom you owe no reciprocal obligation and whom you treat as a virtual enemy." This phrase of Evans-Pritchard regarding the Nuers can be applied to all of Black Africa [18].

The individual's place in society is not defined by a series of guide lines which indicate his profession, his educational level, his social class, his income, or his religion but by a family lineage and his place within that line. The individual only exists and is differentiated from others insofar as he belongs to a family line and is situated in relation to the others within that line.

The two family lines, that of the father and that of the mother, are not always equivalent in the family and social organization. There are patrilineal and matrilineal societies, as well as societies where both systems coexist with one or the other predominating.

In patrilineal systems, kinship, hierarchy, and the transmission of property is decided upon according to the masculine line of descent, while the woman remains a stranger within the family.

In matrilineal systems, it is the uterine line which is the deciding factor; the family head is the representative of the eldest woman of the eldest generation. The surname, the property, the chieftancy are handed down by the women, but through man to man, from uterine uncle to nephew. Within this system, the mother's brother wields the real authority over the child. When the child is grown up, he goes to live with his maternal uncle[5] who will pay the matrimonial sum at the time of his marriage and from whom the child will inherit. The predominating lineage determines the roles and the status of each person and shapes intrafamily relationships.

The family line (going back to the mythical ancestor), implicit in daily life, finds expression above all at the high points of existence: birth, marriage, exploitation of a new field, death. Cut off from his family line, the individual no longer exists, just as he cannot conceive of himself as existing without having children and leaving descendants.

The family line is not only experienced on a quasi-biological level by the collective body, but is also a veritable institution of social security. In order to fulfill its functions efficiently, it is organized according to the principles of solidarity rather than of authority. While the main role is played by the eldest, the wisest, and the one most filled with the strength of his ancestors, from whom he is but barely removed, all the adult men who act as heads of their households can give their opinon. The eldest is the one to whom they listen most, but he does not really command. Ancestral family

[5] In African languages there are four words to designate uncle, corresponding to four different positions and roles depending on which lineage predominates: (a) in patrilineal systems, the subject owes respect and obedience to the father's brother and cannot marry his daughters (incest); in exchange, he will receive property and will be taken care of if he becomes an orphan; he is intimate, even impertinent, with his mother's brother and he can marry his daughters; (b) in the matrilineal system, everything is reversed; the mother's brother plays an important role, the father's brother a small one.

decisions are never dictatorial or sanctioned by physical means. The strict dependence of the individual upon the group brings him to accept its decisions quite as a matter of course.

In addition to the lineage, whose trace dims after four or five generations, kinship is the basis for the constitution of larger and wider groups: the clan groups together individuals who share a common ancestor, the same taboos and the same totem; the tribe, as a wider community whose common ancestor is hypothetical, groups together individuals who share the same customs, the same language, a similar vision of the world, and an always vital feeling of belonging together. Less than lineage but more than the tribe, the clan symbolizes the importance of kinship in daily life and in social structures.

Although the importance of lineage has not been profoundly modified in barely acculturated animist societies, it has been somewhat weakened by Islam which, by introducing patrilineal consanguinity in a direct line, has strengthened the authority of the father over the women and children. Modernization fragments the lineage principle and separates the generations one from the other; but the cohesion of the basic group always manifests itself at life's difficult moments.

MARRIAGE

By definition, marriage unites two family lines and two different clans. The aim of marriage is twofold: on the one hand to assure the continuity of the lineage and, on the other, to form an alliance with another family line so as to enrich one's own and increase its strength. The future marriage partner must be someone outside the line (exogamic marriage). The union between descendants of a common ancestor can be defined as incestuous although in reality, many marriages are formed within the same family line (endogamic marriage).

Incest is a universal conception whose limits within a given kinship are extremely variable. Rules exist which specify the restrictions relating to *endogamy* while at the same time favoring it: some marriages are prohibited, others recommended. Among the Wolof of Senegal, for example, preferential marriages are those between crossed cousins (children of the paternal aunt or of the maternal uncle). Marriages between parallel cousins (children of the maternal aunt or of the paternal uncle), which were formerly forbidden, have since been authorized by Islam. Preferential marriages (endogamic) strengthen the cohesion of the family line; they are also thought to be dangerous because their breakdown causes the dislocation of the group.[6]

An extremely rigorous caste endogamy also exists among certain societies. Among the Serer of Senegal, the nobles (*guelwar, diambur*), the descendants of warriors (*tiedo*), the artisans (*nienyl*), the *griots* (*guewel*), marry only within their own group; the same is also the case with civil and war prisoners. Finally, there is an ethnic endogamy, wherein marriages seem to be conceivable only within the same ethnic group: 92 percent of Toucouleur women in the region of the Senegal River have married a Toucouleur.

Exogamic marriage, which may have been the preferential marriage of small groups in the past (exchange of women), is becoming more and more frequent with increased Islamization and modernity.

Traditionally, marriage is not an individual affair; it concerns all "the fathers and mothers" and all "the brothers and sisters" of the two partners (consanguine fathers and mothers, fathers and mothers by classificatory extension, brothers and sisters of the father and mother). The family line of the woman must receive compensation for the loss of one of its active members – from the economic point of view – and for the loss of a source of fecundity (the possibility of increasing the strength of the line). This is the origin of the *dowry.* The dowry complicates the marriage system: it signifies not the purchasing of the woman but an exchange. The terms and conditions as well as the size of the dowry are extremely variable; it makes marriage prohibitive for those young people who do not have the means to offer the sum demanded, which is sometimes very high. So long as the dowry has not been paid, the children belong to the mother's kinship group. In matrilineal societies the matrimonial compensation always operates in the same way.

The best interests of the family line guide the *choice of the partner*; personal taste must take a back seat. However, accommodations do exist. In cases of conflict, unwritten laws permit the boy or girl to win acceptance for their wishes if they have sufficient energy

[6] This is a very generalized idea. Each favorable or advantageous situation is dangerous; it elicits envy and intimidation and must be protected by special rites. This is the case with pregnancy, for example.

to resist family pressures. In the case of separation, the younger children remain with the mother and the older ones with the father, if the dowry has been completely paid up.

Although *polygamy* is accepted or even recommended in most ethnic groups, in fact many unions are monogamous; but a man's prestige is still measured by the number of wives he has. In rural tradition, where each wife (and her children) constitutes a unit of agricultural production, a polygamous marriage represents several economic units. In the cities, the situation is reversed: only the husband works, and he must give the same income to each of his "households" so as not to cause rivalry between them, a rivalry which is liable to break out at any time on any pretext.

Divorce is very frequent, and the considerable conjugal mobility which results does not generally have serious consequences for the children of extended families. They are taken in charge by relations, and educated by older age groups and initiation societies.

The evolution of African societies is altering the traditional terms of alliances and marriage. Marriage is becoming a more personal affair; the rules of endogamy are losing their force; group cohesion is no longer the desired objective. Many adjustments have been brought about by Islamization, the advent of Christianity, the pressure of modernity, and the outcome of legislation. The public authorities are also taking over more and more responsibility for the codification of family regulations.[7]

KINSHIP

The idea of kinship is both precise and vague: precise, because it assigns to each individual his place in the system of descent and marriage at the same time that it defines roles, status, and attitudes; vague, because it goes beyond blood relationship to other groups (classificatory kinship). This extension singularly complicates the clinician's task of getting the familial constellation in perspective when it becomes necessary to locate an individual within his family setting and understand his relationships.

[7]The government of Senegal has set up a family code which has established rules for giving or not giving the dowry, regulating the expenses relating to familial ceremonies (engagement, marriage), limiting or abolishing polygamy, condemning repudiation of the wife, codifying divorce and alimony laws, and freeing the woman to become her own mistress.

Although there are several words to designate a parental function, designated in other parts of the world by a single word (e.g., "uncle"), a single word can also be used to designate individuals far removed from the direct line, or even totally outside it, who nevertheless play similar roles. The latter is the case for the designation father, mother, brother, sister, grandfather, and grandmother. These "multiple fathers and mothers" include not only the parallels of the parents of the subject but also men or women who have only a remote kinship with the actual parents of the subject or who have in common with them only age or generation.

On the whole, consanguine kinship (1) extends, on the one hand, to the blood relations of the subject's marital partner and, on the other hand, to the partners of the subject's blood relations; and (2) extends horizontally to increasingly vague blood relatives or those belonging to the same age group, and vertically to increasingly distant ancestors reaching back to mythical ones.

Thus, the African lives within a kinship network which is widely extensive, very tightly woven, and very complex, and in which, for each function and for each situation, attitude and behavior are defined by tradition. In each society, the boy or girl learns progressively during childhood about the rights and obligations of each kinship role they will have to assume. Nothing is left to improvisation. This social organization ensures an extraordinary solidarity. There is no place for solitude. Each member of the group is duty-bound to give mutual aid and protection. The complement to this is a quasi-total investment in relationships with others, a rigidity of behavior, an absence of liberty and autonomy, and an extreme dependence on the human environment.

Contemporary changes are causing these ties to lose some of their vitality, but they still remain tenacious, dictating conduct which may at times seem incomprehensible to an outsider.

TRADITIONAL EDUCATION AND AGE CATEGORIES

Traditional education aims at the harmonious integration of the individual into the group, in keeping with the status assigned to him by his sex and by his rank in the brotherhood and, contingently, by his caste, the objective being to make of the individual a unit comparable to all others, if not identical [16]. In traditionally defined societies (according to Riesman's terminology), in which competition does not exist and roles are limited and defined by factors which do not take the individual personality into account, education aims essentially at adaptation. This involves teaching both the elementary techniques necessary to individual and collective life (agricultural techniques, stock farming, fishing, warfare, and even love-making) as well as the intangible elements of culture (historical and cosmological myths, genealogy, codes for human relations, dancing, music, everyday magic practices).

Up until weaning, which occurs between 18 months and two years, education is the mother's responsibility. After weaning, the division according to sex becomes progressively accentuated; boys and girls are educated earlier by their older brothers and sisters, and later by adults of the same sex.

The entire group, therefore, participates in education, which is a continuous process integrated into everyday life. All the older individuals "teach" the younger ones, an entire age category taking responsibility for the younger age group. This system also assumes more ritualized or specialized forms: groups of educators indoctrinating groups of children of the same sex and age; initiation societies preparing the adolescent for adult life after circumcision, the instruction taking place in the bush.

Except for the Koranic school, there is nothing comparable to the European system with its specialized personnel whose sole activity is that of teaching.

Education continues until adulthood is reached, and even later; it is a progressive initiation into a way of life. Each step towards knowledge and progression towards the adult status corresponds to "*age categories.*" To be more precise, an age category includes all individuals of the same village or several neighboring villages who are going through those different stages determined by their age which, as much as their generation category, defines position, rights, and obligations.

The passage from one stage to another is celebrated by "passage rites" which serve to mark the progression and to more closely integrate the individual into the group.

Among the Wolof of Senegal, a man's development takes place by way of the following categories:

Lyr, the fragile infant carried on the back who must be protected against the evil spirits and jealousy on the part of others by means of numerous protection rites.[8]

Perlitte, at the time of weaning (2 years of age), celebrated by a ceremony which separates the child from the mother's breast and back, but leaves him under her close supervision.

Goune, from 4 to 7 years, left alone or with children of his own age within the limits of the concession.

Khale, from 7 to 15 years, henceforth responsible and ready to be educated, to participate in work.

Aate, from 15 to 20 years, not yet adult but no longer a child, enduring the teasing and the humiliations inflicted by the adults, especially by the women.

Djouli, that is to say "wounded," circumcised, re-born (death of childhood, birth to adulthood), with all the weaknesses relating to this birth and all the apprenticeship necessary for a new life. He goes off into the bush with the others in his age category to learn to become a man by enduring a series of ordeals which prepare him for the basic ideas that guide the existence of his people.

Beurlotte, a "completely new man" when he leaves the circumcision camp; and then rapidly, *Wakhambane,* that is to say, a man like the others, not yet married; *Borom-Keur,* head of his household but still obedient to the chief of the family; and finally *Kilifa,* the peak of the hierarchy, who possesses supreme wisdom and authority in the eyes of his milieu.

With regard to women, starting at the age of 7, the different stages prepare her for her roles of wife and mother.

The age categories, which come into effect at adolescence, constitute a family whose solidarity is as powerful as that of blood. Their social functions are complex, covering the economic, the military, the political, and the religious. They meet on certain occasions, either to organize the work requested by the community or a family chief, or to discuss village affairs and make decisions.

Traditional education has been affected first by Islam and then by scholarization. A part of the collective authority constituted by the age hierarchy has been displaced by Islam in favor of the Marabout.

[8] The stages of the early years are still more diversified: *Nar* before baptism, *Lyr* from the ninth day to the third month, *Supintel,* that is to say, able to move about, from 8 months to 2 years.

At the age of 7, the child, on becoming *talibé,* is entrusted for a number of years to the *Marabout* who, after God, possesses power of life and death over him. While studying and reciting the Koran, he also works for his master, thereby learning submission and courage.

In a more far-reaching way, traditional education has been affected by scholarization which has impoverished it and simplified it without causing it to disappear altogether. The authority of age is no longer recognized; the child is no longer integrated into the age categories where essential virtues are developed. All that was collective duty has now become a matter of individual choice. Competition and solitude have taken the place of solidarity and fraternity. Reactons against this evolution are setting in, and the African governments are giving their attention to the problem of reconciling the demands of the modern world with African cultural values.

Family Organization And Intrafamily Relationships

The individual is situated at the center of a network of relationships which stretches out horizontally to constitute society as a whole and vertically from his position in the lineage back to his mythical ancestors. How can a design be carved out of this continuum experienced in its totality, and according to what criteria can the limits of the particular, smaller network, constituting "the family" be drawn on the pattern of Occidental culture?

One may apply either a biological criterion which is universally recognized (the family nucleus, consisting of genitors and children), or a geographical-residential criterion, that is, a group which lives in the same place (the home, the concession, or the neighborhood). Neither one of these criteria is entirely satisfactory. The family as nucleus remains an exception, and in many cases the wife does not join her husband in his home until after her first pregnancy or after the baby has been weaned. As for polygamy in its modern urban form, the various subunits of the family, consisting of mothers and children, no longer live together in the same dwelling place but are dispersed throughout the town or among several towns.

It will, therefore, be necessary to clearly define what is meant by the family and family residence, using the above criteria, and it is also important to try and understand the organizational basis for relationships and interchanges between individuals.

TYPE OF FAMILY

In Africa, the usual Occidental type of family (or family nucleus) is supplemented by two others: the extended family and the polygamous family; these may exist simultaneously.

1. *The extended family* is comprised not only of the nucleus (husband, wife, unmarried children), but also of ascendants (parents and parental relatives), brothers and sisters of the couple (whether bachelors, married, or widowed), and nieces and nephews living with the group temporarily or indefinitely. This is especially so in matrilineal families. There are two sub-types, depending on whether it is age or authority that counts. In the first sub-type, prevalent in rural environments, it is the ancestor who constitutes the central point of reference for the entire family group which may consist of several households (all the ancestor's sons and grandsons in patrilineal systems; in matrilineal systems, power lies equally in male hands). In the second sub-type, the family is headed by the children's father; the group is made up essentially of the father's younger brothers and sisters and his nieces and nephews. In both cases, production and consumption are shared. Living together means making common property of what is produced and sharing dishes prepared for a common meal.

2. *The multinuclear family* consists of several nuclei, pivoting around one man, but not cohabiting. However, in the villages, the huts belonging to each subunit (made up of wife and children) are grouped together on the same concession. Each group of nuclei constitutes an economic unit, owns its own land, and has an autonomous kitchen. The husband takes his meals and spends the night with each wife in turn, according to a well-regulated system of rotation.

In the cities, and even in certain rural areas, the extended families tend to become reduced in size or dislocated as a result of changes in living conditions (industrialization, the introduction of currency, migrations). Within the boundaries of an extended family, the households take on individual characteristics, the concession becomes more and more divided, and an evolution towards nuclear development appears.

When a family is founded, the residence is established near the place of origin of either spouse. The rule varies with the dominant lineage and in different ethnic groups. It carries more weight than the principle of descent in determining the status of the wife and the upbringing of the children. Where residence is established near the father's place of origin, the wife finds herself isolated in alien surroundings, whereas in the opposite case, that of residence near the mother's place of origin, she enjoys the support of her own family.[9]

ECONOMIC AND SOCIAL ORGANIZATION

In rural circles, the economic and social organization is generally centered around a chief who is the oldest male, either patrilineally or matrilineally.

We will take as an example the rural Wolof family in Senegal [8]. Each family lives on a community basis and farms its land collectively; the harvests are administered by the patrilineal head who supports the family, pays the taxes, settles conflicts, and represents the family in dealing with the outside world (neighbors, village chief, political and administrative authorities). The women take turns preparing the meals, but this system, which is a sign of solidarity, seems to be slowly disappearing.

Household and individual land are gaining in importance at the expense of communal land. The women own the produce of their land and buy clothes, jewelry, or cattle; the young boys, who own their own land from the age of 12 or 13, are buying transistor-radio sets, or clothes or are saving up for their dowry; the girls have no field of their own, but they receive a part of their mother's harvest. The authority of the lineal chief is diminishing in favor of the head of the household and the wife is acquiring more autonomy.

The slowness with which these changes are occurring in rural environments helps to avoid crises in family life. But in the city things are different: the autonomy of the head of household is increased, the wife hankers after more freedom but rarely has resources of her own, while the children drift away from the parents.

FAMILY LIFE AND INTRAFAMILIAL RELATIONSHIPS

Family life is responsible for the organization of the personality and the integration of the individual into the group: the aim is fusion

[9] The system is more complex than this and traditionally allows for six possibilities: patrilocality (residence determined by the husband's family), matrilocality (residence determined by the wife's family), virilocality (residence determined by the husband's residence before marriage if he was living apart from his family), avunculocality (residence determined by the residence of the husband's maternal uncle), neolocality, biolocality.

with the group, solidarity, and loyalty to ancestors rather than autonomy, competition, and change.

1. *A first characteristic is the density and physical quality of contacts between individuals.* Limited to those who live on the same concession, the family is composed of 15 to 20 individuals or even more. Even in the cities the number is very high: in Dakar 70 percent of all families number between 10 and 20 people. These figures vary as members come and go or settle down for a few days or several months. The family dwelling is wide open, and its most favored spot is the threshold; relatives and visitors cross it at all hours of the day.

The need to be together is expressed in the close mutual contact between bodies, living on top of one another and a quasi-collective moving about (fluidity of gestures, dovetailing of movement, rhythmical activities, dancing in groups) as if they were one and the same body.

The child is initiated into this communal life at a very early age by those close contacts and relationships within the boundaries of increasingly larger groups. To begin with, there is very close contact with the mother's body or even those of "the mothers". As soon as the umbilical cord drops off, the child is carried during the daytime on its mother's back for several hours (at least four hours); in this position he goes with her to do errands, to travel, to dance, or to work. These various movements and relationships provide a veritable symbiosis which paves the way towards perceiving the other through one's own physical experience. The baby is carried on the back of all the women belonging to the maternal line; [10] the girls begin to carry infants at the age of 6 or 7. The image of a multiple and ever-present mother becomes deep-rooted as a result of these physical experiences which, besides the purpose of child-carrying, touch upon the lives and personalities of all adults.

At night, the child is never alone; he sleeps closely pressed to the mother who answers every need by giving him her breast. Later, when he has been weaned, he sleeps with others (grandmother and after that with brothers and sisters) thus continuing the experience of permanent proximity to other bodies.

As the child grows, no obstacles are put in the way of this freedom of bodily contact. The physical contacts have little erotic meaning,

[10] Babies are carried by others after they have been weaned, but by their actual mother only until weaning.

and sexual restrictions are unrelated to the body. Playing with the mother's breast is permitted for quite a long time, even when it is not connected with nursing; the touching of genital organs is neither prohibited nor sanctioned.

2. Another characteristic is *the plurality of personal exchanges* which are never limited to a two-sided, privileged, and exclusive relationship.

   a. It is rather significant that the mother's milk is symbolic of the family line, and yet that neither the mother's breast nor her back are used exclusively by her own offspring.

Apart from its function as nourishment, the milk carries with it a vertical relationship with the ancestors; it is an uninterrupted channel for which the family line is as much responsible as the mother. The milk is good for the child if the mother conforms to what is expected of her by tradition.

The child may nurse at breasts other than the mother's: the maternal grandmother, maternal aunts, maternal relations within the matrilineal group also participate in feeding him and, in other cases, women of either lineage can also do so. The breast is not only an organ of nourishment; essentially, it provides contact. As it is permanently at the child's disposal, and is a means of reassurance for the mother, it establishes between the child and others a plural, permanent, and confident relationship that knows no disappointment. After weaning, the child has breasts other than his mother's at his disposal, and hers are forbidden to him for feeding purposes. The solid foods which are introduced by the eighth month also have an essentially symbolic function: they prepare the way for food taken in common and for collective living around the family table.

   b. At a very early stage, the actual mother and father are superseded or replaced as parents by other members of the group.

In Wolof societies, the parents have doubles or counterparts in the persons of another couple[11] whose sex is the reverse of their own: the mother's brother (*Nidiaye*) and the father's sister (*Badiane*) are active in the child's official as well as everyday life within his social territory. The *Nidiaye* takes over from the mother when the boy

[11] We may wonder what becomes of the Oedipal situation in the face of these two opposing couples, and how identification with the parent of the same sex comes about.

enters upon the masculine cycle (age 6 or 7), and on the girl's wedding day ("the uncle is the mother"). The *Badiane* or paternal aunt has an equally ambivalent function of man-woman; she plays a role in the baptism rite and also throughout other high points of existence (weaning day, circumcision, sexual education, and marriage), when the individual is introduced into a new phase bringing with it a new relationship to the group.

Older and younger brothers and sisters of the same sex as the parents have less well-defined roles that are wholly physical. They are so many mother-father substitutes.

Above and beyond immediate kinship, every man and woman has a share in parental roles. All the child's "fathers and mothers" belong to the domain of the elders, that is, the generation of grandparents or even further back. The ideal model is still the elder, whether male or female, who is closest to the ancestors from whom strength and wisdom are derived.

3. A third characteristic, which complements the first two, is the *rigid codification of the role and status* of each member in keeping with tradition.

a. Ritual pervades all of existence. Rites begin at birth and give form and meaning to all relationship exchanges: body rites, such as massages, baths, washing of the newborn baby, as practiced by the mother or grandmother according to carefully prescribed techniques; – food rites, which establish the protocol for the manner of preparing and consuming food; – sleeping rites, which dictate not the length of time but the place; – cleanliness rites, which have a great influence on the child's development and on the organization of individual defenses. Toilet control is acquired early and easily. The physical symbiosis resulting from being carried on the back brings about a dialogue between every need and its response, so that the child becomes rapidly conditioned to satisfactory conduct. The mother reacts promptly each time the child soils himself, but without aggressiveness or compulsion. The prohibitions summon up collective images but never emotion or anger, and they are often canceled out by compensations (the child's excretions are replaced by the breast – "I give him my breast whenever he urinates").

There are also integration rites, at the time of each passage into a new phase of existence: baptism, the first time the baby is carried, first outing, weaning, entry into an age category, circumcision; – protection rites, against all dangers which are particularly threatening at certain moments of the day or night, or in certain situations (pregnancy, menstruation); or as defense against illness, evil spirits, casting of spells, man-eating sorcerers; and protection of certain more vulnerable parts of the body; – prohibition, against many kinds of behavior which give rise to evil encounters or provoke threats.

Everything is prescribed for what may be done and what may not be done.[12] Failure to follow these protection rites and prescribed behavior patterns may have serious consequences, not only for those responsible for them but for the whole group.

> b. The techniques of upbringing and education seek to transmit the content of an impersonal culture through multiple and well-defined channels. The mother hands down to her child what her mother has handed down to her; the image she has of the ideal mother remains her own mother. The young woman who enters the maternity cycle loses her autonomy as well as her identity to become blended into the image of the good mother, which is to say that of her own mother as well as that of all other mothers of the culture. This is the "ultimate common channel" by and through which all these collective representations, attitudes, gestures, and language are transmitted. There is no room for actions and conduct of an individual nature.

Punishments, gifts, and rewards do not depend upon the mother's disposition or generosity but rather on kinsmen of all degrees, taken within the code of relationships, defined and limited by established rules.

[12] Here are some examples of prohibitions for the child as well as for the mother among the Wolof of Senegal.

For the child: to run toward the house yelling, carry his hands on top of his head, play with water, dig holes, wear one shoe, go out between 6 and 8 at night, weep too loudly, laugh too loudly, lie down on his belly, knock on a jar during the rainy season, sit with crossed legs, wear his father's nightcap, look at himself in the mirror, suck his thumb, cry during the night, urinate on his father, eat with his left hand.

For the mother: to wash the child on Wednesdays and Saturdays, put him down to sleep in the shade, leave him alone under a tree, eat while nursing him, send his linen to be washed outside the home, feed him eggs or fish, have him massaged by a woman of a different caste, show him something black, let him sleep on his face, mention his weight, praise him, say how many children she has.

This system of collective education might also be deemed impersonal. There is not only a stability of content, but also a stability of form which is independent of individual whims. A good mother is one who faithfully transmits the culture, and whose purpose is not to make the child attached to *her* but rather to integrate him into the group. The fact that the educational task is divided among the adults is a further guarantee that the risk of an exclusive dual and personalized relationship, resulting from bad mothering and disposing to non-integration, will be avoided.

Similarly, the father's importance lies less in the symbolic interaction of the Oedipal triangle than in the link he provides with the family line, which is essentially as follows: "not to have a father is not to exist." He is active at the high points of existence whenever the group confirms and relives its myths: he makes decisions about baptism and the child's name, circumcision, initiation, and all the "rebirths." He represents collective authority and transmits the ancestral law by codified gestures and acts.

Thus, rigidity of conduct and complete codification of rules for education and relationships between individuals prevent a collective congealing, which would be the result of the individual's blending too completely into the anonymous group. Individuality is made possible by these pairs: permissiveness/rigidity, autonomy/dependence, change/tradition. But there is hardly much room for personal adventure, deviation, or singularity. Conformity is obtained by means of a conditioning which provokes neither revolt nor individual defense; the African man is never isolated and remains both submissive and receptive to his environment.

Social Change And Mental Pathology

A. Development and modernity are accompanied not only by new institutional models, new types of behavior, and new values, but they also threaten to disorganize family life.

Whenever a way of life becomes disorganized (or contested), this very fact contains the germ of a possible reorganization of the family which would constitute its better adaptation to the realities of the modern world. But before this new equilibrium can be acquired, whether it be rooted or not in the traditional culture, there is bound to be chaos and anxiety provoking pathological defenses on the part of individuals and of society as a whole.

Africa is not only currently in the midst of technical progress, but it is also being threatened today by a foundering of its fundamental way of life due to the pressure of massive acculturation.

The introduction of modern techniques is radically changing human relations as well as the relationship between man and a world that is still basking in the warmth of myth.[13] Modern techniques separate the generations and lead to individuation through competence, competition, and the need to excel.

School imposes other masters besides the father, an authority other than that of the ancestor. New messages are transmitted through new channels. The continuum of education is broken; the gulf between the generations becomes apparent.

Unifying rites and institutions are losing their strength and meaning. Passage rites are becoming empty forms that no longer fulfill their reassuring and integrating roles. Age groups are disappearing; the old gods are being abandoned, family altars deserted, and traditional worship impoverished.

The Family Council and all other counsel or advice in general, which serve as communication links as well as frames of reference,[14] are losing their hold and are no longer listened to. By the time they reach adolescence, the men realize that they are individuals, concerned only with themselves and for themselves, responsible for their own destiny and in opposition to others.

The village, the traditional structure that was a natural extension of the family, in the past organized the social life and provided the frame of reference for individual identity; it is now undergoing transformations which are profoundly modifying it so that it is gradually losing its function and its meaning.

> Even though, in its physical aspect, this village may still be composed of huts . . . it no longer really has the same soul, and it no longer defines itself in the same way. How then can the parents themselves continue to live in the fullness of their culture and remain certain of the models it is their duty to hand down and transmit (to their children) [1].

[13]The man of myth, inseparable from other men and from the world, is integrated by definition. "He does not yet feel the need to oppose in order to impose, to struggle in order to be recognized by others...He does not dream of mastering and possessing nature" [9].

[14]"When one speaks to a child, he does not hear, he communicates. He does not take in truths, he lives them at the moment you are speaking to him" [12]

In the city, individual relationships become intermingled and blurred in an ethnic cosmopolitanism in which the migrant no longer recognizes his fellowman, his kinsman, his brother from the village; families and households are dispersed.

The family nucleus becomes the standard model. The father and mother are the proprietors of the child as object, bearer of hopes and new values. The relationship between mother and child is disturbed by the anxiety of the mother who, alone and torn between tradition and modernization, can no longer rely on her own family. The breast has become "quantitative"; contacts are impoverished; excellence in performance is demanded very early.

The notion of plural "fathers and mothers" has no longer any connection with reality; the child no longer belongs to the group. He must rapidly confront competition and solitude and be responsible for himself and his freedom.

The individual, the family, and the group are seeking a new identity, a new reciprocal equilibrium. The human continuum, which heretofore provided unity and solidarity, is broken. Relationship to the group has lost its strength and has been replaced by other narrower and more narcissistic investments.

A number of different forms of behavior have been found to compensate for the emptiness and confusion caused by this loss of culture. One is satisfaction in personal success and in the possession of wealth; "to do" and "to have" fill the void left by the loss of being or personality. There is also at times a return to certain traditional ways, a call for magical practices and to ancient gods to help in surmounting family conflicts or personal difficulties.

While the religions of the past have lost hold, new cults flourish everywhere. These blend the past with the imported religions and rapidly prosper, feeding on hope as well as on the need to be together and to belong.

Other phenomena also indicate a resistance to individuation and a desire to take up again with tradition: youth associations, clubs, and neighborhoods, which lack particular aims but which correspond to the need to be together and to give each member a well-defined status [3]. Thcsc transformations are especially noticeable in the cities; with the new generations, they will deepen and become more widespread.

B. The disorganization of the family acts to the disadvantage of two other units of the continuum: individual – family – group; it is accompanied by the autonomization of the individual and it brings about a faceless society under the control of the political State. The community is henceforth experienced on the level of large abstract institutions (Administration, Government, State).

As existence becomes on the one hand individualized and on the other hand socialized, a new mental pathology appears similar to that observed in Occidental societies.

1. In traditional African societies, collective existence, experienced on an almost biological level and reinforced throughout life by integration rites which have a prophylactic function, probably reduces the possibility of conflictual situations.

a. As a complement to group participation there exists a badly-defined ego (or self) whose limits are vague. While this type of social organization prevents isolation and solitude and provides protection and security, it also facilitates confusions of identity: "Am I me, am I the other, am I an animal, a spirit, a tree, am I one, many, am I the world?"

This extraordinary tendency towards secondary identifications, resulting possibly from early nursing experiences which facilitate and prolong primary identifications, is perceived to be a sign of strength and is valued by the culture. It can be easily discerned in everyday behavior, dances of possession, and in African literature and poetry.[15]

But it also facilitates the loss of personal identity which is defined above all by one's place in the human environment rather than by personal history. When this environment becomes threatening and unfamiliar, and especially if the change is abrupt, anxiety sets in and with this the risk of acute psychotic decompensation. The submissiveness and receptivity to the environment make it possible to understand the reactive character of the mental pathology. However, it is due to a pathological reaction against the here-and-now rather than a pathology whose roots lie in the earliest stages of the individual's history.

b. Traditional societies have their own systems for regulating tensions, and these systems also prevent the expression of

[15] "The weakness of many men lies in the fact that they are incapable of becoming either a stone or a tree", as A. Cesaire states in his *Une Saison au Congo, Théâtre.*

aggressiveness within the group. Constant care is taken to ensure group cohesion.

Psychoanalytic interpretations of mental illness throw light on certain protective and prophylactic mechanisms directed simultaneously towards individual mental disorder, the illness itself, social disorder, and aggressiveness inside the group [21]. The illness is held to be due to spirits: ancestral spirits or spirits introduced by Islam. When it is held to be due to other individuals, the aggression which might follow from it is reduced or canceled out either by neutral links in the chain (the medicine-man) or by a collective act which reintegrates the aggressor (this is the case with man-eating sorcerers).

c. The educational techniques reduce conflictual situations which only appear at a late stage and do not leave any profound marks on the individual. After an unhampered oral phase which more than satisfies the child's needs and desires, the period that follows is very permissive and elicits neither anal investment nor anal defenses. The Oedipal situation is not clearly manifested. The showdown with the father, who represents the ancestor, is difficult if not impossible; instead there is a transference to the brotherhood [14].

However, conflicts do exist which are externalized by pathology; these originate in the difficulty of establishing personal autonomy. There are conflicts resulting from the impossibility of standing up to the father, the older brother or, beyond them, to the ancestor who cannot be equalled; – conflicts resulting from situations of rivalry, competition, outstripping, individuation; – conflicts resulting from group pressures which limit individuation and imprison individuals within a given status and in given roles for the rest of their lives. There are two pathological examples rather characteristic of this situation: the outburst of delirium and the child *Nit-Ku-Bon*.

If the outburst of delirium implies a temporary loss of identity, it also expresses an attempt to escape from the character inside which the individual is imprisoned [4].

In another psychopathological tableau, the child *Nit-Ku-Bon* also suffers from what can be called identity illness. He refuses to be situated within the lineage or the group. He enjoys the supreme liberty of being alone and guiding his own movements. He is intro-determined and in fact is the perfect example of intro-determination [20].

Outbursts of delirium and the child *Nit-Ku-Bon* express what is repressed. On the individual level, the outburst of delirium constitutes an attempt to become someone other than the personality inside which society has imprisoned the individual since birth. On the collective level, the child *Nit-Ku-Bon* is the expression of the desire for ambiguity, the desire not to be situated or identified; he expresses the group's unconscious wish for intro-determination and freedom [5].

The transformations undergone by family structures shift the conflicts and modify mental pathology [6]. The frequency and the form of these phenomena are changing. The individual who escapes from his traditional status and who outstrips his father or brother is threatened both from inside and outside. Guilt makes its appearance and persecution increases. Intellectual, sexual, and physical inhibitions and conduct leading to failure are the expression of the difficulty of bypassing the father, of attracting attention as an individual, and of becoming "other". These manifestations are very frequent among schoolchildren, adolescents, and civil servants.

The structure of depressive states of mind is evolving. In traditional cultures, melancholy is the exception; this is due to the multiple mothers who are ever-available and good-natured, as well as to the lack of conflict during the oral phase. With the new intrafamilial relationships, depression sets in, brought about by feelings of guilt, indignation, and devaluation. It is no longer the spirit which is bad because the law of the group has been transgressed, it is no longer the "other" on whom one projects one's own aggressiveness, it is "I am bad." Guilt replaces shame.

The breaking up and disorganization of collective identification models, the dislocation of the group, the gap between the generations, the contradictions of education, and the solitude within the lineage and the brotherhood pave the way for schizophrenia which is increasing in the cities [7].

The disintegration of the family makes it no longer possible for it to fulfill its functions; there is no longer any continuity between the demands made on the child and those made on the adult. Authority generates conflicts and separates individuals rather than uniting them.

A social pathology develops. The need to be together in order to combat solitude leads not only to the organization of "youth groups" but also to the formation of gangs of delinquents and drug addicts. The incidence of problem children and adolescents is beginning to make itself felt [15, 13, 11]. Prostitution is invading the cities.

Both family and society are becoming less tolerant of useless and cumbersome members. The mentally ill are relegated to insane asylums and the phenomenon of alienation is making its appearance; the problem child is sent away from home; no doubt there will soon be a pathology of old age.

All these phenomena are manifestations of the difficulty of making a painful transition for which no preparation could have been conceived.

It is by no means self-evident that it is necessary to abandon the traditional values, accepted and transmitted as a responsibility by the African family, in order to achieve modernity and succeed in the technical race towards industrialization. It is not inevitable for progress to be accompanied by the "lonely crowd" of Occidental cultures. It is something to think about.

Bibliography

1. Agblemagnon, F.N. Sougan, La famille Africaine à l'épreuve, Colloque International sur les relations familiales en Afrique, Dakar 1967.
2. Balandier, G. and Maquet, J., *Dictionnaire des civilisatons* Fernand Hazan édit., Paris, 1968.
3. Billen, M., N. Le Guerinel, and J.-P. Moreigne, Les associations de jeunes à Dakar (Approche d'un fait social objectif), *Psychopathologie Africaine,* III (1967), 3, 373-400.
4. Collomb, H., Bouffées délirantes en psychiatrie africaine, *Psychopathologie Africaine,* I (1965), 2, 167-239.
5. Collomb, H., Psychiatrie et cultures (Quelques considérations générales), *Psychopathologie Africaine,* II (1966), 2, 259-271.
6. Collomb, H., La position du conflit et les structures familiales en voie de transformation, *Canadian Psychiatric Association Journal,* 12 (1967), 5, 451-464.
7. Centre Hospitalier de Fann, Service de Neuro-Psychiatrie (Dakar), Psychopathologie et environnement familial en Afrique, *Psychopathologie Africaine,* IV (1968), 2, 173-226.
8. Diop, A.B., Parents et famille rurale en milieu wolof, *Psychopathologie Africaine,* V (1969), I.
9. Gusdorf, G., *Mythe et métaphysique,* Flammarion édit., Paris, 1953.
10. Garique, Ph., La famille – Essai d'interprétation, *Canadian Psychiatric Association Journal,* 12 (1967), 15-25.
11. Hugot, S., Le problème de la délinquance juvénile à Dakar. Mémoire de Doctorat de 3ème Cycle de Psychologie, Faculté des Lettres et Sciences Humaines de Dakar, June 1968.

12. Le Guerinel, N., M.-C. Ortigues, M. N'Diaye, C. Berne, and B. Delbard, *La conception de l'autorité et son évolution dans les relations parents enfants à Dakar,* Fédération Internationale de parents et d'éducateurs, Paris, 1968.
13. Ortigues, M.-C., A. Colot, and M.-T. Montagnier, – La délinquance juvénile à Dakar, Etude psychologique de 14 cas, *Psychopathologie Africaine,* I (1965), 1, 85-129.
14. Ortigues, M.-C. and E. Ortigues, – *Oedipe africain,* Plon édit., Paris, 1966.
15. Pierre, E., J.-P. Flammand, and H. Collomb. – Délinquance juvénile à Dakar, *Revue internationale de politique criminelle,* 20 (1962). 27-34.
16. Sadji, A., *Education africaine et civilisation,* S.A.F.E.P., A. DIOP, Dakar, 1964.
17. Sankale, M., *Médecins et action sanitaire en Afrique Noire,* Présence Africaine édit., Paris, 1969.
18. Thomas, L.V., Analyse dynamique de la parenté sénégalaise, *Bulletin de l'I.F.A.N.* série B, XXX (1968), 3, 1005-1061.
19. Valantin, S., Le développement de la fonction manipulatoire ches l'enfant sénégalais au cours de 2 premières années de la vie. Thèse de 3ème Cycle, Faculté des Lettres et des Sciences Humaines, Paris, 1969.
20. Zempleni – Rabain, J., Modes fondamentaux de relations chez l'enfant Wolof, du sevrage à l'intégration dans la classe d'âge, *Psychopathologie Africaine,* II (1966), 2, 143-177.
21. Zempleni, A., L'interprétation et la thérapie traditionnelles du désordre mental chez les Wolof et Lebou du Sénégal. 2 vol. ronéo-typés, Thèse de la Faculté des Lettres et des Sciences Humaines, Paris, 1968.

Personality and Mental Health of Indians (Hindus) in the Context of Their Changing Family Organization

A. A. KHATRI* (INDIA)

Introduction

There are many forms of family organization in India with its teeming millions. Out of this multiplicity of family forms, two broad types may be culled. One is a patrilineal joint family in which generations of patrilineally related family members stay with their spouses and children (predominantly in North India) and the other is the matrilineal family in which the daughters continue to stay with their mothers and inherit the property while their husbands are brought in to stay with them (prevalent in some parts of South India). We will concern ourselves primarily with the Hindu patrilineal family, its impact on personality and mental health, social change taking place in this family organization, and its repercussions on personality and mental health. Despite our primary concern with Hindus who constitute the majority in India, many of the propositions concerning personality and mental health would also be

*The author thanks his psychiatrist colleagues, Dr. Erna Hoch, Visiting Consultant, and Dr. B. K. Ramanujam for making available their unpublished material and for making many useful comments. He also acknowledges his debt to the B. M. Institute which has provided clinical experience, clinical data, and an intellectually stimulating atmosphere without which this chapter could not have been written in its present form.

applicable to non-Hindu Indians, most of whom had Hindu ancestry before conversion and who share the same "ideal" type of family (to be described later), the same network of role-governed, hierarchical family relations, common child-rearing practices, and similar familistic orientation.

Before we endeavor to trace the relationships between the family, personality and mental health, and impact of social change on them, we draw attention to the paucity of published literature in the broad field of the Indian family in general and its impact on personality and mental health in particular. This has been repeatedly pointed out by a number of workers [44, 23, 28]. The published literature on the Indian family has shown concern mainly for the study of the family as an institution in general and opinions-attitudes with respect to joint family and certain issues in particular. Very few studies have focused on primary aim of relating personality and mental health of Indians to their family organization and social change therein [24, 25, 27].

Rationale for Hindu Basic Personality Structure

We may ask the question: In a vast country like India with many regional variations even in the patrilineal family, how can one speak of the Hindu family and postulate personality of Hindus reared under these conditions? The present investigator has made this attempt despite diversity of prevalent family forms on the basis of the following considerations:

Behind the apparent diversity, one can broadly discern in all types of Hindu family, the same patterning of family relations characterized by dominance-submission, warmth-detachment, and approach-avoidance, attitudes and expectations based on role positions; similarity in child rearing practices, commitment to an "ideal" type of joint family with consequent familistic orientation and lack of concern with individuality.

This "ideal type" can be briefly described as follows. The traditional joint family consists of patrilineally related males with spouses and children (e.g., A, his father and mother, his grandfather and grandmother, his uncles, aunts, and their married sons with their wives and children, their unmarried sons and daughters, his sons with their spouses and children), who stay under the same roof, have a common kitchen, share property in common, pool their earnings and are considered as a single unit in their caste and society at large, and worship the same family deity. Major family decisions are made by the *pater familias,* and there is a clear-cut hierarchy of intrafamilial relations in terms of dominance-submission patterns. Obedience to family elders, respect for them, and joint pursuit of family-centered goals rather than individualistic ones are characteristic of the joint family in India. Parent-adult son relationships dominate over husband-wife relations. Any demonstration of affection between husband and wife and parents and their children in the presence of family elders is tabooed in traditional joint families.

They are perceived as one family unit by themselves as well as by the community. This "ideal type" appears to be internalized by most Indians and affects their family living and relations in various ways.

Child-rearing environment in general and child-rearing practices in particular provide a basic framework for certain dispositions, unconscious assumptions, basic expectancy sets, broad attitudes of relating to persons in general and to certain role occupants in particular. According to Kardiner and Linton [20], a definite groundwork is laid for the basic personality structure. In the opinion of the writer [27], these early experiences of Indian children in family living provide a scaffolding for positive mental health and/or vulnerability to mental disturbances in later life.

Having made our assumptions explicit, we now proceed to deal with the traditional Indian family and its impact on the personality and mental health of the family members. We will then deal with social change occurring in the Indian family and its repercussions on the personality and mental health of family members caught in this whirlpool of social change.

Attitudes Towards Childbirth

In the Hindu culture,, children, particularly male children, are highly valued, and a woman who is childless is looked down upon. Her face should not be seen in the morning, otherwise the whole day might turn out to be bad. When a Hindu married woman becomes pregnant, certain ceremonies are usually held during the fifth month or soon after. These ceremonies, called *Simant,* enact symbolically the meaning that pregnancy is a gift from God. A pregnant woman gains considerable prestige and status in the eyes of her family. After the fifth month or so, she goes to her parents' home for delivery, particularly for the first delivery. This practice thus removes the hardworking daughter-in-law from the pressures and conflicts of the family of in-laws and from the sexual demands of her husband, and places her in the familiar, less stressful, and more accepting milieu of her childhood home where she continues to stay until 3 to 5 months after delivery. In this way, a congenial climate is provided for the birth of her child.

It is a conviction of the author that in the orthodox Hindu family the child-rearing environment for the male children is radically different from the child-rearing environment of the female children although more in terms of attitudes than rearing methods; therefore, the two sexes have been considered separately in this presentation.

The Hindu Male in the Traditional Family

For various culture-specific reasons, the birth of a male child in the traditional Hindu joint family is greeted with considerable acclaim, especially if he happens to be the first child. A very intimate relationship, both physical and emotional, develops between the mother and the infant whose every cry is immediately responded to either by the mother or a female surrogate. He is breast-fed on demand for an average of 3 years and sleeps with his mother during that time.

In a predominantly rural country with no built-in lavatories and with unfurnished dwellings, toilet training is gradual and very permissive. However, the Indian practice of cleaning by water rather than toilet paper may lead to socialization conflicts concerning the use of the left hand for cleaning and the right hand for eating.

This physical closeness to the mother by day and by night, her continuous ministration to his needs, and the prolonged breast feeding on demand are all theoretically conducive to the development of basic trust, a sense of security, a positive self-image, a capacity to receive and give affection, and a conception of the world as good; however, they can also generate feelings of omnipotence and dependency strivings.

There are other negative features of this "childhood paradise." Sleeping with the mother opens up the possibility of exposure to the "primal scene" which, theoretically, may prove to be traumatic.

Furthermore, in spite of the intimate contact permitted when alone with the mother, demonstrations of affection by either parent in the presence of family elders is strictly tabooed. The mother is also not accessible to the boy during the period of menstruation because of the taboo forbidding all interpersonal physical contacts. These several prohibitions, to some extent, mitigate the almost suffocating symbiotic union that is culturally permitted to develop but, in addition, they carry, for the sensitive child, a traumatic potential. The presence of other female members in the family may also help to relieve the intensity of this closeness.

The end of the symbiosis is often sudden with weaning brought about by the application of a bitter paste to the nipples. Ramanujam has referred to the abrupt change from the blissful state to the subsequent one in which, with every passing year, more is expected in dutiful behavior of the child [45].

In this developmental drama, as in many other childhood episodes, the socialization of the male child is accomplished largely by the mother and the other female members of the household, so that the main models for identification are women, and it is their attitudes and behavior that tend to get internalized.

Talcott Parsons has postulated that it is the nuclear family that provides the child with his psychological development through an internalization of roles played by both father and mother, the identifications being pointed and specific [50]. In families, such as in Samoa, where the children are reared in an environment of multiple mothering and fathering, not only are identifications multiple but a diffuse dependence results with some flattening of affect [35].

As the male child grows older and another sibling appears, he becomes subject to certain prescriptions and proscriptions. Leaving the predominantly female environment in which he has passed the early crucial years, he is slowly inducted into the world of men, although his contacts at this time remain essentially peripheral. The sudden weaning and dethronement by the new sibling can lay the foundations of ambivalence and distrust, at the same time shattering to some extent the small boy's feelings of omnipotence. A certain independence in matters of dressing and in looking after some of his own needs is now expected. He is exposed to a family atmosphere that is traditionally authoritarian, demanding obedience to family elders and conformity to the family's rules and regulations. He begins to experience a variety of disciplining agents; he is given immediate negative reinforcement for family-disapproved behavior, and this is further reinforced when he is witness to the system of negative reinforcement operating in the case of other children. Repeated exposures of this sort are likely to generate a strong sense of conformity and provide the basis for anxiety reactions to nonconformity. The authoritarian family climate encourages dependence and passivity and stifles the strivings for autonomy. Firmly embedded conformity and built-in anxiety about nonconformity become additional barriers to the emergence of independent and creative activity. (In this context, it is worth noting that in a study of large American families, Bossard and Boll found that conformity was valued above self-expression [2]. This type of family atmosphere is likely to develop rigid controls over positive impulses in the service of sexual taboos and strong suppressions of negative impulses for the sake of conformity. On the other hand, the family elders cater to the child's physical needs, provide him with shelter, decide on his occupation, and choose a mate for him. In such ways, it gives him a stable constellation of roles for purposes of identification and, most significantly, a sense of security.[1]

In summary, the familial environment of the Hindu male from childhood to adulthood develops in him trust, security, a capacity to give and receive affection, and a positive self-image. Due to his acceptance of roles assigned to him by the family and to the predictability of his environment, he is likely to develop few intrapersonal and interpersonal conflicts [24, 25]. Thus, it would seem that the traditional family conduces to positive mental health as reflected in our postulated indices (to be described later).

The Hindu adult male, with an occupation and a mate provided for him by the family, continues to grow in the stable familial and extrafamilial environment. His orientation remains familistic; he helps and is helped by his siblings and other family members. His rank in the family hierarchy gives him certain rights over persons lower than him from whom he expects respect and obedience but not overt expression of affection. In times to come he may be the eldest surviving male and may thus attain the position of *pater familias* with the authority for making important family decisions.

[1]Erik H. Erikson has questioned the author's assumption of security emanating from a culturally prescribed constellation of roles (personal communication).

Whether he becomes *pater familias* or not, with increasing age, he continues to gain the respect of the other members of the joint family. Throughout his life, therefore, he remains a valued individual within this special setting with no risk of ending his days as an isolated, helpless, old man left to his own miserable devices.

The personality of the Hindu male thus helps him to adapt to his culture with minimal frustration and maximal gratification providing a close "fit" between culture and personality. However, the price that he has to pay for this adaptability is low initiative, prolonged dependency, and a restricted range of autonomy and creativity for most of his life.

The Hindu Female in the Traditional Family

Whereas the birth of a male child is received with zest and delight in a traditional Hindu household, the birth of a girl is resented and rationalized. The proverbs current in Hindu society refer to her as being "a bundle of serpents" or an "alien property." This partly stems from the custom of dowry and other economic liabilities that are incurred in getting a girl married in many castes and sub-castes. Even the mother giving birth to a girl is accorded negative treatment and is often abused, prompting her, in turn, to perceive the baby daughter in a negative light.

In the traditional Hindu family, open favoritism is shown to the brothers who are given better food, better clothes, and overall better treatment. Because of these aspects of the child-rearing environment, the ground is laid for the development of a negative self-image, envy and jealousy with regard to males, and a perception of the world as basically unfair. At the same time, this differential treatment may raise her threshold for the tolerance of tensions and frustrations. It is true that many child-rearing practices for the girls are the same as for boys, but they take place in the overall context of a more negative attitude. This may be to some extent tempered by the consideration that the girls are "guests in their own home" and that it is important to find suitable mates for them as part of the family's responsibility.

In contrast to her brother, she is unlikely to develop any difficulties in the sphere of sexual identity, her strong feminine identification, encouraged by the other females in the household, ensuring her a clear conception and acceptance of her role as a woman.

As she grows older, her personal mobility is more restricted than that of her brothers, and an early induction to domestic work takes place. She is fed with religious concepts that decree that her future husband must be treated as God and is exposed to the cultural ideal of *Sati,* symbolizing lifelong self-sacrifice, complete submergence of her own individuality within the family, acceptance of a subservient position, commitment to her major task of gratifying her husband's needs, and complete conformity to the standards traditionally imposed upon her. The child-rearing environment helps to foster those dimensions of personality which prepare her for living as a wife and a daughter-in-law in the family of her in-laws, once more illustrating the "fit" between culture and personality. It does not, however, prepare her adequately for her role as a woman, since she is given very little information about menstruation and sexual aspects of marriage. Both of these may come as a profound shock. By tradition, she will be deflowered by her husband, whom she will meet alone for the first time (in many cases) on the day of her marriage and who is in all significant respects a stranger to her. She cannot but view herself as an alien in the new family of in-laws where she may have visited on a few brief ceremonial occasions. Even when married, she is not permitted to interact with her husband openly during the day, and whatever contact she may have is vitiated by the numerous domestic chores that make up her day from early morning until night. Her husband, for his part, continues to invest emotionally in his peers and finds his recreations extramurally. His relationship with his wife is, therefore, formal, distant, and sex-centered.

For many years, the life of the Hindu wife is characterized by feelings of isolation, by multifarious frustrations and tensions which she learns to bear as she continues to perform her role as kitchen robot, domestic servant, a sex-fulfilling partner, and reproductive agent. Failure to perform as expected in any of these roles, especially reproductivity, adds to her many difficulties. A childless Hindu woman, as stated earlier, is despised and considered an ill omen.

Redeeming features in this otherwise bleak existence may be the joking relationship with her husband's younger brother, brief visits to her family of origin, the birth of a son (which boosts her prestige), and the close, clinging tie to her children. It is still a matter for careful investigation as to what happens in the millions of families in predominantly rural India as a result of these immature, unprepared teenagers becoming mothers so prematurely [17]. It may be that the mother surrogate activity as girls in their own families may help them on a practical level, and they are no doubt often assisted by older females in the household in the discharge of maternal duties.

When a young Hindu woman becomes a widow, she is at once exposed to considerable abuse specific to Hindu culture. Her ornaments are taken away, her head is shaven, and she is compelled to wear a widow's dress for the rest of her life. She is regarded superstitiously as the bearer of ill luck and is avoided. She cannot attend any festive occasion, and it is improper for her to laugh or show any signs of joy. In some vague sense, she is even considered responsible for the death of her husband. As a widow, she becomes a scapegoat for the frustrations of the family and a target for the aggression of members higher in the "pecking order." As a consequence, she is burdened with shame (for being made ugly), guilt (for "killing" her husband), and loneliness (from being isolated). Her negative woman's self-image is made more negative by widowhood. Her new circumstances demand that she control her sexual as well as her aggressive impulses. Preoccupation with the rites and rituals of the Hindu religion may provide some relief for her otherwise dismal existence. An autobiography by a remarried widow, given by Karve, illustrates in more detail the aspects of life during widowhood [21]. The reference to widows as mental health risks by the W.H.O. Research Committee [54] would be specifically applicable to young widows in traditional Hindu families.

The treatment given to the Hindu female from birth to widowhood lays the foundation, in the opinion of the author, for vulnerability to mental health disturbances, like hysteria, anxiety state, psychosomatic illness, schizophrenia, or maladaptive behavior in the form of prostitution or suicide. It connects the risk to mental health with the culturally derived tensions induced by particular family practices in particular cultures and it varies with the balance of gratification and frustration [26]. This raises the important question as to what the consequences on personality development would be for children who are clung to by an emotionally unsatisfied widowed mother who might also make them the object of her aggression.

However, for the Hindu woman who does not become a widow in early married life, circumstances continue to improve and her lot is bettered with each son that she produces and with the appearance of each younger female who enters the family through marriage with a younger brother of her husband. She not only dominates these younger women who take over domestic chores from her, but she also makes use of them to vent her pent-up aggression. Furthermore, If her husband in time becomes *pater familias,* she will wield considerable control over all the other female members of the family and also gain in importance because of her dominance over her adult sons and daughters-in-law. Her relationship with her aging husband is often characterized by the affection that results from years of married living and sharing of common concerns. She is no longer the tortured, isolated, helpless, alienated daughter-in-law of early life. Apart from the importance that she has achieved and the power that she wields, she now has free access to the children of the family with whom she can pass her time pleasantly and affectionately.

Personality Dimensions in the Traditional Family

The salient personality characteristics of boys and girls reared in the traditional Hindu family can be summarized as follows:

CHARACTERISTICS COMMON TO BOTH SEXES

1. Dependency.
2. A firm sense of identity with a clear conception of the roles to be occupied.
3. A sense of security.
4. Conformity and anxiety over nonconformity.
5. An interpersonal orientation characterized by a relative ease with strangers, a deferential submissiveness to people in superordinate positions, a tendency to dominate people in subordinate positions, a firmly entrenched hierarchical conception of human beings with a concomitant rejection of democratic values, a need to placate authority figures or deal with them by suppressing aggression, "leaving the field," or psychosomatization, a tolerance for ambiguous interpersonal cues ("double bind"), a preference for role relations over individual ones, an intolerance for being alone coupled with a dread of loneliness, resulting in clinging behavior.
6. A low drive for achievement, initiative, and creativity.
7. A relative invulnerability to separation from or rejection by significant adults.
8. A world view in which destiny (Karve) is all important and human strivings futile.

CHARACTERISTICS DIFFERENT FOR BOTH SEXES

	Males		Females
1.	A predominantly positive (although vacillating) self-image.	1.	A predominantly negative self-image.
2.	A predominantly positive attitude to people in superordinate positions.	2.	A predominantly negative attitude to family members in superordinate positions (especially an ambivalent attitude to the husband during the early years of marriage).
3.	Extension of self beyond the nuclear family to include other joint family figures.	3.	Extension of self limited to husband, children, and in-laws.
4.	Less vulnerable to mental health disturbances.	4.	More vulnerable to mental health disturbances.

Though some of these personality characteristics come to fruition in the "ideal type" of joint family described earlier, they would all develop to varying degrees in families characterized by familistic values, a dominance-submission hierarchy, differential treatment based on sex, and a subservient position for women, even though they may not be typically joint.

Social Change and Mental Health

Hindu society has never been a static society, and gradual change in its institutions in general and in the family organization in particular has been taking place for centuries. However, the exposure to Western education and ideology, the development of industry leading to urbanization and migration from rural areas, the introduction of democratic principles and methods at the federal, state, district, and village levels, the increased educational possibilities for girls as well as boys, the rigorous campaign for family planning, the widespread use of mass media such as radio, newspapers—these and other factors have brought about radical changes in the political, economic, cultural, social, and family institutions in the new India. There is, however, great variability in the exposure to and assimilation of the various facets of change and in the degree of cultural conflict that results [26].

Some aspects of the social changes that have been taking place in the family are summarized in the following chart.

SOCIAL CHANGE IN THE HINDU FAMILY

Aspects of the Traditional Hindu Family	Emergent Trends in the Hindu Family
1. Preferred mode of living is in the traditional joint family consisting of the propositus, his parents, uncles, aunts (uncles' wives and father's sisters), cousins, their wives and children, his own spouse and sons—married and unmarried—his unmarried daughters, and at times his grandparents or grandsons.	1. Preferred mode of living is in (A) the nuclear family consisting of the propositus, his wife, and unmarried children, or (B) three-generation lineal joint family consisting of the propositus, his wife, his parents, his sons, and unmarried daughters [30].
2. The head of the family functions as *pater familias* wielding all authority, making, on his own, all major decisions which concern the family and its individual members and which are binding on them.	2. Consultation of individual members and democratic decision-making are increasingly being adopted.
3. There is a hierarchy of intrafamily relationships in terms of dominance-submission, usually based on age and sex. Elders in the family are looked	3. The hierarchy is tempered by intimacy and increasingly free and spontaneous interaction between family members.

upon with deference, and interaction with them is respectful, minimal, and formal.	
4. The mother-in-law and other elderly women in the household of the joint family and her husband's sisters can and often do dominate and even torment a young daughter-in-law. The husband cannot rescue his wife from these assaults—usually verbal. The parent-child relationships prevail over husband-wife relationships. In other words, the husband is more influenced by his filial duty to his family of orientation than by his relationship to his wife. Demonstrations of affection and even verbal interactions between husband and wife in the presence of family members is tabooed.	4. In a family with educated family members, domination over the daughter-in-law is less, and her husband would take her side. He is also likely to interact freely with his wife in the presence of family members. The husband-wife relationship increasingly assumes more importance and often prevails over the parent-child relationship.
5. The rule of avoidance (as expressed in the woman concealing her face with the edge of her saree, no direct face-to-face interaction, etc.) is to be observed between (1) father-in-law, (2) husband's older brother and wife, (3) brothers of father-in-law and daughter-in-law, and between other specified relatives and adults.	5. In modern families, interaction among family members is not affected by the rule of avoidance and becomes increasingly free, less formal, and more spontaneous.

6.	Socialization of the child is mainly in the hands of the family elders—particularly women members in early and late childhood (up to 10 years or so) and not in the hands of the child's parents. Demonstration of affection to the child by his parents is not permitted before family elders. +3,	6.	Socialization of the child becomes increasingly the primary concern of the parents, usually both of them. In the case of the joint family, there is increasing acceptance of parental demonstration of affection to their child in the presence of family elders.
7.	The birth of a girl is not warmly accepted as that of a boy. Open favoritism is shown to boys. Education is not considered necessary for girls. The place of women is in the kitchen—either in her family of orientation or in her in-laws' family. She cannot seek or secure gainful employment outside the family. After 10 years of age, she is not expected or allowed to mix with members of the opposite sex outside the permitted circle of near relatives. Usually she is married off in her teens.	7.	The birth of a child of either sex is warmly accepted. Equal treatment is meted out to all children. More and more girls are receiving education—even college education. Both married as well as unmarried women can take up jobs. Inter-sex mixing is on the increase and much more accepted. The age at which girls marry is steadily rising.
8.	Marriage partners are selected by family elders, without consultation of mates. Sub-caste endogamy and geographic endogamy, family status, and often bride or bridegroom dowries are major determinants in mate selection. Reasons for marriage are	8.	There is increasing involvement of the young people themselves, often at their own initiative, in the mate-selection process. Often potential mates have a preview of each other and interact briefly. Considerations of endogamy, family status, and dowry are being replaced by

	social duty or economic gain (for one of the parties). Personal happiness of the mates is not a determining factor.		considerations of personal happiness, levels of education, earning power, and personality characteristics in the boy and physical appearance and personality characteristics in the girl. There is also an emergent trend of selection of the marriage partner by the person concerned, based on love, with or without the consent of the family elders.
9.	After marriage, the couple stays with the bridegroom's family of orientation.	9.	There is increasing tendency on the part of newly married couples to establish an independent household of their own.
10.	After the death of her husband, a widow is deprived of her ornaments and the hair on her head. She is not allowed to remarry. She is considered an ill omen on festive occasions and is believed to have brought about the death of her husband because of her destiny.	10.	More and more widows continue to wear pre-widowhood ornamentation and seek employment. They are considered neither an ill omen on festive occasions nor responsible for the death of their husbands. Widow remarriages are on the increase.

In summary, it would appear that important changes are taking place in the direction of smaller family groups, of less tyrannical relationships between the family elders and the youngsters, of more equalitarian treatment of women (as manifested by increased education, extramural gainful employment, and more enlightened attitudes toward widows, widow remarriages, etc.), and of freer relationships between the sexes with autonomy in mate selection [24].

Evidence supporting many of the statements made so far can be found in a number of studies. Contrary or conflicting evidence may also be found for some of the statements. This is partly because there are certain subcultural groups within the vast Hindu community and certain specific situations where global descriptions of behavior, attitudes, and relations of family members may not be applicable.

A number of investigators [1, 4, 6-17, 19, 21, 22, 24, 27, 30, 32-34, 36-43, 45-47, 51, 52] have attempted to shed light on diverse aspects of the Indian family and/ or the personality and mental health of its members. Attempts to relate certain dimensions of personality and mental health to family organization in other Oriental countries have also been made [48, 53]. Bronfenbrenner has discussed, on the basis of empirical evidence, how changes in child-rearing practices have been accompanied by changes in certain dimensions of personality of American children [3].

Crises in Adjustment Brought About by Social Change

As social change takes place on an uneven plane and is often desired by the young people against the wishes of the family elders, it seems to increase the vulnerability to mental health disturbances.

Let us consider the Hindu male from the traditional family who, nevertheless, gets educated because of the high premium placed on education in upwardly mobile groups. He enters college and becomes emotionally involved with a girl from a different caste. This relationship breeds a number of intrapersonality conflicts with respect to the expression or inhibition of his sexual urges, and the problem of making an autonomous decision to marry a mate of his own choice who belongs to a different caste against the disapproval of his family. Even without bringing this matter to the attention of the family elders, he may rupture his relationship with the girl, the effect of which may disturb his emotional balance as well as that of the girl. If, on the other hand, he pursues the matter further with the family elders, a number of interpersonal conflicts may result which may prove to be traumatic for him and also precipitate a mental disturbance. And finally, if in spite of these intrapersonality and interpersonal conflicts, he should decide to enter into what is called in India a "love marriage," both the partners may be overcome by guilt as a result of disregarding the internalized prohibitions of parental figures. If these unconscious, parental images are both nurturant and powerful, thus evoking intense ambivalence, basic conflicts at a deeper level may be generated and may bring about divorce or mental disorder.

Let us envisage another situation. Having been to college, the highly educated youth secures a responsible executive position in an organization. This position, however, demands initiative, independence of thinking, and decision-making for which he is psychologically unprepared due to his "culture of infancy and childhood." This inability on the part of the Hindu youth to fulfill the requirements of modern society has been described by the author as a "personality lag," which may also have repercussions on the mental health of the individual [24].

In still another situation, a wide disparity in the educational levels between this youth and older males in the family may also create problems both for him as well as for them. He is no longer able to respect them to the same extent as before, and he may prefer the companionship of his wife to the resentment of other female members of the joint household. He may even elect to stay in a residential nuclear family and no longer feel it his duty to earmark a considerable portion of his income for the joint family. When he does undertake some of these responsibilities, his wife on her side may resent these and respond with psychosomatic or other mental disorders. He may thus be caught in quite a conflictual bind. His patrilineally related joint family members may feel "cheated" and may consider him ungrateful, or his wife may feel isolated and helpless in the face of traditional pressures. It is not surprising that he sometimes breaks down in the middle of these opposing forces.

In what way does social change affect the personality development and mental health of the Hindu female? In the nontraditional family setting, her birth is welcomed, she is treated like her brothers and receives an education. She thus develops a positive self-image, made up of self-respect, self-confidence, and poise. She is not resentful or envious of males, so that she can enter into nonrivalrous relationships with them. At the same time, she does not develop an adequate capacity for tolerating frustrations which is conducive to vulnerability.

In many households, where these changed attitudes and perceptions prevail, restrictions of personal mobility and autonomy still persist leading to conflicts concerning modes of dress, freedom of movement, heterosexual mixing, and autonomous mate selection. If she is gainfully employed, she may come into conflict for this reason with other female members of the household who are confined to the house. This, in turn, may stimulate conflicts within herself regarding her role expectations. As a working wife and mother, she also encounters pressures in industry for which she has not been prepared in her earlier life [27].

If this educated girl with a positive self-image (accustomed to a fair amount of personal mobility, tolerance for her likes and dislikes, respect for her individuality and privacy, and encouragement for her autonomy) gets married into a traditional family (as happens nowadays in many cases), conflict, again, is almost inevitable and may be serious both for her and for the adjustment of the family.

In the discussion so far we have presumed uniform family organization, well-defined, hierarchically established, intrafamily relationships, strict conformity to prescribed and proscribed relations, modes of conduct and values, and deduced sex-specific uniform models of personality. We have ignored intracultural variability, idiosyncratic adaptations and responses to unique stressor conditions, individual differences in terms of variant genetically transmitted thresholds, as well as divergent ontogenetic experiences—all those factors which are involved in the variability of individuals in a given culture. It is also a fact that not all parents and family elders use the same child-rearing practices to which they themselves were exposed and consequently do not always produce the same basic personality presumed to be shaped by them. Inkeles has shown that parents do show awareness to social change and its requirements and modify their child-rearing practices "for better adapting" their children "to changed social conditions they may meet as adults" [18]. Sophisticated parents of children investigated in the Longitudinal Project of the B. M. Institute have been found to be doing the same thing. At the same time it must be emphasized that despite diversity of prevalent personality configurations among individuals of the Hindu society, various approximations to the models presented here are likely to be found in their basic personality structure.

Indices of Positive Mental Health and Vulnerability to Mental Illness

Certain assumptions have been made in this presentation about factors contributory to positive mental health, to vulnerability to mental health disturbances, and to mental illness. For clarity of comprehension, these are presented here in the following schematic form [24].

	Indices of Positive Mental Health		Indices of Vulnerability to Mental Health Disturbances
1.	A positive self-image associated with the feeling that one is a worthy person and a valued member of one's social group.	1.	A negative self-image associated with the feeling that one is useless, inadequate, and likely to be rejected by one's social group.
2.	A firm sense of identity so that one clearly knows what one is, what roles one occupies in one's social group, and what one would like to be.	2.	Role confusion so that one does not know what one is, what one's roles are and ought to be in one's social group, or what one would like to be.
3.	Optimal work involvement; neither obsessional preoccupation with work nor lethargy.	3.	Either or obsessional preoccupation with work or shirking of work.
4.	Acceptance of one's sex role associated with the feeling of sexual adequacy, an acceptance of a heterosexual partner, and the role of being mother or father with a capacity to give and receive affection.	4.	Rejection of one's sex role associated with sexual impotence, frigidity, and perverse modes of sexual gratification; an impaired capacity to give and receive affection and to assume a parental role.
5.	A capacity for comfortable interpersonal relationships; sufficient attachment to family members, peers, etc.; neither quarrelsome nor paranoid in one's interactions.	5.	Disturbed interpersonal relationships as evident in over— or underattachments to family members; quarrelsome or paranoid.
6.	An optimal tolerance of tensions, neither courting them masochistically nor avoiding them at all costs;	6.	A masochistic tendency to suffer; a low threshold for aggression.

	a moderate threshold for aggression.		
7.	Mild intrapersonality conflicts.	7.	Serious intrapersonality conflicts.
8.	A sense of trust and security that one is not in danger or that if one is, that one can deal adequately with it.	8.	A chronic sense of insecurity and mistrust associated with feelings of anxiety and apprehension that one is in danger and that one cannot grapple with it as and when it arises.

Social Change and the Incidence of Mental Illness

Because of the increased stresses and strains of modern everyday living, a crucial question confronting psychiatrists today is whether mental illness is on the increase throughout the world and is this particularly so in developing countries where traditional institutions are being rapidly modernized. There are many hazards in making cross-cultural comparisons of the incidence of mental illness by means of epidemiological studies, and these involve the use of different diagnostic criteria, the use of different methods of detecting mental illness, and problems of verbalizing, reluctance to communicate, and distortions of interpreters in the case of foreign investigators [5, 14, 31].

This was resulted in a wide divergence in reported incidence figures ranging from 6.8 to 233 per 1000. However, Lin's carefully controlled study revealed an increase in the incidence of mental illness in his sample over a period of 15 years which he attributed to increase in stress and strain of social change [31].

Some reported increase in India can be attributed to an increasing availability of treatment facilities; to their increasing use due to the spread of education making for more awareness and acceptance of "nonindigenous" treatment modes; to increasing transport facilities enabling villagers to get to treatment; to the exposure of "weak" persons hitherto sheltered by joint families within a simple pastoral-agricultural economy to the complex demands of urban living; to lesser opportunities for seclusion-seeking and psychologically weak individuals to lead supported lives as religious mendicants because of diminishing veneration for such roles in a more secular world [15]; to the saving by modern medicine of mentally and physically handicapped children; to the reduction in infant mortality and to the increase in longevity, this latter bringing more "degenerated" old persons for psychiatric treatment; and to the sick role no longer being accepted by the changing society [14].

In their study of 160 schizophrenic and 160 hysterical Indian patients, Sukhathanker and Vahia found that the most common precipitating factors for both disorders lay in family disharmony in the joint or traditionally arranged marriage [49]. According to them, schizophrenia and hysteria were common among migrant industrial workers. Cormack refers to her discussion with Bhatia and Gore who have indicated an increase in mental illness in India due to social change, though with some reservations [6].

Another development which has considerable consequences for personality development and mental health is the widespread movement for family planning and the resulting emergence of families with small numbers of children, adequately spaced, changed husband-wife relations, nutritional adequacy, and increasing utilization of educational opportunities [54].

There are also, of course, positive consequences of social change on personality developments and mental health. Planning, economic development, improved sanitation, medical treatment, large-scale introduction of welfare activities of the State and increase in amenities of life—all these appear to have reduced the stresses and strains and to have expanded the zone of felt security, sensitivity to aesthetic experiences, creativity, and so on.

Concluding Remarks

This chapter contains many hunches and broad hypotheses. To psychiatrists and psychologists trained in statistically sophisticated and rigorous methodology and to social scientists seeking precision and definite relationships backed by empirical research, the armchair type of speculation attempted here and mainly based on impressionistic and clinical evidence may appear unscientific.

Justification for the approach undertaken here, despite the many pitfalls, comes from the fact that attempts to understand the Hindu personality and mental health in the context of changing Indian family have been scanty.

It is hoped that researchers in the field of Indian family life would work out operationally defined conceptual schemata rather than the crude ones presented in this chapter, state in definite terms the incidence and range of family forms, and outline in due course a body of knowledge in which the hypotheses and hunches developed here and by other investigators can be verified or refuted.

Bibliography

1. Asthana, H. S., Some aspects of personality structuring in Indian (Hindu) social organization. *J. Soc. Psychol.*, 44 (1956), 155.
2. Bossard, J. H. S. and E. S. Boll, Security in the large family, *Mental Hygiene*, 38 (1954), 4.
3. Broffenbrenner, U., The Changing American child: a speculative analysis, *J. Soc. Issues*, 17 (1961), 6.
4. Carstairs, M., *Twice Born*, Indiana Univ. Press, Indiana, (1958).
5. Chance, N. A. et al., Modernization, value identification and mental health: A cross-cultural study anthropologica 8:2 Abstracted in *Transcultural Psychiatric Research*, 4 (1961), 108.
6. Cormark, M., *She Who Rides a Peacock*, Praeger, New York, (1960).
7. Desai, I. P., *Some Aspects of Family in Mahuva*, Asia Pub. House, Bombay, (1964).
8. Devanandan, P. D. and M. M. Thomas, *The Changing Pattern of Family in India*, Christian Institute of Study or Religion and Society, Bangalore, (1966).
9. Ghurye, G. S., *Family and Kin in Indo-European Culture*, Oxford University Press, Bombay, (1955).
10. Goode, W. J., *World Revolution and Family Patterns*, Free Press, New York, (1963).
11. Gore, M. S., *Urbanization and Family Change*, Popular Prakashan, Bombay, (1968).
12. Hate, C. A., *Changing Status of Woman: In Post-Independence India*, Allied Publishers, Bombay, (1969).
13. Hoch, E. M., Mental health services for students, an unpublished paper, (1965).
14. Hoch, E. M., Transcultural psychiatry, *J. Soc. Res.*, 11 (1966), 64.
15. Hoch, E. M., Family Mental Health Risks in P. D. Devanandan and M. M. Thomas, *The Changing Pattern of Family in India*, Christian Institute of study of Religion and Society, Bangalore, (1966).
16. Hoch, E. M., Why the body as a scapegoat for psychiatric symptoms? an unpublished paper, (1966).
17. Hoch, E. M., *Indian Children On a Psychiatrist's Playground*, Indian Council of Medical Research, New Delhi, (1967).
18. Inkeles, A., Social change and social character; The role of parental mediation, *J. Soc. Issues*, 11 (1955), 12.

19. Kapadia, K. M., *Marriage and Family in India,* Oxford University Press, Bombay, (1966).
20. Kardiner, A. and R. Linton, *Individual and His Society,* Columbia University Press, New York, (1939).
21. Karve, D. D., *The New Brahmans: Five Maharashtrian Families,* University of California Press, Berkeley, (1963).
22. Karve, I. C., *Kinship Organization in India,* Asia Publishing House, Bombay, (1965).
23. Khatri, A. A., Some neglected problems and approaches to the study of family in India, *Sociological Bull.*, 10 (1961), 75.
24. Khatri, A. A., Social change in the caste Hindu family and its possible impact on personality and mental health, *Sociological Bull.*, 11 (1962), 145.
25. Khatri, A. A., Social change in the Hindu family and its possible impact on mental health, *Vidya, J. Gujarat University,* 6 (1963), 65.
26. Khatri, A. A., Cultural conflict and mental health, *Vidya, J. Gujarat University,* 6 (1963), 84.
27. Khatri, A. A., Changing family and personality of Hindus – A few broad hypotheses, *Vidya, J. Gujarat Univ.* 8 (1965), 112.
28. Khatri, A. A., Marriage and family in India. An overview of researches, Part II of *Researches in Child Development, Marriage and Family Relations Done in Indian Institutions of teaching and Research,* Department of Child Development, Faculty of Home, Science, University of Baroda, Baroda, (1966).
29. Khatri, A. A. and B. B. Siddiqui, A boy or a girl? Preference of parents for sex of the offspring as perceived by East Indian and American children: A cross-cultural *J. Marr. Fam.*, 31 (1969), 388.
30. Khatri, A. A., The Indian family: An empirically derived analysis of shifts in size and types (1969). To be read before the family session of Seventh World Congress of Sociology, scheduled for meeting at Varna, Bulgaria, Sept. 1970.
31. Lin, T. Epidemiological study of mental disorders, *W. H. O. Chronicle,* 21 (1967), 509.
32. Mandelbaum, D. G., The World and the world view of the Kota, in Y. A. Cohen, Ed., *Social Structure and Personality,* A Casebook, Holt, Rinehart and Winston, New York, (1961).
33. Mandelbaum, D. G., The Family in India, In R. N. Anshen, Ed., *The Family: Its Function and Destiny.* Harper & Bros., New York, (1959).
34. Marfatia, J. C., *Psychiatric Problems of Children,* Popular Prakashan, Bombay, (1963).
35. Mead, M., *Coming of Age in Samoa,* New American Library, New York, (1951).
36. Minturn, L. and J. T. Hitchcock, The Rajputs of Khalapur, India, in B. B. Whiting, Ed., *Six Cultures,* John Wiley & Sons, New York, (1963).
37. Minturn, L. and W. W. Lambert, *Mothers of Six Cultures: Antecedents of Child Rearing,* John Wiley & Sons, New York, (1964).
38. Mitra, S. K., A Study of personality of school-leaving boys by T. A. T. method. An unpublished paper.
39. Morris, C., *Varieties of Human Values,* University of Chicago Press, Chicago, (1956).

40. Murphy, L. B., Roots of tolerance and tensions in Indian child development in G. Murphy, *In the Minds of Men,* Basic Books, New York, (1953).
41. Narain, D., Growing up in India, *Family Process,* 3 (1964), 127.
42. Narain, D., *Hindu Character,* Bombay University, Bombay, (1957).
43. Prabhu, P. N., *Hindu Social Organization – A Study In Social Psychological and Ideological Foundations,* Popular Book Depot, Bombay, (1963).
44. Poffenberger, T. et al., *A Preliminary survey of Indian Institutions teaching and conducting research in child development and family relationships,* Dept. of Child Development, Faculty of Home Science, M. S. University of Baroda, Boroda.
45. Ramanujam, B. K., Relevance of psychological implications of family relations in India, unpublished paper, (1966).
46. Ramanujam, B. K., Some thoughts on psychological problems of families in India, *Ind. J. Psychiat,* 9 (1967), 9.
47. Ross, A. D., *The Hindu Family In Its Urban Setting,* Oxford University Press, Toronto, (1961).
48. Straus, M. A., Childhood experience and emotional security in the context of Sinhalese social organization, *Social Forces,* 33 (1954), 152.
49. Sukhathanker, H. C. and N. S. Vahia, Influence of social cultural factors in Schizophrenia and Hysteria in Bombay (India). Abstracted in *Transcultural Psychiatric Research,* 2 (1965), 34.
50. Talcott, Parsons, The Incest taboo in relation to social structure and the socialization of the child in *Personality and Social Systems,* N. J. Smelser and W. T. Smelser, Eds., John Wiley & Sons, New York, (1963).
51. Taylor, W. S., Behaviour disorders and the breakdown of the orthodox Hindu family system, *Ind. J. of Social Work,* 4 (1943), 162.
52. Taylor, W. S., Basic personality in orthodox Hindu culture patterns. *J. Abnorm. Soc. Psychol.* 43 (1948), 3.
53. Vogel, E. F. and S. H. Vogel, Family security, personal immaturity and emotional health in a Japanese sample, *Marr. Fam. Liv.* 23 (1961), 161.
54. W. H. O. Scientific Group on Mental Health Research Meeting (64): A Report, Mental health and research, *W. H. O. Chronicle,* 18, 380.
55. Winch, R. F., Some observations on personality structure in Japan, in R. F. Winch and R. McGinnis, Eds., *Selected Studies in Marriage and Family,* Holt, Rinehart, Winston, New York, (1960).

Changing Dynamic Aspects of the Turkish Culture and Its Significance for Child Training

EMEL A. SÜMER (TURKEY)

Introduction

Present-day Turkey is definitely changing in its dynamic process of growth and modernization. Since Ataturk's great revolution in the early twenties, this movement, which had already started among the young Turks, has continued to accelerate. Lerner points out that Turkey is the outstanding example of this modernization in the Middle East [6]. If the changes in the Middle East countries between 1927 to 1957 are taken into consideration, it becomes clear that Turkey moves at a faster speed than the other countries. Perhaps with the exception of Israel, Turkey seems to be much more culturally dynamic than any other country of the Middle East. Therefore, a single family type or a unique way of child training cannot be taken as the prototype of a typical Turkish family. One can only speak in terms of dynamic changes in Turkish families which correspond to cultural changes occurring in Turkey.

The views offered in this chapter are based on intensive psychiatric work with large numbers of families who have either applied to the out-patient service of the Istanbul University hospital or to private clinics. Our findings have been corroborated by other psychiatrists and psychologists working in the same area which lends some sort of clinical validity to them.

The first Turkish settlements were in central Asia. There are no definite data pertaining to the family structure of the ancient Turks, but it is highly probable that it was patriarchal due to the influence of other Asian tribes like the ones mentioned by Takeyoshi Kawashima in his book, *Japanese Character and Culture* [5].

According to Findikoglu's studies, Turks in the early seventh century, before accepting the Islamic religion, lived in large family groups. They were not polygamous and did not divorce. Marriage was considered to be a very serious and important institution. If men left their wives they were ostracized and punished by being hanged [3].

The tribes were nomadic, hunting and herding cattle. The men fought courageously and the women shared the family responsibilities with their husbands. This also applied to the rulers. After the king's death the queen governed the tribe and remained as queen until her death, retaining legislative power on state affairs. The change of climate in central Asia and the disappearance of the central Asian sea, caused the migration of Turkish tribes. This movement started about 3000 B.C. and documented migration to Anatolia occurred about 1000 years ago. On arrival in Asia Minor, the Turks found other tribes among them such as Greeks, Arabs, Persians, and Caucasians. They did not attempt to destroy these native groups but integrated with them.

In the seventh century, under the influence of the Arabs, they accepted the Islamic religion. The effect of this showed itself in further changes in the family life and structure. Following the Crusades from the eleventh to the thirteenth centuries, they developed stronger territorial feelings and defended their land against successive Christian invasions. From then on, until Ataturk's nationalist movement, the Turks more and more assumed an Islamic identity. However, in this century there are still remnants of scattered nomadic tribes called the *Yoruk* in the southern part of Anatolia who continue to live much like the ancient Turks. Under the influence of the Islamic religion, the patriarchal family structure intensified the masculine predominance and thrust the women into a passive role bordering on slavery. Men assumed complete control of the family's affairs and left women with little influence beyond the raising of children. Islamic law supported this subjugation: a man could marry four women; a male witness was worth two female witnesses; sons inherited twice as much as daughters; and men could divorce their wives by simply stating it three times. These laws were taken from the Koran and the system of justice was called *Mecelle* (*Sharia*). These rules gradually became part of the Turkish culture, especially after the Turks settled down as farmers in Anatolia. Centuries of settlement stabilized the cultural structure.

However, different sections of Anatolia show differences in the customs, temperament, and personality of the people inhabiting them. For example, those living in central Anatolia are in many ways unlike those living on the Black Sea coast, so that the so-called "static groups" of Turkey are far from homogeneous. The Central Anatolians are generally noncommunicative, evasive, shy, introverted, conservative, and uninterested in anything outside their daily routine. It is difficult for them to adapt to change. They lead encapsulated lives, dominated by religion, reacting slowly to external events and suspiciously to all strangers. When they become ill, they generally develop schizophrenia. It would seem as if this culture predisposed them to this type of response.

The Black Sea people, in contrast, are lively and are generally called *Laz*. They live in the coastal area which is heavily wooded and their economy depends largely on fishing, tobacco, and nut crops. They are energetic, outgoing, aggressive, and they express their emotions freely. Adaption to new situations is easier for them than it is for their Central Anatolian brothers. Their psychiatric illnesses are mostly diagnosed as manic depressions and conversion hysterias[8].

People from the Aegean section are hard-working farmers, fishermen, and landowners. Most of them have acquired a higher standard of living than is prevalent in the rest of Turkey. The men of this section are called *Efe*. They are brave, highly competitive, interested, and curious. Psychosomatic disorders and conversion hysterias are very common among patients from this area.

On the Marmara coast, the local inhabitants show a complex ethnological structure. There are many immigrants, from other sections of Turkey, and mental hospital admissions parallel the ethnological structure very closely. Industrial centers such as Istanbul, Izmir, Izmit, and Bursa tend to attract families from rural areas, who have not yet been assimilated and who function ethnically as a "transitional group."

Eastern Anatolia is the most secluded area, having little communication with the rest of the country through a lack of transportation and communication facilities. There are parts where the natives, even today, do not speak proper Turkish but "Kurdish," the regional language, and their way of living is extremely primitive. Houses are still built of mud and clay. Until quite recently, men were laws unto themselves and lived in constant threat of murder by their enemies in a form of "vendetta." Like the Central Anatolians they are inclined to be suspicious, hostile, uncommunicative, and action-oriented. Admissions to psychiatric hospitals from this area display mostly paranoid and schizophrenic reactions.

Although all these sections show cultural differences as reflected in their music, dancing, and customs, there are certain general similarities that still exist. In common, all these people have a respect for tradition ("traditionalists" in Lerner's classification), a proclivity for the sedentary life, a very religious outlook, and a disinclination to transact with those outside their territory. Until a few years ago, they did not listen to radios or read the newspapers and most of them were unable to either read or write. Only after Ataturk's revolution, were these remote inhabitants of Anatolia encouraged to become literate and, for the first time, they were exposed to the mass media. However, the problem of illiteracy although decreasing, is still far from being resolved, especially among women.

As an example of the conservatism of these people, Morrison describes how the peasants of Alisar, a central Anatolian village of 58 households comprising 292 individuals, were still living in the year 1922 like the *Hüyük* of 3000 years ago [7]. This situation was regarded by the Alisar villagers as quite normal since they knew no other. The road connections to the metropolitan areas were almost nonexistent so that isolation was virtually complete. The concept of distance was measured by travel on foot, prolonged time by the harvesting of crops, and daily time by phases of the sun. Change was identified with evil and feared. They seemed to be totally lacking in curiosity and drive. Superstitions helped to relieve their primitive anxieties.

The adults in this traditional culture have to fit themselves to a certain rigid pattern of conduct. The children have even less choice as to what they are, and what they are going to be. The life style and the life cycle are predetermined and deviancy is not well tolerated. Under such conditions, the personality becomes stereotyped and constricted. In such traditional cultures there is only one way of life and only one way of looking at life. All boundaries are within walking distance and the villagers live and die within them. What goes on beyond these is irrelevant and, when confronted with communications from the outside, withdrawal ensues. Every novelty is by definition threatening and so to be rejected. The children accept their father's point of view without question and unconditional respect and obedience is built into the family system. The younger generation are therefore without initiative and take their orders automatically from the older people. There is no push to self-realization and personal achievement. They are content with the little they have in accordance with the Anatolian saying: "Just a bit to eat and something to wear" (*Bir lokma bir hirka*). They are usually gloomy-looking and depressed people, who react helplessly in the face of major problems. They are not accustomed to express ideas about events outside their daily routine. Anatolian man is called *Mehmetçik* which signifies the heroic man. He goes to battle bravely while his woman waits at home in prayer. The man is conceived of as courageous, honest, and loyal and the woman as passive, helpful, unselfish and self-sacrificing. Her daily duty is to deny her own interests, wishes, and needs.

The Traditional Family Group

The families live in large groups that are patriarchal in structure comprising young fathers and the parents and grandparents of these young fathers. The grandfather is in charge of the household, and he is the unquestionable authority. Second in the hierarchy is the paternal grandmother. They are usually farmers and they need people to work on the farm. The young man at a very young age is married off to a girl of his grandmother's choice, usually a healthy and strong girl who can work on the farm. The young woman does not have much choice. She is trained to be obedient and makes no objection to the decision of her parents.

The wedding ceremony shows slight differences from section to section in Anatolia, but the nuclear ritual usually symbolizes the loss of the girl to the boy's family. In fact, before the marriage the boy's family has to pay the girl's family a sum of money or goods which is called *başlik*. This *başlik* can be considered as the purchase price of the girl as a commodity. However, another interpretation of the transaction sees the money as a contribution toward the wedding expenses incurred by the bride's father. The latter may even speak of "selling" his daughter when he is marrying her off. Although the young man's mother manipulates the whole arrangement, she still cannot help feeling, like every other mother, that she is losing her son to another woman. In one section of Anatolia, for example, in the village of Balikesir, after the wedding ceremony, the mother makes the son pass between her legs before entering the bride's room on the wedding night, which is an interesting symbolic variant of the *rites de passage.*

The young woman is without power or prestige in the home. In the Eastern sections of Anatolia she cannot speak or even sit in the presence of her in-laws. She does most of the housework and, in addition to this, she also goes to work in the fields. When the husband leaves for military service, he writes home to his parents and not to his wife whom he cannot mention by name in his letters. The young wife's pregnancy is hardly her own business. She has no say as to whether she wants a child or not and no control over conception. Even in the later stages of pregnancy, she continues to work both inside and outside the house. The delivery usually takes place at home with the help of the most experienced old woman in the village, and it is the grandmother who announces the birth and arranges a feast in the baby's honor. For economic reasons, the women's fertility is of the greatest importance to the family, especially her ability to bear male children. After the birth of a child, the young mother gains some status in the household, especially if she has a boy but, although her situation improves with each subsequent birth, she can never hope to become as powerful as the grandmother. Neither parent, in Eastern Anatolia, is allowed to show affection to the child in the presence of the grandparents.

Under the cultural mask, the young woman not infrequently resents her passive and exploited position, but frustration and anger seldom get expression except in the form of some hysterical of psychosomatic manifestation. However, as she gets older, especially after the menopause, her status improves. She becomes freer with her in-laws if they are still alive and, when her husband dies, she takes complete control of the household so that a striking metamorphosis takes place from what she was – a passive, fearful girl – to what she becomes – a powerful, authoritarian old woman taking revenge from her early sufferings and treating the new bride as herself was once treated. The sinister figure of the old woman is well known in Turkish folklore where she appears as an omnipotent character who can do either good or harm, who gets involved as a go-between in the love affairs of the young, and who is to be feared, respected, and consulted on every difficult subject including illness. They practice a type of "old wives" medicine based on herbal prescriptions and referred to in the vernacular as *koca kari ilaci.*

CHILD REARING

Breast feeding starts when the baby is a day old and continues, on an average, until the child is 3 to 4 years old, on demand. Not only can he have the breast when he wants it but he is permitted to play with it at will. Boys are nursed longer, particularly the first son, because of the entrenched belief that the mother's milk makes for strength. After this very indulgent, sensual, and dependent relationship with the mother, the intimacy suddenly ends with the grandmother taking over the care of the children. Socialization with peers is encouraged and no doubt helps the separation process.

During the dependent phase, the baby is tightly swaddled and carried by the mothers on their backs as they work in the fields. It has been suggested that this immobilization may be responsible in part for the aggressive heroism and warmth of the Anatolian male.

Eating is an important activity in Turkish culture and to eat with someone signifies friendship. One is expected to eat what one is given, no less and no more. If one refuses to eat what is given, one is rejecting the offer of friendship. To eat more than one's share is to be impolite. Much of this is summed up in the old Turkish saying that "a cup of coffee is worth forty years' consideration."

TOILET TRAINING

In the mose secluded villages of Eastern Anatolia, diapers are not used, the child being put to sleep in his cradle bundled up with a type of soil that soaks up the urine. Erikson has described similar customs among Indian tribes [2]. In the morning, the wet soil is dried in the sun and used again in the same way. Occasionally a kind of wooden apparatus is fitted to the child's genital area, the urine passing through a pipe to a receiving cup on the floór. This is called *sübek.*

During the daytime, the child wears a dress without underwear so as to make it easy for him to urinate. Defecation is a private function which is performed privately but urination is performed casually and publicly. As soon as he can walk, the toddler is taken by the older children to places defined for purposes of defecation. Appropriate toilet behavior is regulated by shaming, and the children seem to learn quickly and sensitively about what is required of them. Here too, as observed by anthropologists, bodily possessions carry the bodily identity which it is superstitiously believed can be used for evil purposes by their enemies.

SEXUAL EDUCATION

Even though children are given much freedom with regard to sensual satisfaction in the initial years, sex is generally not discussed too much and is rigidly controlled by religion. Sexual training of the girls shows major differences from that of the boys. Until the boy is 5 or 6 years of age, his penis is a matter of great pride to the father who will often encourage the boy to expose his genital among the father's friends to demonstrate his masculinity. Of course, in so behaving, the fathers are also seeking reassurance about their own potency.

As the boy gets older, he is warned repeatedly against homosexual assaults. There is a very strong taboo on homosexual relationships. However, the culture provides sublimated outlets for homosexual drives in the form of homosocial closeness, such as kissing and hugging, *hamams* (Turkish baths), and so forth. It has been postulated that these rigidly repressed homosexual tends are, to some degree, responsible for the frequent crimes of jealousy in Turkey, but this needs further investigation.

The boy is trained to be brave, intrusive, and proud of his masculinity, but after the prolonged dependency on his mother, he often experiences great difficulty in separating from her so that his sexual identity becomes blurred. As a result he develops various techniques to compensate for his feminine identification and enhance his masculine ego. As anthropologists have pointed out, the ritual circumcision at the critical age of 6 years is a culturally sanctioned method of breaking the boy away from his mother. Following circumcision, the boys enter the men's world. However, since this problem of masculine identity is not always solved satisfactorily, many men remain extremely sensitive to any challenge to their masculinity and may even go as far as murder to prove themselves. It is not uncommon to read in the daily papers of the murder of a woman who has triggered this hypersensitive aggressive response simply by saying "Are you a man?" At a less intensive level, the boys become boisterous and competitive as wrestlers, a national sport, and equally competitive in a popular game played with the short bones of cattle called *aşik*. The good-humored rivalry stimulates closeness among the boys in general, but especially among brothers who tend to be extremely close to one another. The oldest brother is next in line to the grandfather and father in terms of prestige and power and there is a descending "pecking order" with regard to the rest.

Girls, on the other hand, are made aware of their difference from boys from the early age of 5 years. She has to stay at home and take care of the younger ones. She is trained to be shy, bashful, afraid of men, and afraid of rape without knowing what is meant by it. Virginity is of vital importance and valued as much as life itself. Like her mother, the girl modestly covers her pubic hair and at puberty she learns from the same source how to hide her menstruation, which she is taught to regard as dirty. She receives intensive instruction on domestic matters, such as sewing, embroidering, cooking, and working alongside her mother in the fields. It is not culturally acceptable for her to imitate or emulate boys or participate tomboyishly in their sports.

DISCIPLINE

Discipline is obtained by techniques of frightening and shaming. The mother frightens the child with stories of superhuman punishing agents or by the display of vengeful objects of which she herself is superstitiously afraid. At times, however, she will simply spank the child. To some extent, the entire village participates in disciplining. Every adult female is an aunt, and every adult male an uncle and all have responsibilities in promoting good behavior. The child's grandparents are traditionally lenient and permissive with their grandchild. Thus the child is brought up in a large and loving family circle, the members of which are sufficiently involved in his welfare to maintain a constant check on his conduct. As a result, delinquency is rarely seen in the villages. Responsibility comes at an early age and from 7 years on, the boy drives the village herd to the meadows when his turn comes, and the girl takes care of the younger children and helps her mother in the house and in the field.

In short, after 6 years of age, the girl is disciplined to become passive, fearful, reticent, and industrious like the older women, while the boy is disciplined to become responsible, reliable, and self-sufficient like the older men so he can go out and do things for himself on his own.

RELIGION

Religion is a major influence on the functioning of the Turkish family and on its structure. Prior to the seventh century, the Turks believed in two gods – an "earth god," and a "heaven god" – which tended to further a more "democratic" family pattern. After accepting Islamic monotheism, family structure changed and the women were pushed into the background and hidden behind the veil. The Sultan became the earthly representative of the prophet, Mohammed, and supernatural powers were projected on to him.

Today religion is extremely necessary for the villagers to compensate for their earthly frustrations. They are comforted with the prospect of a better life after death, and are preoccupied with the necessity of not doing anything to conflict with a religious system that punctiliously delineates the good and the bad. Religion also requires the men to go into the army and it is believed that those killed in the war go directly to heaven.

The Moslem man goes to prayers five times a day, and he meets his friends in the mosque at least once a week on Fridays, after which they have group discussions on religious matters. The occasion is thus both religious and social.

The religion also inculcates a fatalistic point of view and a belief in *kismet*. The future is in the hands of God. It is this that engenders passivity and resignation in the face of disasters. This outlook stems from an interpretation of the Koran which is understood as saying that one should "do one's best and leave the rest to god." This provides much release from anxiety as compared with the Christian dogmas.

Aside from religion, superstitions and supernatural powers are seen as causal so that misunderstood natural events are explained by the interventions of *cins*, demons, and other evil spirits. The authentic Moslem religion offers a complete and satisfying philosophy of life but, when misinterpreted, it can be misused for any dubious purpose. For example, under the influence of powerful but ignorant clergymen, printing machines could not be imported into Turkey because of the superstitious excuse that sacred words like "God" might be written. Behind all such irrational prohibitions lay the fear that priestly dominance might be undermined. Thus the first Turkish printing machine was installed in 1729, three centuries after printing was invented in Europe, with the result that the West failed to make its cultural impact, so that nothing comparable to the Renaissance took place. The artistic efflorescence in any case could not have been transmitted since religion also prohibited the portrayal of God in any fashion.

The Transitional Family Group

Utilizing Lerner's classification, the "transitional" urban groups are immigrants from rural areas. They are born in the rural sections, and migrate gradually, first to small towns, and then to larger metropolitan areas like Istanbul, Ankara, and Izmir. After the revolution, Atatürk, in order to further the modernization of the villages and stem the tide of immigration, introduced a special law (March 8, 1924) containing several practical measures. One provided agricultural instruction for the village youth during their military service, and another made provisions for the establishment of agricultural credits through the central Agricultural Bank. The most significant, however, was the setting up of the "Village Institutes" which offered primary education to villagers who would then return to their villages and instruct others. Even though Atatürk's plan was successful in improving local conditions, it did not stop the immigration to the industrial and metropolitan centers. According to the plan, the urbanization of the villages was to progress slowly so as to preserve a cultural balance. Initially it was customary for men to leave their villages and families periodically for work in the cities. After 1950, men started bringing their families with them minus the grandparents to settle in *gecekondu* (overnight house districts) that were privately owned or run by the government. They themselves constructed one-room houses in a single night before the government officials could interfere, and the buildings were therefore under constant threat of being torn down. Since these people were unskilled laborers and frequently unemployed, this threat to their homes engendered a great deal of insecurity.

However, even these unfavorable conditions were better than their lot in the villages, so that rural families continued to invade the towns. According to Karpat's survey, *gecekondus* constitute 39.55 percent of the town residential area of Istanbul and the inhabitants of *gecekondus* make up 45 percent of Istanbul's entire population and 50 percent of Turkey's total population[4]. These figures point to the major importance of this migratory group to the total economy of Turkey.

The peasants that come to the cities usually work at odd jobs requiring no particular skills. The family usually moves into an overnight housing district. Thus, in general, they simply exchange primitive rural conditions for slum life with its gross overcrowding. However, they are able to observe ways of living different to those of the villages and, although they are ambivalent about the new things and nostalgic about the old life to which they try to adhere, they enter into a process of change. The reaction to change is both striking and varied. Some of them become resistive and more entrenched in their conservativism and hyperreligiosity; some become restless and upward striving; but the majority are stimulated to follow the latest news in papers, go to the movies, and listen to the radio. They are interested in knowing what is going on in the country and in the world and, as their knowledge of the world enlarges, they begin to emphatize with the people of the other lands and become less xenophobic. They find explanations for their frustrating lives rather than ascribing it all to "kismet," or "God's doing." But the frustrations of living and the miserable conditions under which they exist take their toll and result either in a higher rate of psychiatric disorder or, when the aggression is channeled into competition, improved standards of living. This latter development constitutes one of the main dynamic forces modernizing Turkey.

The sections where the immigrants live, *gecekondu mahallesi*, are like a boiling cauldron mixing many different values together. Religion, which was a strong force in the family when they were in the village, is now in conflict with the city's free thinking, materialistic attitudes. In place of servitude, the woman has freedom, equal rights, better education, and a wide variety of job opportunities; she may also well become the family breadwinner. In short, the old traditional balance is upset with the woman achieving dominance while she is still far from old. As a consequence, a new type of family conflict comes into existence originating in cultural change. In an investigation carried out by Arkun [1], it was shown that there was a high rate of suicide among married couples in 1927, soon after the declaration of the Civil Code. Arkun concluded that women preferred suicide to divorce – the latter not yet being acceptable to society. In 1960, the divorce rate increased and the suicide rate among marked couples decreased. One might infer that couples were now ready to solve their neurotic conflicts through more realistic modes of behavior. It is also worth mentioning that adultery was the primary cause of divorces signifying perhaps that the Turkish woman was rebelling against the "shame" culture which compelled her for so long to deny her own needs and wishes in deference to those of the male[1].

This transitional society was not geared to the needs of the children. While the mother went to work, the children were left to their own devices on the streets, unsupervised with a key tied around their necks. In the city there were no aunts and uncles to whom the child could turn for help or guidance. The close personal relationships of the traditional group were replaced by the impersonal contacts of the city. Maternal deprivation and lack of parental control began to show their effects with a rise in delinquency. Some of the mothers, as if revenging themselves for centuries of exploitation, abandoned their families in order to go to work in Germany. On the opposite side to desertion are the overindulgent mothers, in both transitional and modern types of families, whose children remain delinquent and immature. In our own clinical studies, we found these Turkish mothers to be egotistical, controlling and demanding of the child in a way that bore no relationship to the child's needs at his particular stage of development [9]. This type of overprotective and overstimulating mother impedes the normal process of separation and individuation so that not only is the mother unable to leave the child alone but the child becomes unable to let the mother go. As a group, these women are hypochondriacal, preoccupied with somatic concerns, sexually immature and frigid, and very threatened by their child's developing sexuality. Even though they dress themselves in a very feminine manner and behave seductively, inwardly they are extremely hostile toward men. Today they have equal legal rights, but this does not prevent their having a poor self-concept associated with marked feelings of inferiority. The possessive behavior with the children, particularly their sons, is to some extent an effort to compensate for this sense of inadquacy. The new feministic outlook also creates conflict with the older women since the younger women in the city, unlike their counterparts in the village, resist dominance and exploitation.

The transitional situation, therefore, brings strife between husband and wife, mother and child, and daughter-in-law and mother-in-law. This can frequently end in sexual maladjustment between the partners, divorce, the misuse of children for libidinal satisfactions, and emotional disturbances in the children who run away or remain tied to the mother. These women raise their children to feel a deep sense of obligation which they must repay even into old age.

The transitional family shows all stages in the admixture of traditional and modern ways and is, therefore, culturally the most heterogenous of the different group. Having lost its earlier values and having not quite assimulated the modern ones, the life of the immigrant is often in a state of turmoil and confusion. The families are chronically anxious and apprehensive, and the children insecure and uncertain. There are more neurotic referrals from this group of children than from any other. Whereas psychiatric disturbances in the traditional group are explained by the influence of "evil spirts" and the "evil eye" and patients are taken to an old lady or *hoca* to be cured by prayers, in the transitional group, although they may sometimes go to the *hoca*, nevertheless they also come to the doctor for advice.

As they become more secure economically, they move to better sections of the city and rent their *gecekondus* to newcomers, who then pass through a similar cycle.

The Modern Family Group

"Transitionals" comprise only half of Turkey's population, and the "moderns" a minority of perhaps 15 percent. These latter people are born in large metropolitan cities, are generally well educated, and come from well-to-do families. They have wholly integrated Western thoughts and ways into their personalities and lives and are chiefly responsible for shaping the character of contemporary life in Turkey.

In this group, girls are encouraged to receive education as much as the boys, and the women have equal job opportunities. There is an increasing number of professional working women. The members of this group as a whole are achievement-oriented and highly competitive. Emphasis is placed on individuality and they are much more egocentric than traditionals or transitionals. The transitional groups are disliked by both traditionalists and moderns for the reason that they have changed the structure and outlook of the family. The modern group, on the other hand, although integrated with Western culture, still maintains the traditional patriarchal structure. However, in place of the subservient traditional relationship, there is a system of rights and obligations under the supervision of the father. In addition, there are an increasing number of marriages that are based on love, mutual respect, equal rights, and self-determination.

There is no doubt that Turkey owes a huge debt to Atatürk whose revolutionary legislation between the years 1924 and 1927 included the separation of Church and State, equal rights for women, the uncovering of the female face, and the alphabetic shift from Arabic to Latin (thus facilitating the reading and writing of the Turkish language). These are just a few of the profound changes that Ataturk brought about that were to have endless repercussions in the economic, social, and psychological spheres. It was logical that a society with such a long history of traditions could not change overnight. However, the process of change continues in Turkish society as is evident in the political and psychosocial growing pains currently being experienced. Freud once said that "in order to have a new construction there must first be a dissolution." In fact, what we are witnessing in present-day Turkey is the dissolution of the traditional and the search for a new Turkish identity that will fit better with the new conditions. Predictably, there is a phase of diffusion so that the Turkish people today are restless and troubled at all generational levels. It is, perhaps, a little exaggerated to say that Turkey has entered a stage of mass neurosis which is the price one is said to pay for civilization.

Summary

This chapter paper dealt with the cultural changes taking place in modern Turkey. The social structure is explained in three groups, that is, traditional, transitional, and modern.

A detailed description of the multiple variables entering into those changes are considered and tentative analytical explanations are offered. Emphasis is specially given to child training.

Bibliography

1. Arkun, Nezahat, Türkiyede evlenme ve bosanmalar hakkinda psiko-sosyal bir araştirma, *Istanbul Matbaasi,* Istanbul, 1965.
2. Erikson, Erik Homburger, Childhood and Tradition in Two American Indian Tribes. *The Psychoanalytic Study of the Child.* Vol. 1, International Universities Press, New York, 1945.
3. Findikoğlu, F, *Essai sur la Transformation du Code* Familial en Turquie (Etude de Sociologie Jurisdiqe Applique), Berger-Levrault, Paris, 1936.
4. Karpat, Keml H., Sosyal yapi değismeleri acisindan turkiyede gecekonu sorunu. *Milliyet Gazetesi,* 15-28 Haziran, Istanbul, 1969.
5. Kawashima, Takeyoshi, *Japanese Character and Culture.* Bernard S. Silberman, Ed., University of Arizona Press, Tucson, 1962.
6. Lerner, Daniel, *The Passing of Traditional Society,* The Free Press of Glencoe, Cambridge, Mass., 1962.
7. Morrison, J. A., Alisar, A Unit of Land Occupance, Ph.D. Thesis, University of Chicago, 1939.
8. Songar, Ayhan, Turkish Character, Istanbul Conference at Bakirköy Akil Hastahanesi, 1969.
9. Sümer, E., R. Cebiroğlu, H. Yavuz, Disturbances related to prolonged dependency in Turkish children. Paper read at the International Conference of Child Psychiatry, Edinburgh, Scotland, 1966. *Acta-Paedopsyiatrica*, in press.

On Aspects of Child Rearing in Greece

George Vassiliou and Vasso Vassiliou (Greece)

If one can assume that methods of child-rearing influence all the other transactions that shape a milieu, one should equally assume that any alteration in these transactions can result in changes of child-rearing.

In the past it seemed natural to suppose that in a given milieu the interplay of variables contributing to its development would lead to the formation of child-rearing patterns highly appropriate to the conditions. It also seemed self-evident that these patterns would be conducive to the fullest realization of the human potential and that they would lead in general to the new generation's participation in the life that evolves with benefit to both individual and milieu.

These suppositions were based on the facts that in the "pre-industrial" era exchanges between different milieux were limited, and alterations tended to synchronize so that people were normally responsive and adaptive to the social environment. With the coming of the "industrial era," alterations in the social, economic, and technological fields started to accelerate and change abruptly under controlled conditions, while alterations in psychological and cultural areas continued slowly, gradually and indirected. This gave rise to a crucial asynchronism, at times completely without rhythm, thus disrupting transactions. Under such circumstances, the established child-rearing patterns no longer appeared pertinent to the changing demands of the milieu and were out of keeping with the needs of the newer generation. Furthermore, in response to the massive technological transformations around them, they also became subjected to uncontrolled, unguided, "blind" alterations which made them even more discrepant with the new environment. In short, it had become increasingly difficult for the child to become, in an adequate way, the father to the man.

The transactional study of child-rearing within each milieu in terms of its historical aspects, its impact on within-milieu variables and its similarities with and differences from other milieux is only just beginning [9].* Since the foundation of the Institute of Anthropos (1963), the authors and their associates have conducted a number of interrelated but diversified studies related to the present topic. We will attempt to summarize our main findings.

Patterns of feeding and toilet training were investigated among the urban Greek population [1]. Representative samples of mothers in Athens and Thessalonike (towns containing approximately 30 percent of Greece's population) were asked questions similar to those relating to feeding and toilet training asked in the Sears, Maccoby and Levin [4] study in the United States. We have described Athens (population 2.1 million) as a "high complexity milieu (HCM)" and Thessalonike (population 350,000) as a "lower complexity milieu (LCM)" for Greece, and considered the findings of Sears et al. as relating to an even higher complexity milieu.

Breast-Feeding and Weaning

A total of 90 percent of Greek mothers report having breast-fed their children as opposed to 39 percent of American mothers. Frequency of breast-feeding tends to be inversely related to milieu complexity in Greece. The 10 percent of Greek mothers who report not having breast-fed their children give physical-medical reasons, indicating that they had "no choice." Among mothers with less than eight years of schooling, breast-feeding is reported by 93 percent of them, a figure which drops to 69 percent among mothers with more than eight years of education. Higher education correlates with increased involvement of mothers in activities outside the home; both education and outside involvement correlate with higher income; and all three variables are related to a lower number of children. All the above variables correlate with changes in the traditional value orientation of mothers.

A tendency can be detected to favor boys (91 percent of boys breast-fed versus 87 percent of girls). Breast-feeding frequency increases with the number of children. While 80 percent of first-borns are breast-fed, 90 and 95 percent of second- and third-borns are breast-fed, respectively. This may be a result of economic factors (less money available for bottle feeding) or a need for increased birth control, which is practiced by means of prolonged breast-feeding. It may also mean that mothers who cannot breast-feed avoid having more children. Among American mothers neither sex nor order of birth of the child seem to differentiate feeding practices.

The length of breast-feeding tends to decrease with increases in milieu complexity. By 15 months of age, only 66 percent of boys and 64 percent of girls are reported to have stopped breast-feeding, while by 9 months almost all United States infants have done so. Characteristically, in the Greek sample, 2 percent of children continued to be breast-fed up to 4 years of age. Furthermore, even when the Greek child stops being breast-fed, he is likely to continue on the bottle.

It is interesting to note that 26 percent of children in both milieux were weaned "suddenly" and harshly with such methods as putting pepper, quinine, or soap on the nipple or by putting a brush on the breast. It would seem that some mothers cannot or will not go through the successive stages of gradual weaning and, given the sociocultural sanction, they terminate abruptly.

Only 26 percent of children in Thessalonike and 35 percent in Athens shift gradually from breast-feeding to cup and spoon. When we move to the LCM, we find that a greater percentage of children are left to stop sucking on their own initiative (19 percent in Thessalonike vs. 13 percent in Athens). On the other hand, sucking is more often dealt with by "harsh" methods (17 percent in Thessalonike vs. 7 percent in Athens). Athenian mothers appear to be more "manipulative" (15 percent of children are weaned by having the mother either disappear physically or refuse in different ways to give her breast).

In both milieux girls are found to be treated more harshly than boys (16 percent vs. 10 percent), and when the child is a girl, mothers give up breast-feeding for physical reasons more readily (23 percent for girls vs. 16 percent for boys). Sears et al. [1] report that in the United States the mother is likely to be warmer toward her infant if it is a girl.

The duration of weaning is directly related to milieu complexity. While in Athens 38 percent of children are weaned over a period of two weeks, in Thessalonike this is accomplished in 56 percent of the cases. In both milieux, the sex of the child and the order of birth play no role; with increasing education of mothers, the frequency of children weaned in two weeks time decreases (58 percent with illiterate mother, 29 percent with mother of elementary education, and 22 percent with mother of higher education). The more educated mothers appear to be more "permissive." Characteristically, a good 7 percent of mothers are unable or unwilling to recall and report on their weaning methods.

With regard to regularity of feeding, 69 percent of children in Athens are fed according to a schedule, while in Thessalonike the same proportion of children (68 percent) are fed on self-demand. In both milieux, from a total of 45 percent of children fed on self-demand, 47 percent are boys and 42 percent girls, a finding which again indicates a tendency for a differential treatment of boys. As the mother's educational standard rises, it becomes more likely for the baby to be fed according to schedule.

With the cessation of breast-feeding, the majority of mothers in Athens (83 percent) report using canned milk, while only 45 percent of mothers in Thessalonike do so. Sucking, however, continues for prolonged periods. By the age of 16 months only 47 percent of children are reported as having been weaned. After the second year of life, 30 percent of the children are still sucking. Birth order of the child and education of the mother do not seem to play a role in weaning, whereas the sex of the child does. Somehow boys tend to be weaned earlier than girls. Mothers do not report any difficulties or emotional reactions in the child connected with weaning.

To summarize, a comparison of Greek findings concerning breast-feeding with those of a higher complexity milieu in the United States indicate that most Greek mothers breast-feed their children, while in the United States the majority of mothers report not doing so. The Greek mothers also report breast-feeding and/or bottle-feeding for considerably longer periods of time. Findings suggest that there is differential treatment of children, and that boys are favored over girls. Within Greece, comparing findings from LCM and HCM, we detect an evolution of practices along lines followed in other more developed, "modernized" milieux during the earlier phases of their development.

Toilet Training

In view of the above it is surprising to discover that with regard to toilet training, Greek findings are quite comparable with the findings of other developed milieux, such as the United States.

Our data indicate that in both milieux, Greece and the United States, the average age for the beginning of bowel training is the same, between the tenth and eleventh month, while completion occurs on an average between the eighteenth and twentieth month. Nearly half of our Athenian mothers, however, report that they began bowel training before the child was 9 months old and completed it by the age of 16 months. The Thessalonike mothers report beginning of bowel training by the twelfth month and completion by the twentieth month (United States completion age, 18 months). Generally speaking, the total time required to complete bowel training is somewhat longer in Greece than in the United States.

The sex differences of children are worth noticing. Average age for the beginning of training is 9 months for boys, and 12 months for girls. In other words, mothers tend to start bowel training earlier for boys than for girls and to complete it earlier.

Greek mothers, like American mothers, are not able to be specific regarding bladder training and bed-wetting. Our results show a large percentage of "not ascertained" cases. Toilet training is associated with punishment in about one-fifth of the cases. Punishment in Thessalonike is physical, while in Athens mothers report verbal as well as physical punishment.

Conclusions on Feeding and Toilet-Training Practices

It should be noted that in answering the questionnaire, while all mothers gave answers about feeding practices, 12% of Athenian and 15% of Thessalonikean mothers avoided answering questions concerning toilet training under different pretexts. One forms the impression that mothers, in the milieu under study, associate feeding with love and toilet training with shame; consequently, they are eager to talk about the former and are evasive about the latter.

Reviewing the above findings we draw the conclusion that in practicing breast-feeding and toilet training Greek mothers are primarily concerned with fulfilling the sociocultural requirements of "mothering" which prevail in their milieu. They do not take as their first consideration the psychological and biological needs of the child. They appear to fulfill these needs only to the extent dictated by their role requirements, at times overfulfilling them and at times underfulfilling them.

Parents' Perceptions of Their Child-Rearing Role

A pilot study [3] investigating the perceptions of Athenian parents concerning their child rearing role[1] provides the following findings. Both fathers and mothers report that they "very often" do "something that pleases the child." Following that, however, they report that they allow the child to interfere with their work "very little." Qualitative observation shows that it is actually the mother who decides what "pleases" the child. Parents praise the child only "a little" when he does things right (for the fear he might otherwise relax his efforts for continuous improvement).

Parents report playing "little" with their children and this tends to decrease as the children grow older. Qualitative observation shows that mothers have a tendency to interfere with the spontaneous playing of children. When their infants and toddlers spontaneously develop some play activity, mothers tend to participate, introducing and imposing their variations of it. At other times they interfere to protect them or prevent them from upsetting things or people around and this continues throughout childhood. "Doing things" for children is the preferred way of expressing love to them (feeding them, protecting them, buying things for them).

Fathers report being only "a little" expressive with their children. Mothers report being "a lot" expressive in early childhood but perceive that this behavior decreases as the child grows. Parents tend to admire the child "a lot" in infancy and childhood and less later, with the exception of fathers who report admiring their pre-adolescent boys more.

[1] In a representative sample of Athenian households, selected on the basis of a modified probability technique, parents of both sexes were interviewed with an extensive questionnaire.

ATTITUDE TOWARD AGGRESSIVE BEHAVIOR (INCLUDING DISCIPLINE)

Parent-directed aggression is not tolerated by either parent irrespective of the age and the sex of the child. Both parents perceive themselves as tending to punish the child for parent-directed aggression—mothers more so when children are younger and fathers when children are in pre-adolescence.

Among disciplinary measures that parents report applying are spanking, scolding, withdrawal of privileges, threat of punishment, withdrawal of love and advice and supportive explanation of what the child did wrong. While mothers say that they tend to favor spanking over advice, fathers mention the reverse.

Qualitative observation shows that other directed aggression is controlled within the in-group. If it concerns the out-group, it is excused in many ways. In fact, both parents report that they punish their children only "a little" for fighting with other children or attacking animals, and they tend to do so "very little" when fighting occurs in self-defense.

It seems that the sharp differentiation of behavior between in-group and out-group which characterizes the surrounding social reality is strong enough to shape both actual and perceived parental behavior. Parents are inclined to accept "explanations" that "prove" that their child was actually the "victim" or that he had to do it in self-defense or in defense of a friend, and so forth.

Following this, one is surprised to find the same parents disagreeing with the statement that "since life is a struggle, children should learn how to fight." It appears to be a contradiction. But one should keep in mind that the matter this time is presented as a moral axiom. And Greeks tend to be quite moralistic in their answers to items relating to ideologies [2]. Their basic assumption though is that normative behavior concerning morals is operational mainly within the in-group. Outside of the in-group it ceases to be operational because the "others" are not going to follow "fair play," or they are going to take advantage of one's lack of "flexibility" and readiness to "manipulate" the situation.

DISCIPLINE AND THE "PROBLEM" CHILD

Concerning children's "misbehavior" in general, qualitative observation supported by data [6] shows that the things which are not tolerated are mainly:

Behavior defiant of parental authority

Underachievement at school

Social misbehavior which could bring shame to the family

Such misbehavior according to qualitative observation is punished inconsistently and usually with some kind of corporal punishment and restriction of privileges. However, when the situation demands socially acceptable answers, as in responses to public opinion surveys, Athenian parents report that they use more verbal means such as scolding, reprimanding, explaining, or threatening. They report that the most effective way of punishing a child is to tell him "he has no *philotimo*," he is not liked by his parents as he is," and that "God is going to punish him." Restriction of privileges, threat of withdrawal of parental love, and physical punishment follow.

Philotimo is the highest Greek value. Literally *philotimo* means "love of honor" but it has acquired the meaning of the generalized "loftiest value." It was found [8] to be polysemantic, a kind of abstract frame which acquires a subtly different specific content for each primary and secondary group. Following this, it is common to find parents, when quarreling, to label each other's families or communities as *aphilotimoi* (lacking *philotimo*), basing this on sets of behaviors which are considered by the one as implying that the other has no *philotimo*. The fact is that the growing child is subjected to different definitions of *philotimo* even within the frame of his family. It is through the formation of his in-group of which we will talk later, that the child finally enters a social unit with a relatively uniform definition of *philotimo*.

Regarding overall discipline, parental responses indicate that both fathers and mothers are quite demanding. They think their children do not obey as quickly as they should. They report scolding them "a lot" and spanking them "a little." Mothers tend to report more corporal punishment than fathers.

Concerning consistency of parental punishments and rewards, both parents perceive themselves as "little or very little" inconsistent while actual observation and findings from other studies reveal considerable inconsistency, the factor mainly determining parental reaction to the child being parental mood and emotional needs of the moment.

SEX EDUCATION

Concerning sexual education of children, a study [6] based on a representative sample of Athenians reveals that the large majority of Athenians (6 out of 10) feel that proper sexual education is not offered to children. Only 3 percent reported having received information about sex before adolescence and 74 percent in adolescence (12-19 years old). Friends and classmates were the source of information for the majority. And to indicate more the prevailing contradictory attitudes on the matter, while most respondents felt that sexual education is necessary, 9 out of 10 said that this should be offered after the tenth year. Adolescence is considered as the proper age for sexual education by the majority, while 14 percent believe that the proper age is after the eighteenth year.

Regarding the person who is most appropriate to provide sexual education, 37 percent of the respondents propose both parents, 26 percent the mother, with women respondents overwhelmingly prevailing, and 14 percent the father, with men overwhelmingly prevailing, while no significant differences were found according to the other demographic variables (age, education, and income). Finally, 12 percent of the respondents proposed a teacher as the most appropriate agent, with male respondents prevailing.

It seems that (a) each respondent tends to consider the parent of his own sex as the most appropriate agent of the sexual education of children, and (b) among the respondents who want to shift the responsibility to teachers, men prevail. This is an indication that men, while reluctant to see the woman undertaking the task, are at the same time inclined to relay it to an authority outside of the family. The unpreparedness of parents to deal with sexual education of children is indicated by their responses concerning the best methods of sexual education; 45 percent propose special classes for parents, 40 percent propose special classes for children at school, 20 percent propose the use of educational pamphlets. It is interesting to note that while sex and age do not differentiate, respondents of higher income and education tend to favor special classes for parents. When a representative sample of Athenian mothers was asked to respond on a 5-point scale whether a mother should permit her children to satisfy their curiosity concerning the other sex, 2 in 6 "disagreed absolutely " and one "disagreed partly," while 1 in 6 was undecisive, 1 agreed absolutely and 1 partly. When the same mothers were asked the loaded question: "Should a mother teach her children that it is not proper to be curious about sex?" almost 4 out of 6 said that they agree absolutely.

Given the above it is not surprising that 73 percent of respondents "never dared" to ask their father and 65 percent their mother about sex. The most hesitant was the generation that grew up between the two world wars – 12 percent reported having asked their fathers and 25 percent their mothers. Half of the people in each subgroup were punished or misled with inaccurate information or lies. Mothers are reported to react more strongly and punitively than fathers.

However, there are clear indications that parents feel that things "should be" different. For instance, in the previously mentioned study of self-perceived child-rearing practices, Athenian parents reported that they lie only "a little" or "very little" to their children about sex. Only mothers of pre-adolescent girls admitted that they lie "extremely" to them on sexual matters.

RESPONSIBILITY

Throughout our studies parents have not been found to train their children consistently to responsibility. Their attitude ranges inconsistently from extreme demands to permissiveness depending on the situation. If something concerns the in-group, the child is expected to behave very responsibly, otherwise he might be excused to follow his whims.

Athenian parents report [3] asking their children to perform only a few chores with the exception of mothers concerning their 6- to 12-year-old daughters, who report demanding of them "a lot of chores," obviously in an attempt to train them in their future role requirements.

PEER GROUPS

Qualitative observation and research data [6] indicate that parents tend to control and supervise closely peer-group relations. The child is discouraged from associating with "everybody," the term including practically all children except those approved by parents or even selected by them. Playing "out of the house" with peers is supervised by mothers as much as possible. Direct visual supervision is considered necessary so "things could be prevented," which means, of course, that mothers interfere constantly in children's activities. It is quite characteristic that permission to "play with peers" is considered a special reward.

THE NATURE AND EXTENT OF PARENTAL INTRUSIVENESS

Athenian parents express the view that they know more about child-rearing than their grandparents do [3]. However, this is contradicted by studies [7] and qualitative observation which shows that grandparents, and mainly grandmothers, are getting very much involved in child-rearing. And this is despite a structural change of the Greek family, from the extended to the nuclear type (about 7 out of 10 Athenian families are presently found to be nuclear).

All findings indicate that mothers intervene for prolonged periods of time in the child-milieu transaction, functioning as "modifiers," "transformers," and "mediators." This is intensified in relation to the future achievement of the child and the pursuit of it.

Parents closely supervise the child's school life. The overwhelming majority of mothers, with additional assistance from fathers, are found to work with their children during homework (in many cases for hours). Thus the whole family invests in the child's schoolwork. It becomes a joint endeavor and mothers give a personal meaning to the child's success in school.[2] It is actually this success which is considered as determining *their* success in mothering.

In group discussions with mothers, when we asked them to examine textbooks used in other countries for first-graders, mothers insisted to the end that "it is impossible for a first-grader to complete such work and if our schools use them it is only natural that mothers have to do the work, with the children only watching them learning." Their most frequently voiced complaint is that teachers "load children with hours of homework so mothers and fathers have to spend all their free time assisting their children."

On the other hand group discussions with teachers reveal that one of the main complaints of the teachers is the close control that parents exercise over teaching. According to teachers parents ask persistently that homework assignments be both extensive and demanding so "children have something useful to do at home."

[2] Here is a characteristic case. A mother with high school education says to the startled interviewer, "well, Doctor, I got straight A's at the Medical School, straight A's at the Polytechnic Institute and I succeeded with honors at the Academy of Arts." She then explained what she meant. She did it by working *with* each one of her three children throughout their undergraduate studies "preparing them for such successes."

It seems that the limits of the optimal homework that parents desire for their children fluctuate without any clear rationale. One could speculate that in these cases it is not the child who really counts. Maternal, parental in general, plans for the child's future achievement require that he receives the maximum of education in the minimum of time. But given that this has to be a joint effort, it reaches the limits of parental endurance at times. These two, then – parental endurance and plans – seem to be the primary determining factors.

Frequently the child's achievements are told and retold to in-group members and, with more satisfaction, conveyed directly or indirectly to out-group members. They are purposely "redescribed" and "interpreted" to enhance the family's prestige. In this way these children are presented with stories "rewritten" by mother "really telling" of their achievements and predicting "for sure" their future "success." When the child encounters difficulties and obstacles (even as late as adolescence or early adulthood), the majority of mothers consider it their job to alert fathers, relatives, their whole in-group if necessary – mobilize, in other words, every conceivable source of help, in order to "open the way" for the child.

Consequently the growing child is not transacting with milieu directly. Mothers (parents) constantly intervene and mediate, transforming and modifying the developing transaction.

Vignette of the Greek Family

The reviewed findings strengthen the conclusions that emerge from other studies concerning the Greek family [6]. Mothers are assigned and assume a primary role concerning child-rearing. It isnot simply a matter of being assigned this role. They seem to seek it out and compete with other potential sources of child-rearing (fathers, grandparents, other relatives, teachers, etc.) in order to perform it exclusively. This is quite consistent with the fact that "Mother" represents the only totally respectable female social role. Outside of motherhood, the woman has a negative stereotype, no significant social role and, if married, her role involves mainly "house activities." But once a mother, the woman becomes holy. Almost unconditional love and respect are due to her. Naturally then, "mothering" for her becomes as all-important and inclusive as life itself.

Fathers are assigned a superordinate role. They are the "household providers" and supporters of the family. They assume a kind of a stand-by role in child-rearing. Assigned the role of the provider of socioeconomic security for the family and of the overall disciplinarian, fathers have considerably fewer opportunities to be with the child. Even when they are, the role of the overall supervisor and controller does not leave them as many chances for an affective spontaneous exchange with the child. Family roles are kept clearly delineated and complementary with little overlapping.

Through the traditional patterns of "mothering" a number of sociocultural demands are imposed on mothers forcefully enough to make them primarily concerned with their fulfillment. The psychobiological needs of the child do not seem to be the primary determining factor.

From breast-feeding and toilet training to sexual education, peer-group relations, and schoolwork, all findings reviewed above indicate that the needs of the child tend to be overfulfilled or underfulfilled depending on the sociocultural demands imposed on mother's role. The family functions more or less as a system providing the child with dependence-interdependence [10] and nurturance [5] in expectation of achievement and fulfillment of "shared" plans and ambitions. Parents perceive themselves as permissive, loving, and admiring the child but maintain their superordinate role and are cautious in praising the child's efforts.

Mother, securing if necessary the father's and the in-group's assistance, intervenes actively in the child-milieu transaction and continues to do so for prolonged periods of the child's life (up to adolescence and early adulthood in certain matters).

The whole family is future-oriented and achievement-oriented. Milieu conditions fluctuating always from difficult to extreme, being stably unstable, have made the hopes and dreams for tomorrow a fundamental element for survival. It is only natural then that the child becomes the personification of such hopes and dreams, the main vehicle for family achievement, and consequently the focus of parental feelings, thoughts, and efforts.

For socioeconomic and sociocultural reasons, a son has more chances to fulfill the family's ambitions and needs for achievement and social mobility, and he is preferred over a daughter. In his absence, though, a daughter is expected to substitute either directly by studying and developing a career or indirectly through a successful marriage.

The Function of the In-Group in Greece

For centuries in Greece, in the middle of all the conditions, plans, and efforts, parents and children have had one social institution to reply upon for assistance, achievement, or even sheer survival: their *in-group,* defined as "people concerned with me, members of my family (not necessarily all), friends, and friends of friends." And, despite the quickly accelerating socioeconomic and sociocultural developments described as "modernization" in the Greek milieu, the in-group maintains almost fully its operational potential.

Raised in this way the child, specifically a son, is inclined to feel that in a sense he is "chosen," a very special task (in exceptional cases a kind of a mission) is bestowed on him, and it is intimately related to his family's or his in-group's and (through it) his country's future.

He grows up with people who feel in harmony with nature, who love life and enjoy the present with all available means, but he is taught that this should be proportional and not at the expense of achievement in the future.

On the other hand, he is taught explicitly or implicitly that the kind of linear and collateral relations he develops depend on where the other belongs. If he belongs to the in-group he is due unlimited respect, concern, and loyalty, collaterally and, in addition obedience linearly. Relations are cooperative. If he belongs to the out-group he is treated in ways that do not fall into any fixed rules. Both collaterally and linearly he can be antagonized, defied, cheated, misled, outmaneuvered. Relations are competitive.

Conclusions

The mental health practitioner, the educator, the group or community worker, the managerial or industrial consultant, as well as the manager or the businessman, the civic leader, the political observer and the politician, the student of social issues as well as the social planner, the reader in general who is familiar with aspects of the milieu under study will have the feeling that even such a summarized review of child-rearing patterns contributes to the clarification of puzzling questions. To repeat, it is old-fashioned and simplistic to assume that there is a linear, cause and effect relationship between child-rearing patterns and the milieu. It is closer to the evidence to assume that the transactions involved are highly complex, multivariate and ramified within the environment. With rapid industrial developments, a "cultural lag" may occur so that the child-rearing generates an outmoded type of adult. This is what is happening in Greece. The Greek patterns we have described were developed and institutionalized in a slowly changing "pre-industrial" milieu where alterations along all variables were both synchronic and syntonic. Currently the socioeconomic-technological developments are being accelerated. This forces individuals and their families to enter into qualitatively and quantitatively different frames of transaction. Under the circumstances, the old child-rearing patterns prove not to be operationally relevant. They generate conflicts that strain human relations and overtax the personality's synthetic capacities. Their overall negative impact on individual, family, and communal life is intensified and they interfere seriously with the further development of the milieu. This is another important illustration of the way in which people, as human beings, fall behind their own technological advances.

Bibliography

1. Karatsioli, Litsa and Vasso Vassiliou, *Patterns of Feeding and Toilet Training in Urban Greece,* Technical Report No. XI, The Athenian Institute of Anthropos, Athens, 1969.
2. Katz, Daniel and Vasso Vassiliou, unpublished research findings.
3. Papadopoulou, Elli and Vasso Vassiliou, *Athenian Parents Perceptions Concerning Their Child-Rearing Role,* Technical Report No. VII, The Athenian Institute of Anthropos, Athens, 1969.
4. Sears, R. R., E. E. Maccoby, and H. Levin, *Patterns of Child Rearing,* Row Petterson and Co., New York, 1957.
5. Triandis, H. C., H. McGuire, Tulsi Saral, Kuo-Shu Yang, W. Loh, and Vasso Vassiliou, *A Cross-Cultural Study of Role Perceptions,* Technical Report, Group Effectiveness Research Laboratory, Illinois University, 1969.
6. Vassiliou, G., *A Preliminary Exploration of Variables Related to Family Transaction in Greece,* Technical Report No. V, The Athenian Institute of Anthropos, Athens, 1966.
7. Vassiliou, G., Milieu-Specificity in Family Therapy in *Family Therapy in Transition,* ed. by G. J. Pearce and J. Lieb, Little, Brown and Co., Boston, in press.

8. Vassiliou, G. and Vasso Vassiliou, Preliminary Exploration of the Semantics of *Philotimo*, *Acta Neurologica et Psychiatrica Hellenika*, Vol. 5, No. 2, 1966.
9. Vassiliou, G. and Vasso Vassiliou, A Transactional Approach to Mental Health in *New Directions in Mental Health*, ed. by Bernard Riess, Grune and Stratton, New York, 1968.
10. Vassiliou, Vasso, Harris Katakis, and G. Vassiliou, Milieu Variations of Motivational Patterns of Pre-adolescents in Greece as Revealed by Story Sequence Analysis, Paper read at the Seventh International Congress of Rorschach and Other Projective Techniques (London Aug. 5-9, 1968), to appear in the proceedings.

A Child Psychiatric Study of Sudanese Arab Children

MARIANNE CEDERBLAD (SWEDEN)

Problems of Method

Cross-cultural studies of mental phenomena are subject to serious methodological difficulties. As in all epidemiological studies, the definitions of the variables and the experimental instruments must be the same in the populations compared. But when groups in greatly differing civilizations are to be studied, there is a risk that a variable may be experienced differently in the groups compared, and that, therefore, a question worded in the same way may be conceived differently in the two populations. So, for example, can an interviewer's judgment of the intensity of aggressiveness or depression vary greatly, due to what is judged to be "normal." In the same way, differences in the ability to observe mental phenomena and the habit of describing feelings as well as capacity for introspection vary between cultural groups. Differences in language comprehension in the respondents is also of importance, as well as the interviewer's ability to establish contacts with the respondents. It has been pointed out earlier that great differences between respondents and interviewers in respect to such factors as race, status, and values make contacts difficult and thereby probably also impair the reliability of interviews. It is extremely important that this is borne in mind when such interviews are to be made.

Taboos may also affect willingness to collaborate at interviews as, for example, in the Sudan, where it is believed that the "evil eye" (i.e., disease, injury, bad luck) may overtake a child if anyone knows too much about it – length and weight, for instance.

The question has been discussed whether, in other civilizations, there are mental diseases and symptoms which are not found in the Western world and vice versa. Most descriptions of symptoms from various African and Asian countries that seem curious and foreign may be explained on the basis of accepted diagnostic categories, such as states of anxiety and hysterical manifestations, although the picture of the disease is formed pathoplastically by different cultural elements [3, 5, 19]. It is now assumed, therefore, that the psychiatric nomenclature is universally valid.

In some mental deviations it may be difficult to decide whether a pathological symptom is present or whether one is concerned with an accepted phenomenon. This refers mainly to the delusions, phobias, rituals, and so forth. Leighton, in a psychiatric field study of 262 persons in Nigeria, considered, however, that only twelve interviews were difficult to interpret on account of cultural singularities. In two of these cases it was the behavior of the respondents that was difficult to judge [18].

In the present study, I chose to compare a population of children living in three villages near Khartoum, the Sudan, with the same investigation blank as had been used earlier on groups of children in San Francisco, California, by Macfarlane [20] and in Stockholm, Sweden, by Jonsson [14]. The same operational definitions of the behavior variables studied were used.

Growing Up in a Sudanese Village

The total situation of the Sudanese children and the two other populations differs widely. Although it cannot be claimed that the villages and the two other populations differs widely. Although it cannot be claimed that the villages and the two cities represent statistically greater regions than those studied, it may be said that in many ways, the Sudanese village environment is typical of that of a large group of children outside the Western civilization, while the cities undoubtedly contain many environmental elements typical of the experience of city children in the West.

The villages studied are 8 miles east of Khartoum on a flat steppe. The climate is dry and hot, with temperatures around 30 to 35° C in April through November. The nights are cool, and in winter a cold north wind blows continuously.

The people, about 5000 in number, 2500 of them under the age of 15, are Arabic-speaking Mohammedans. Ninety percent of them belong to a former nomadic tribe, Batahein. Earlier they lived on animal husbandry, but now most of the men work in Khartoum or its suburbs as unskilled manual laborers. The average income was 25 piastres a day (6 English shillings). The women never work outside the home except as midwives. The dwellings are square buildings of sun-dried clay with earth floors. Usually a whole family of four to six persons shares a room. Half of the children shared a bed with at least one other.

The diet is very monotonous. The main meal is of *kisra,* thin, unleavened bread baked of unpolished millet meal. This is dipped in *mulah,* a kind of meat-vegetable broth with tomatoes and onions as the main ingredients. Only little broth is eaten, and the nutritional value is therefore doubtful. Beans and wheat bread are also eaten. Sweet tea and coffee are the main beverages. During certain periods, bananas, mango, dates, and lemon juice are consumed. Nevertheless, the diet is unsatisfactory in respect to the supply of calories, proteins, and vitamins.

Marriages are contracted when girls are in their lower and boys in their upper teens. Marriages between cousins are preferred, and people marry within the same subsection of the tribe. Polygamy still exists, 18 percent of the children in the sample being from polygamous families, in which the man usually had two wives. A girl has very little opportunity of influencing the choice of her husband. While polygamy is a kind of status symbol (a sign that one's financial situation is strong), it also gives rise to tension and problems within the family. Of the mothers in the sample living in polygamous families, only 35 percent considered that this did not cause problems. In the others, the mothers disapproved of the new marriage; the children disapproved, too, or there was much antagonism between the half-brothers and sisters. (This is encouraged traditionally by the mothers – probably a way of giving vent to aggressiveness vicariously.) Divorces are very unusual (1 percent) and can, generally speaking, be demanded by the man only.

People in the villages live in an extended family system. Several generations and siblings and their families often live in adjacent houses, and many household tasks, cooking and baking, for example, are performed in common. The upbringing of the children is also spread beyond the nuclear family; the member of the group who happens to be nearest intervenes with protection, punishment, and reward. The open village communion with intensive relationships between the individuals gives maximal social control as well as strong emotional support, since people participate intimately in each other's lives and share difficulties and privation. The members of these extended families also support each other financially, so that when one gets a job he shares his income with those of the clan who are without means of support. The village culture is homogeneous and at the same time static, which implies that practically all persons, regardless of generation and social status, have the same system of norms in respect to fundamental values in social behavior, sex roles, and desirable characteristics. This means that, on the one hand, a growing individual is spared the insecurity of value relativism and norm conflicts between adults in their surroundings, while on the other hand it gives little scope for the development of those misfits who cannot, on account of temperament or constitutional idiosyncrasies, adapt themselves to the prevailing patterns. The social pressure probably facilitates the social adjustment of some weak individuals by external constraint, while it causes low tolerance towards those who nevertheless become social deviants or who are ejected from the society.

Upbringing gives rise to a tendency towards traditional conformism with fear of deviation even in modern ideas, such as, education for girls, more modern methods of midwifery, new dishes. Morals are preserved by the help of feelings of "shame" rather than by feelings of guilt from an internalized superego. The creation of such feelings is impaired because parents are inconsistent in bringing up their children, they react more according to their own temporary feelings of irritation than according to conscious, consistent rewards and punishments of the child's conduct. The emotional ties between a child (after the first 2 years) and its parents are also less exclusive, since the child lives surrounded by several adults in the extended family situation. This probably makes the process of identification with parents more difficult.

The goal of socialization is partly to teach an acceptable external behavior, for example, to show respect for older people, to be generous and hospitable towards strangers – a traditional virtue in a nomadic system. It is desired to form the child according to certain traditional virtues and sex role patterns. Of the former, family honor is important. This is maintained by sexual decency in the female members of the family and the dignity of the male members, which is dependent on the respect he enjoys from others, and which implies that he must refuse to tolerate insults.

Physical courage and self-control are also valued highly in both sexes. This leads to a high degree of self-restraint when in pain, at circumcision, for instance.

Parents tolerate and encourage aggressiveness in boys, for the male role is to be *shediid* (strong). The girls are trained never to show anger. Instead they should be *tageela* (heavy), that is, calm, retiring, mild, dignified, and silent.

The emotional needs of small children are satisfied in full during the first 1½ to 2 years. During these years the mother carries the child with her wherever she goes, and sleeps with it in her bed. Unlimited suckling is the rule – the child is given the breast as soon as it cries. But the supply of mother's milk is, naturally, often far too small. Infection and diarrhea are very common among weaning children, for the new food they are given is contaminated and consists mainly of carbohydrates, which causes fermentation in the intestines. After 1½ to 2 years children are weaned abruptly, are no longer allowed to sleep in their mothers' beds, and are left more or less to manage with the help of older sisters. The mother's main interest is already often centered around a new child.

Stool and bladder training are started early, in 60 percent at the age of 6 to 8 weeks. This is probably because diapers are not used. Most mothers, therefore, study their children's behavior and learn when they are about to urinate or defecate, otherwise their clothes or the bed would often be soiled. Training is performed by very mild methods; the child is held between the mother's knees and learns to make a smacking noise to indicate that it needs help. No formal training was found in 33 percent of the cases; the children learned spontaneously to imitate their older brothers or sisters.

Demands made on children below the age of 7 years are very small, except that they are expected to fend for themselves to a great extent. From the age of 7 or 8 years, greater demands are made on the children; they must help in the house, work with their fathers, or attend school. The father begins showing an interest in his sons when they are 9 or 10 years old, when they begin helping him with his work. His contacts with his daughters, on the other hand, consist mainly in ensuring that they behave respectably. Neither of the parents show much interest in stimulating the intellectual development of their children or in playing with them. Even expressions of affection are rare after the children are 4 or 5 years of age, for that would, it is thought, "spoil" them.

Boys and girls are not allowed to play together after they have reached the age of 9 or 10 years, and the girls are watched carefully. This is associated with the taboo on premarital intercourse, the ultimate consequence of which is the female circumcision practised (Pharaonic circumcision or infibulation). This is performed when the girls are 7 to 9 years of age; the labia minora and parts of the labia majora and mons veneris are cut away with a razor, without anaesthetic. After the operation the girl must lie in bed for one or two weeks with her legs bound together until the edges of the sores have grown together. The boys are circumcised at the age of 8 to 10 years according to Mohammedan tradition. While the latter operation has no sex-inhibiting purpose, one of the reasons for infibulation is that it makes girls less sexually excitable, and thereby reduces the risk of premarital intercourse.

One sign that this trauma and the conflict-loaded attitude towards sex in the civilization causes fear and feelings of shame to be associated with the sex organs of girls were the strikingly frequent embarrassed reactions in the somatic examinations I made. The girls often refused to uncover their stomachs and thighs. They were stiff and tense when their leg reflexes and their hip joints were to be examined, which contrasted strongly with their calm cooperation during other parts of the examination.

The children receive intellectual stimulus only through school. As a rule, neither books, newspapers, nor radio are found in the homes. There is a four-year elementary school for boys in the village and about 50 percent of the boys attend school for one year or more. Of the girls, only 18 percent had attended school in a neighboring village. This is partly because many parents think education unnecessary for girls – they will get married anyway – or harmful; it makes them more independent and self-assertive, which is contrary to the rest of their upbringing.

The general situation in the life of the children is characterized by a high frequency of somatic illness. Repeated acute or chronic infections in the gastrointestinal channel, the organs of respiration, and the urinary tracts were very common. Signs of undernourishment were present in each fifth child. Length and weight curves reflect the nourishment situation in a population of children [7], and when nourishment is inadequate both length and weight are below normal [8, 9]. The Sudanese village children were 10 to 15 centimeters shorter and 5 to 10 kilograms lighter than Swedish children of the same age. Only slightly more than half of them were judged to be quite healthy or had only less severe, transient diseases.

Methods and Subjects

By preparatory interviews made by Sudanese students of medicine, all the 1716 children in the villages aged 3 to 15 years were studied in respect to stuttering, disturbed sleep, somnambulism, enuresis nocturna, and encopresis during the previous year. From this population a stratified sample was taken for an intensive study. All the children with more than one of the symptoms or encopresis were included. Each seventh child with one symptom and each fifteenth of those not noted for any symptoms were taken. The selection was made in the two latter strata in proportion to sex and age. The sample consisted of 214 children, 17 of whom dropped out. Of the 197 children studied, 113 were boys.

The advantage of a stratified sample was that the chances of finding children with several behavioral deviations might be expected to be greatest among those who, in the total examination, had one of the behavioral symptoms studied. Thus, this mode of procedure made it possible to examine relatively more of the disturbed children than if a random sample had been taken. It was particularly important in this population, where it was to be suspected that the frequency of disturbed children would be low.

A form with 296 questions in English dealt with the following variables: socioeconomic factors, intrafamilial relationships, cultural phenomena, the child's early development, its previous and present somatic status, and its current behavior. The last-named treated the occurrence of disturbed sleep, problems of feeding, enuresis nocturna and diurna, encopresis, psychosomatic headache, hypo- and hyperactivity, tics, nail-biting, thumb-sucking, stuttering, overt and suppressed aggressiveness, depression, anxiety, phobias, compulsion symptoms, certain hysterical conversion symptoms, lying, pilfering, truancy, and vagabondage. Only symptoms prevailing on the occasion of the examination were included. These were divided into four grades except aggressiveness, anxiety, and depression which were divided into three because of the difficulty in judging them. Thumb-sucking, nail-biting, and phobias were registered without grading.

The interviews took about one hour each and were made in the homes by Sudanese psychiatrists and medical students together with the author. In 95 percent of the cases, the mother answered the questions. I made the somatic-neurological examinations of the children. The material was collected between 1 March and 15 June 1965.

The anthropological data were collected by interviews with a number of persons in the village – mothers, old and young men, one of the sheikhs, the headmaster of the school, the head of the dispensary, a religious faith-healer, and a midwife.

Results

LOAD OF SYMPTOMS

The children were divided into four groups according to burden of symptoms, which were defined operationally in the same way as in the Stockholm study mentioned earlier [14].

Grade 0. Symptom free. No symptoms observed at all, or only nail-biting or the like.

Grade 1. Slight symptoms. One or more symptoms of such a nature and degree that they do not disturb the surroundings. ("Coping well with symptoms.")

Grade 2. Moderate symptoms. One or more symptoms which clearly place the child in a special situation, but which do not cause any acute problems, the child is able to cope with the symptoms. No immediate need of treatment.

Grade 3. Pronounced symptoms. Several symptoms of such gravity that immediate treatment should be given, if available.

The grading was based mainly on how much the symptoms disturb the child's social adjustment, but was not concerned directly with whether the child was regarded as a "problem child" by its mother. Several of the symptoms registered cause suffering in the child (e.g., anxiety, depression, headache), or cause uneasiness and stress in the parents (e.g. certain manifestations of aggressiveness, antisocial symptoms, enuresis). The children in "Grade 3" must therefore be regarded as mentally insufficient or maladjusted. On the other hand, individual behavior disturbances cannot be regarded as signs of maladjustment. Several studies [13, 15, – 17, 20, 22] have shown that behavioral disturbances often appear in children as a reaction to temporary environmental situations, or as transient developmental phenomena in essentially normal children, and that they have a tendency to appear and disappear without treatment.

Of the total population of children in the villages studied (calculated from findings in the sample), 63 percent were without symptoms, 8 percent had slight symptoms, 20 percent moderate, and 8 percent had pronounced symptoms. In addition, 1 percent was judged to be mentally deficient; these children were not included in the symptom groups above, for it was difficult to determine whether their symptoms were due only to defects in intelligence or also to emotional disturbances. No significant difference in frequency of symptom loadings appeared between boys and girls or between young (3–6 years) and older (7–15 years) children. That the frequency of children with heavy burdens of symptoms was low is shown very clearly if the group of boys aged 7 to 15 years is compared with the 222 Stockholm boys aged 8 to 16 years, studied by the same methods (see Table 1).

Table 1 Comparison of Loads of Symptoms in 222 Stockholm Boys and Boys in the Sudanese Villages

	Percent			
	0	1	2	3
Stockholm boys, 8 to 16 years (n = 222)	21	23	31	25 = 100
Sudanese boys, 7 to 15 years (n = 439*)	55	16	21	8 = 100

*Statistically blown-up figure.

Other studies in Europe and the United States have given frequencies in the same size range as in Jonsson's Stockholm material. The frequency of children with symptoms is usually higher in urban than in rural samples. However, the frequency varies greatly, due probably to different investigation methods and definitions.

The Sudanese children with slight symptoms had, on an average, 1.1 symptoms each, those with moderate symptoms 1.6, and those with pronounced symptoms 4.0. The mentally deficient had 2.4. Thus, only the last two, numerically small groups had high frequencies of symptoms. It seems, therefore, as if the frequency of maladjusted children (Grade 3) was low in the village population studied.

BEHAVIORAL DISTRUBANCES

The individual behavioral disturbances with the highest frequency in the total material were aggressiveness, 17.6 percent, enuresis nocturna, 13.7 percent (age 5–15 years, 11.9 percent), anxiety, 12.6 percent, and phobias, 12.4 percent. Encopresis, tics, hysterical conversion symptoms, and enuresis diurna (all below 0.5 percent) were uncommon.

Among the smaller children (3–6 years), aggressiveness, enuresis nocturna (significant difference, 21 and 8 percent respectively in the older children), anxiety, and phobias were most frequent. Among older children (7–15 years), aggressiveness and phobias were the most frequent. Antisocial symptoms and psychosomatic headaches (significant difference) were found almost exclusively among older children. Frequencies of some behavioral disturbances differed somewhat for boys and girls. Enuresis nocturna and stuttering occurred significantly more often among boys, who also had more extrovert symptoms such as hyperactivity, aggressiveness, and antisocial symptoms. Headache and disturbed sleep were also more frequent among boys. The girls had higher frequencies of introvert symptoms, such as nail-biting, thumb-sucking, anxiety, and depression, but also more phobias. The differences were small, but they show the same tendency as was noted by J.W. Macfarlane [20], for example. She considers that they are partly manifestations of biological sex differences, but also of cultural influence.

The comparable groups of boys in Stockholm and the Sudanese villages also differ. While the most frequent symptoms in the former group were nail-biting, headache, disturbed sleep, and tics, these symptoms were, except for headache, uncommon in my group, in which, apart from headache, enuresis nocturna and aggressiveness were most frequent.

Covariation of certain background factors and symptom loads was also studied. Children without or with slight symptoms (0+1) were compared with groups with moderate and pronounced symptoms (2+3). In the latter group nervousness in the mother during pregnancy, somatic disease in the child, and nervous disturbances in the parents was significantly more frequent. The 7- to 15-year-old boys in the group attended or had attended school to a significantly higher degree. Physical illness in the mother during pregnancy and signs of cerebral lesion in the child during the first year of life were present in almost significantly higher frequencies in group 2+3.

Discussion

THE FREQUENCY OF DIFFERENT BEHAVIORAL DISTURBANCES

The variables occurring more frequently in the Sudanese village population than in the corresponding group in Jonsson's study were aggressiveness and enuresis nocturna. The former is a variable in which it is difficult to determine whether it is to be regarded as a negative deviation or whether it can be regarded as a form of behavior encouraged in upbringing and therefore a positive feature according to the norms prevailing in the culture. It seems very likely that the frequency was affected by the positive attitude to aggressiveness in boys which is part of upbringing. This is also supported by the fact that the girls show a surplus of repressed aggressiveness, which is in line with their upbringing.

Enuresis nocturna is probably one of the variables which gives more reliable responses. Attempts to determine the occurrence of previous and current infections of the urinary tract were made partly by questions on case history and partly by a sample of urine from each child. Owing to examination technical difficulties, the results of the samples of urine are uncertain. It seems as if infection of the urinary tract is very common in the villages. The group with enuresis nocturna showed significantly higher frequencies of pathological finds in the urine (protein, white and red blood corpuscles). Therefore, it is likely that such infections explain part of the high frequency of enuresis. On the other hand, the method of bladder training was without importance for the frequency of enuresis. The lowest frequency was found among those who had received no training at all, while different kinds of punishment gave somewhat higher frequencies than mild methods. The differences were not significant, however. The high frequency of enuresis cannot, therefore, be explained by lack of bladder training. The study supports the view that the process of growth is most important, and bladder training plays a smaller role for the occurrence of enuresis. It is also quite possible that specific genetic situations are of influence, which could not be elucidated by the present study, however. Evidence in favor of this is the high proportion of primary enuresis (13 percent, secondary 1 percent), and possibly also the high frequency of enuresis in siblings. Of 26 pairs of siblings in the sample, enuresis was present in 7. Of these both siblings had the symptom in five cases.

Anxiety and phobias were also among the more common variables in the sample, although the frequencies in the corresponding groups did not differ from those reported by Jonsson. Thus the frequency of phobias was the same as in European studies, but the objects of phobias were quite different; fear of the dark was the most common, followed by animals. Thus the culture is reflected in the content of the symptom. In two European studies [13, 14], it was shown that children are most often afraid of imaginary figures, such as ghosts and witches, and certain groups of people used to frighten children in the service of upbringing – sweeps and policemen, for example; characters found in books, or seen on television – murderers, thieves and villains – but also more abstract dangers such as war, catastrophes, illness, and lightning. The last-named may be classified as "induced objects of anxiety," that is, anxiety transferred from the mother or some other relative. Many of the differences can be explained by the fact that the children in the present study are obviously not fed on fairy tales – television and cinemas do not exist for them either. Wireless, newspapers, and books are found in only few houses. Induced anxiety from parents, who function on a magical level with fear of the "evil eye," jinn, dead relatives who may return to kill children and the like, is probably not reported, since these "phobic objects" are common to most people in the culture and fear of them cannot, therefore, be regarded as deviant. Threats and fright in upbringing – except for concrete things like corporal punishment and circumcision – are probably not resorted to; the child is struck instead.

Among the variables occurring less frequently in the Sudanese villages were disturbed sleep and psychosomatic headaches. Both are implicit items and therefore give, perhaps, somewhat unreliable responses. Disturbed sleep was uncommon in the extensive study, too, so these two findings support each other. Here we are probably concerned with two stress symptoms, which are much more frequent in the overstimulating urban environment of the Western world. The frequency of disturbed sleep is probably also reduced by contacts during the night with the other members of the family sleeping in the same room, which gives a feeling of security. In this context it may be of interest to mention how often pediatricians and child psychiatrists in Sweden are faced with the problem of small children with sleeping difficulties and who also wish to sleep in their parents' beds every night. If they are allowed to do so, sleeping problems often disappear at once! Difficulty in falling asleep has been considered to be associated with separation anxiety [2, 11]. Physical separation (in the present study defined as at least 3 months' separation of mother and child during the first 3 years of the child's life) was almost unknown (1 percent).

The frequency of feeding problems was low, equivalent to only 1 percent. But such problems are very common in Western countries. One important cause of this is probably the shortage of food in the country. This symptom is more usual in affluent societies.

The antisocial symptoms were, not unexpectedly, rather infrequent (ca., 1 percent theft, truancy from school, and vagabondage, 3 percent lying). These figures may be misleadingly low, because parents are either not always aware of their children's thefts and truancy or because they will not mention the symptoms during the interviews, particularly as neighbors were often present. It is probably, however, that antisocial symptoms really are uncommon in the culture studied. As mentioned earlier, the social control is very strong and there are also few things to steal in the villages. Few children attend school, and those who do so are of an age when truancy is uncommon in Europe, too.

The low frequency of thumb-sucking (1.3 percent) and nail-biting (2.4 percent) must be interpreted primarily as evidence that the children's oral urge to suck was adequately satisfied by the prolonged, free suckling period.

DISTRIBUTION OF SYMPTOM GROUPS

It seems rather certain that children with a heavy burden of symptoms are very rare in this culture compared with what is found in Western countries. What may cause this difference?

Genetic factors. It is probable that this population is genetically exceptional because of the high frequency of inbreeding. The small size of the population makes the genetic drift important, too. Since the sheikhs decide, to a certain extent, which people are to be allowed to settle in the villages, the selection may be positive compared with other regions. Many behavioral disturbances, such as stuttering (Andrews [1]), enuresis nocturna (Hallgren [12]), and encopresis (Bellman [4]), may be considered to have genetic disposition, and it is therefore probable that such factors are effective.

Somatic factors. The high frequencies of somatically poor state of health, infections with cerebral symptoms, and signs of possible cerebral injury neonatally or during the first year of life are striking in the case histories. The frequencies are also higher, often significantly higher, in children with various behavioral disturbances and in the groups with moderate and pronounced symptoms. Thus, the cases studied seem often to have been mainly organically conditioned either by general physical weakness and consequent increased vulnerability to mental stress or by factors that may have given rise to cerebral lesions. Since these injuries and disorders are very frequent in the whole child population compared with Sweden, for example, it is all the more remarkable that the frequencies of such behavioral disturbances as are usually attributed partly to brain damage (e.g., aggressiveness, activity disturbances, tics, stuttering, and antisocial conduct), are not high, except for aggressiveness. The frequency of children with pronounced symptoms is, on the contrary, very low. This gives rise to the reflection that if children in an environment where cerebral injury, infections, and general severe physical illness are so frequent do not show a higher prevalence of behavioral disturbances than those found, these causes cannot be very important except for a very small proportion of all the children who reveal various types of behavioral deviations in the Western world.

Psychosocial factors. It seems that the low frequency of behaviorally disturbed children observed can be explained mainly by factors in the psychosocial environment.

To some extent, as already mentioned, this is due to the fact that the children are exposed to few temptations and less provocation than children in other cultures. Theft is uncommon where there is very little to steal.

Another factor may be that the village environment makes such small demands on the functional ability of the children that even rather seriously disturbed individuals can manage to live there without showing overt behavioral symptoms. The increased frequency of symptom-loaded children among those attending school supports this theory (38 percent and 20 percent respectively of the boys). Field [10], in her *Search for Security,* expresses similar theories with reference to schizophrenia and environment in Ghana.

> In any village or small country town, on any morning of the week, are to be seen numerous able-bodied men sitting under trees drinking palmwine or playing draughts while other idlers look on. They are all farmers, but only during planting, harvesting and weeding need they do any active work, and even then, if they feel disinclined, some kinsman or wife will usually take over. No demands are made on these men in the way of regularity or punctuality. Simple schizophrenia may thus go unnoticed. Other potential schizophrenics may never meet any stress severe enough to precipitate an acute attack.

It may also be that the stress factors found in the Sudanese villages are less psychogenically deleterious than those found in a Western urban environment. If so, fewer environmental injuries would occur. Generally speaking, the individuals in the villages studied are exposed to concrete, simple threats from the environment, while the stress factors in a large town are more complex and difficult for the individual to master and, consequently, perhaps they give rise to more anxiety and conflict. Hunger, illness, and poverty cause mental strain for the individual, it is true, but it may be that these external threats arouse less anxiety owing to the experience of group solidarity and the consciousness that one can get both moral and material help and support from the other members of an extended family.

It is also possible that seemingly grave traumatic experiences, such as circumcision, scarification, and illness are tolerated without the same experience of strain because the village environment is a homogeneous culture where all share about the same experiences. Mead [21] wrote as follows.

> In such a setting the child can theoretically prefigure his future experiences for as long as he lives. The homogeneous culture changes so slowly that the past continues to be a reliable guide to the present. This is not to say that development in a homogeneous community insures a smooth, painless or untraumatic socialization process. No matter how traumatic or frustrating experiences may be between infancy and death, life can nevertheless be presented to each individual as viable and to that extent bearable. Thus the homogeneous culture provides protection. In it there should be constant, low frequencies of mental disease in particular individuals who are subject to unique and severe pressures or who are constitutionally more vulnerable to strain than other individuals.

The demands made on the individual in Western communities, particularly in an industrialized urban culture, that he himself must overcome his conflicts and adjust himself during his active life to rapidly changing social roles, the transformation of society, which requires flexibility and ability to act without support of tradition, are hardly found in the Sudanese villages. Nor is the high value placed on individual performance and personal resourcefulness found there. The static, well-defined, and stereotyped role offered an individual by the village culture probably gives rise to far less internal strain and conflict.

Can the low frequency of children with a heavy burden of symptoms then be interpreted to mean that mental disturbances are rare in children in the villages investigated? There are some findings in my study suggesting that this is not necessarily the case. Anxiety, aggressiveness, and phobias are the variables occurring most frequently in the culture in addition to enuresis nocturna. According to psychoanalytical theory, symptoms, in the form of behavioral deviations, for example, may arise as a defense against anxiety. But there are other defense mechanisms which may occur instead of symptoms of disorder. Thus, it is quite possible that cultural sanctions influence the form of defense chosen.

Characteristic of the Sudanese culture are magic theories and the well-developed rites around childbirth, circumcision, and marriage, and the paranoic attitude manifested in the explanation of illness, accident, and bad luck due to the evil eye and *amel* (evil doing, sorcery). Fetishism in the form of *jertik* symbols, to protect the bearer from the evil eye, amulets with verses from the Koran, water and sand from holy places, and the development of phobias of jinn, the evil eye, and the spirits of the dead, are probably other defenses against anxiety. Introjection in the form of the consumption of pieces of paper with texts from the Koran written on them or the inhalation of the smoke from such pieces of paper when burnt is another. The great dependence on support from an extended family and individual lack of independence may be regarded as regressive features. (This may be the case with enuresis nocturna, too.)

The collective, sanctioned use of the defense mechanisms – compulsions, projection, introjection, displacement, regression – perhaps causes fewer symptoms of behavioral disturbance while anxiety and aggressiveness can be noted in the cases where these mechanisms are inadequate. That the latter were observed as frequently as in Jonsson and Kalvesten's study and that parents described themselves as "very nervous, irritable, anxious or very unhappy and depressed" very frequently (30–40 percent) suggests rather that the mental status is not so satisfactory as the low prevalence of behavioral disturbances may lead one to suppose.

The unexpectedly low prevalence of mental reactions after circumcision might be explained in a similar way. (The number of behavioral disturbances in girls seemed to increase during the year following circumcision. The smallness of the investigation population does not allow any definite conclusions to be drawn about the findings.) No increase in the number of symptom-loaded girls (2+3) in higher ages, in which all were circumcised, could be observed, however. It is possible that the trauma causes a powerful repression of sexual impulses and that these are not provoked during the years prior to marriage because boys and girls are never allowed to associate informally, thus, a restraint causes repression to remain effective. The passivity of the girls – which is encouraged by upbringing – might then be explained on the basis of loss of energy due to these powerful defenses against anxiety. That depression and hypoactivity occurred more frequently and that phobias were more common in older girls also supports this theory.

To sum up, the findings may be interpreted to mean that the village environment makes small demands on the functional ability of the children. The homogeneous culture offers the individual a static, well-defined role and strong support through the extended family. The collective forms of defense found in the culture can help the individual to cope with his anxiety. These factors may explain why the number of children with pronounced symptoms is low in spite of the high frequency of organic stress factors such as the illness and infections with cerebral symptoms observed. When it is a question of individual behavioral disturbances, other factors are probably very important: urinary tract infections, the absence of overstimulation and noise, oral gratification, upbringing practice, absence of temptation, strict social control, and genetic factors.

Bibliography

1. Andrews, J. G., The nature of stuttering, *Med. J. Austr.*, II (1964), (23):919.
2. Anthony, E. J., An experimental approach to the psychopathology of childhood: sleep disturbances, *Brit. J. Med. Psychol.*, 32 (1959), (1):19.
3. Baasher, T. A., The influence of culture on psychiatric manifestations, *Transcultural Journal,* 1 (1963).
4. Bellman, M., Studies on Encopresis, *Acta Paediat Scand.* (1966) Suppl. 170.
5. Carothers, J. C., A study of mental derangement in Africans, *Psychiatry,* 11 (1948) :47.
6. Cederblad, M., A Child Psychiatric Study on Sudanese Arab Children, *Acta Psychiat. Scand.*, (1968) Suppl. 200.
7. Collis, W. R. F., I. Dema, and F. E. A. Lesi, Transverse survey of health and nutrition, Pankshin division, Northern Nigeria, *W. Afr. Med. J.* XI (1962) (4):131.
8. Cravioto, J., E. R. De Licardie, and H. G. Birch, Nutrition, growth and neurointegrative development: an experimental and ecologic study, *Pediatrics,* 38 (1966), (2, part II):319.
9. Culwick, G. M., *Diet in the Gezira Irrigated Area, Sudan,* The Sudan Survey Department, Khartoum, 1951.
10. Field, M. J., *Search for Security,* Northwestern University press, Evanston, Ill., 1960.
11. Gottfarb, L., R. Lagercrantz, and A. Lagerdahl, Somnrubbningar hos spada och sma barn, *Nord Med,* 69 (1963) :339.
12. Hallgren, B., Enuresis. A Clinical and Genetic Study, *Acta Psychiat. Neurol. Scand.* (1957), Suppl. 114.
13. v. Harnack, G.-A., *Wesen und soziale Bedingtheit fruhkindlicher Verhaltensstorungen,* Bibl Paediat, Basel, 1953.
14. Jonsson, G. A.-L. Kalvesten, *222 Stockholmspojkar,* Almqvist & Wiksell, Uppsala, 1964.
15. Lapouse, R., M. A. Monk, and E. Street, A method for use in epidemiologic studies of behavior disorders in children, *Amer. J. Public Health,* 54 (1964) :207.
16. Lapouse, R., The relationship of behavior to adjustment in a representative sample of children, *Amer. J. Public Health* 55 (1965) :1130.
17. Lapouse, R., The epidemiology of behavior disorders in children, *Amer. J. Dis. Child* 111 (1966) :594.

18. Leighton, A. H., T. A. Lambo, C. C. Hughes, D. C. Leighton, J. M. Murphy, and D. B. Macklin, *Psychiatric Disorder among the Yoruba*, Cornell University Press, Ithaca, N. Y., 1963.
19. Lin, T. Y., A study of the incidence of mental disorder in Chinese and other cultures, *Psychiatry*, 16 (1953) :313.
20. Macfarlane, J. W., L. Allen, M. P. Honzik, *A Developmental Study of the Behavior Problems of Normal Children between Twenty-one Months and Fourteen Years*, University of California Press, Berkeley-Los Angeles, 1954.
21. Mead, M., The Implications of Culture Change for Personality Development in D. G. Haring, Ed., *Personal Character and Cultural Milieu*, University Press, Syracuse, 1949.
22. Shepherd, M., A. N. Oppenheim, and S. Mitchell, The definition and outcome of deviant behaviour in childhood, *Proc. Roy. Soc. Med.*, 59 (1966) :379.

Isolated Families in the Mountains of Norway

ERNEST A. HAGGARD (U. S. A.) AND
ANNA VON DER LIPPE (NORWAY)

What is it like to grow up on a remote isolated farm? How do such children tend to be reared by their parents? In the absence of peer groups, or even neighbors, how do children learn to view themselves, their parents, their world? With only nominal social and intellectual stimulation, what kind of psychic structures do they develop to deal with impulse, frustration, or conflict? How do they learn to channel their energies, feelings, thoughts, and activities? How do they guard against the regressive pull of the pervasive monotony and understimulation of their social microcosm—and the constant presence of the other family members? What is the nature of their mental life, both fantasy and cognitive? How do they view their future? In short, what kind of people do they become, as compared with persons reared in an urban center?

*This research is part of a larger investigation of the effects of being reared in social isolation, as compared to being reared in small town or urban settings, which was conducted through the Institute for Social Research, Oslo. The research was supported by grants (62-259 and 65-321) from the Foundations' Fund for Research in Psychiatry and by a Public Health Service Career Program Award (MH-K6-9514) from the National Institute of Mental Health to the senior author. Colleagues who participated in this research include: Arvid As, Carl-Martin Borgen, Anne Brekke, Sissel Eide, Claus Fasting, Marida Hollis, and Sita Norum. We wish to thank R. Darrell Bock, Arvid Amundsen, Susan Beal, Jan Ellen Kaderabek, Albert Kilburn, Donald Kolakowski, and Audrone Kublilius for their aid in processing and analyzing our data.

Although we approached the study of social isolates with a host of questions, hunches, and hypotheses in mind, a more general interest had to do with the nature of the child's world and his modes of adaptation to it. That is, we were interested in the congruence of the child's ecologies (psychological, social , and physical—including what they both provided and required of him) and the intrapsychic structures which he developed in order to adapt effectively in those ecologies. For example, since the world of the socially isolated and the world of the urban child are strikingly different in terms of their social and cognitive complexity, we were interested in learning whether the children in each show a corresponding difference in their internalized ego and cognitive structures. It is thus that we viewed Norway, with its isolated areas, towns, and cities, as an appropriate natural laboratory in which to seek answers to our questions.

Because of Norway's geography, with its mountains and fjords and glaciers, only about 3 percent of the countryside can be tilled, so over the centuries families have developed and worked small farms by a mountain lake, in a valley, or on a hillside. Some of these farms have been practically inaccessible, separated by miles of beautiful but rugged terrain—and without public roads.

The nature of the farm, and the way of life on it, is determined largely by the ecology in which it rests. If the elevation is too high, it will not be possible to grow grain or potatoes in the summer; if the farm is by water (the sea or a fjord or lake), fishing will most likely be an important part of the farm's economy, and so on. These farms differ also in the extent of their isolation. If a family or community is very isolated, it is apt to prize and institutionalize the virtues (and rigors) of isolated living, and to deplore life in the town. But if the family or community lies fairly close to society's periphery, where the advantages of urban living are apparent, the adaptations that ease the movement of the young into the main stream of society are apt to be made as a matter of course. Consequently, it is not possible here to discuss "life on the isolated farm" in a general sense; rather, we will consider the farms and individuals which we have studied.

Most of the farms are in a valley, a forest area, or lie around a mountain lake. Since the farms are not large, and only part of the land can be used for growing grass or hay for the animals, fishing and animal husbandry have provided food for the family and a modest source of income. The men may earn money also by gathering moss in the forest, or as lumberjacks during the winter (but they do not like this work, since it takes them away from home). Recently, they have also rented cottages or served as guides to sportsmen or vacationers from the cities. (Even so, the coherence of the family, and how the members of it relate to each other, is hardly affected by the presence of occasional "outsiders.") The women manage the house, do the cooking, and care for the animals, which may include some cattle, sheep, or goats. They also make butter and cheese, and preserve food during the short summer, and the man may sell calves and sheep to the butcher, and butter and cheese to a dealer in the nearest town. The families thus earn the equivalent of less than $2000 per year which, along with what they make or produce, provides a reasonably comfortable existence.

Social life and stimulation on the farm is minimal and is made up primarily of contacts within the immediate family, or extended family if grandparents live on the farm or nearby. Also since the farms have telephones, the women frequently talk with their counterparts (on some pretext of practicality), and the radio, and recently some TV, eases the monotony. The radio is used primarily for weather, news, and folk music; the TV for the evening programs. Nonfamily social contacts occur when the farmers go to town to sell or shop, and may "drop in" on friends en route, or go to church or other events, such as marriages, funerals, or special celebrations, which occur a few times each year, or to help a neighbor with some project that requires cooperative effort. But by and large the isolated farmer manages by himself. He has had to become a "jack of all trades" to run the farm, and self-sufficiency is both a necessity and a primary virtue.

The mother's duties are many and unending, so she has little time to dote on her children. In fact, during the first 6 to 9 months the infant usually is left alone in the parents' bedroom, except for periods of feeding, cleaning, and changing clothes. Later, when the child is old enough to climb about, so that it might fall and hurt itself, it is brought to the kitchen during the daytime. There it is expected to remain quiet and placid while the mother does her work. When the child is able to walk about, it usually tags along with the same-sex parent, doing as much as it can of what the parent does.

The low levels of emotional, social, and perceptual stimulation experienced by the infants on these isolated farms may remind one of "institutionalized children." If so, they are similar to those children who never had much "mothering," rather than those who had but lost it abruptly—at least until they enter a state-run boarding school at the age of 7. Depending on the distance to the farm, the child may spend days or weeks away from home throughout the school year. It would not be surprising, then, to find that isolates develop interpersonal detachment; yet, their experiences during the early moths and years provide an excellent foundation for the kind of life they are expected to lead as adults.[1]

Methods of Studying Social Isolates

We first spent several months locating an area which contained a sufficient number of social isolates and the necessary control groups, which also is relatively homogeneous from the genetic, cultural, and socioeconomic points of view. We then proceeded in two main directions. On the one hand we visited a sample of the isolated families several times to develop a reasonably clear picture of the ecological, historical, political, socioeconomic, and kinship characteristics of the area. On the other hand we developed a battery of tests and measures which was designed to appraise various cognitive, intrapsychic, and interpersonal characteristics of three samples of school children, aged 7 to 14.

After the usual attrition of cases, the 87 children who took the tests were: *40 isolates* (19 boys, 21 girls) from single isolated farms; *28 urban controls* (13 boys, 15 girls) from a large town—or small city—of over 5000 population in the same area; and *19 semi-isolate controls* (10 boys, 9 girls) from two communities of 200 to 500 persons, who live on the outskirts of isolation, but not in a real town. The isolates were selected to cover equally the 7 to 14 year age span,

[1] With the spread of communication and transportation networks, the isolated farms are becoming depopulated. A young man can make a better living (with less work and much more fun) in the town. And a young unmarried woman, who has no place in the economy of the isolated farm, is drawn to the town to find work in a store or factory, and hopefully also to find a mate. In some isolated areas, practically all the young people between, say, 15 and 16 and 30 to 35 have left the farm. Those younger are still in school; those older find it too difficult to adapt to urban ways. By and large the young leave the farm because of some necessity or need, such as employment or further education. Usually, they move the shortest distance possible, and to where they have relatives or friends.

and the children in the two control groups were matched with the isolates on age, sex, sibling position in the family and, as nearly as possible, the father's occupation (to avoid confounding socioeconomic levels with degrees of social isolation). Thus, the fathers of the children in the two control groups worked primarily with things rather than people, for example, as truck drivers or mechanics.

Following our well-laid plans for the research, we soon learned that several considerations exist with respect to the study of social isolates, including the following.

GENERAL IGNORANCE OF ISOLATED LIVING

Little is known with any certainty about isolated individuals or communities, or the kind of lives they lead. There are, of course, accounts written with insight and charm, such as Lewis' [13] description of the "Children of the Cumberland," or a brief glimpse of refugees from some previously unheard-of volcanic island, like Tristan da Cunha, in 1963. But perhaps what insights we have into the isolate come as much or more from novelists like Knut Hamsun, or the ancient teller of folk and fairy tales, as from direct or systematic observation. There are, however, a number of recent studies of primates or lower animals reared in isolation (see Harlow and Harlow [10] and Bronfenbrenner [7]).

INVESTIGATOR BIASES

Our general ignorance of the social isolate leads one (especially if he is a clinical psychologist or a psychiatrist) to suffer from two types of bias. One is the usual clinical bias, specifically, overemphasis on pathology, and the implicit assumption that the meaning of responses to test protocols are to be interpreted as though the subjects were patients in a hospital or clinic. The other bias is that of the urbanite—the implicit assumption that the meaning of responses to test protocols are to be interpreted as though they were from persons reared in urban settings. For example, all members of our research group hypothesized (i.e., "projected") initially that the isolates had a rich and free fantasy life—as urbanites would experience if they were to move to an isolated farm (or, indeed, into a perceptual isolation chamber). This assumption, if held, would lead to the erroneous conclusion that something must be "wrong" with the isolate who engaged seldom if at all in free-floating fantasy.

CONCEPTUAL CONSIDERATIONS

Behavioral scientists have only recently turned their attention to the importance of such factors as space and distance on man's behavior. In this connection, Hall's [9] concept of proxemics, and Barker's [1] interest in ecological psychology are much more pertinent to the study of social isolates than the traditional physicalistic definitions in terms of meters or miles. Simple measures of distance—as the crow flies—ignore such crucial factors as the amount of physical and psychological effort it takes to go from one's own farm to visit a neighbor or the nearest town. In this study we used a criterion of "behavioral distance," namely, the (in)frequency with which adults met with other nonfamily adults, and the (un)availability of playmates for the children—other than their siblings—until they went off to school at age 7.

PRACTICAL CONSIDERATIONS

For a variety of reasons, isolates lead a relatively nonverbal existence and certainly find it hard to talk about sensitive areas involving strong affect or ambivalence. That is, they tend not to discuss (even among themselves) many matters of primary interest to the behavioral scientist. Consequently, if an investigator is insensitive to what the isolate is ready and able to discuss, or if his probes are too rapid or deep, he more likely than not will rupture the interview and may even terminate the relationship. This means, of course, that the investigator cannot set about to collect data with nearly the same speed and efficiency as in an urban setting, but must with patience wait until the isolate is ready (perhaps in a later interview) to talk about what is of interest to the investigator. It also means that indirect methods of data collection, such as projective techniques, may need to be developed and used in order to get at variables, attitudes, or feelings that the isolate just cannot discuss openly.

Research Strategy

We were also faced with a basic question of research strategy. Should we strive to capture the subtle nuances of life in, and adaptation to, social isolation, as we observed or sensed them intuitively—or should we attempt to objectify our findings by the use of explicitely defined, pre-tested scales, with reliance on statistical analysis to ferret out the wheat from the chaff in our thinking? We chose the latter approach, partly because isolates differ in important ways from urbanites (which we irrevocably are) and to employ tests which would prove us wrong, if in fact we were, in our appraisal of the social isolate.

There remains, of course, a large area of ignorance: in the case of those hypotheses or scales which did not "pan out," we cannot tell whether our ideas really were without substance–or whether our scales were inappropriate, or too insensitive, to measure the phenomenon in question. Furthermore, our decision does not preclude occasional regrets. Since impressions from overt behavior may be more vivid (and valid) than those from recorded speech or typed protocols (the source of most of our data), "important findings" may have escaped our procedures. For example, in one test two dolls get into a fight, and the child being tested was required to strike them together and describe what they said to each other. Ratings were made of both the child's verbal response and his vigor in striking the dolls together. For this situation, the ratings based on overt behavior differentiated among the three groups much more clearly ($P = .002$) than did the ratings of the children's verbal behavior ($P = .21$)

Tests and Measures

A battery of tests and measures was used to appraise various cognitive, intrapsychic, and interpersonal characteristics of the three samples of children. Four of the tests were administered and/or scored in the standard manner (see numbers 4, 5, 11, and 12 below). We felt that other available tests or measures either did not probe for the things we were interested in, or they were not sufficiently "urban culture free" for our children, since they tended to use urban scenes and situations and were standardized on urban children. Consequently, eight of our tests or sets of measures were developed for this study, and were pretested on appropriate samples of children with scoring systems developed in accordance with our research interests.[2] The data sources which we will refer to are the following.

[2] Reliabilities (inter-judge agreement) were computed for most of the scales. For the 15 Rorschach scales (R_S), for example, the median r is .85, and the median r for 35 scales from the Bear (B) and Doll Play (DP) tests is .79. Scales were dropped when satisfactory reliabilities could not be established.

1. *The Bear Test* (B) was a series of 10 black-and-white water-color pictures of teddy bears in various situations. The scenes were drawn to elicit responses to areas of particular interest, for example, a young bear sitting alone while others played in the background; or eating with the parents; or seeing the parents embrace; or choosing between the path to a town or to the forest. The test was administered like the Thematic Apperception Test but scored according to our scales and categories.
2. *The Doll Play Test* (DP), adapted from the Lynn and Lynn [14] test, was a model of a small cottage outfitted with furniture and dolls which corresponded to all the family members of the child being tested, with a variety of situations to which the child responded.
3. *Free-Choice Drawings* (D_f) for which the child was given paper and crayons and asked to draw anything he wished.
4. *Drawings of Mother and Father* (D_p) for which the child was given paper and crayons to draw his family, including his parents. The test was scored according to the procedure proposed by Machover [15].
5. *The Embedded Figures Test* (EF) was administered and scored according to the procedure proposed by Karp and Konstadt [11].
6. *Essay: "Myself in 15 Years"* (E) was given as a school assignment to children ages 10 to 14.
7. *The Family Relations Test* (FR) was adapted from the test designed by Bene and Anthony [2] and consisted of short statements which the child assigned as being characteristic of the mother, the father, or other family members. The separate items later were combined to form scales.
8. *A Linguistic Analysis* (L) of the 7310 different words in the Bear Test protocols was made in an attempt to minimize our clinical and urban biases. Each word was precoded in terms of cognitive, affective, or behavioral categories, then a frequency score for each child for each category was obtained, and the categories combined to form scales. For example, the scale "Use of modifiers" is

the proportion of adjectives and adverbs to all the words used by the child and is intended to be a measure of cognitive differentiation. The scales later were transformed to permit statistical analysis.

9. *Rorschach Scales* (R_s), based on all 10 protocols, were developed to reflect dimensions of cognitive and intrapsychic functioning relevant to our research interests.
10. *Scaled Rorschach Determinants* (R_d).[3] In an attempt to minimize our clinical and urban biases, each of the 31 determinants used in the initial scoring of this test, according to Klopfer's [12] system, were assigned to one of 9 scales, which later were transformed to permit statistical analysis. The names of the R_d scales are intended as terse approximations of their psychological meaning.
11. *The Child-Rearing Practices Q-Sort* (Q), developed by Block [3], was administered to samples of socially isolated, semi-isolated, and urban control parents.
12. *The Wechsler Intelligence Scale for Children* (W) was selected as the preferred measure of general intelligence because it provides a variety of measures of intellectual functioning.

General Method of Data Analysis

Table 1 illustrates our general method of data analysis. We were primarily interested in finding out which measures indicate statistically significant differences among the groups of children, on the assumption that they represent different subcultures. But to obtain valid indices of such differences, it was necessary to allow for the following conditions of our measures and designs.

1. *Inter-measure correlations.* Since each child contributed many measures, which are intercorrelated to some degree, we used a mutlivariate analysis of variance procedure

[3]This approach was used initially in a study involving Rorschach and Holtzman inkblot data from normal adolescents by Bock and Haggard, et al. [5]; a description of the procedure is given in Bock [4].

Table 1 Scaled Rorschach Determinants

Scales	Correlation with Age		Group Means		Significance of Difference (*P* value)		
	Isolates (1)	Controls (2)	Isolates $N = 40$ (3)	Controls $N = 29$ (4)	Schools Within Isolation (5)	Sex Groups (6)	Isolation Groups (7)
1. Sum: 0 (Original responses)	.27	.09	1.66	1.25	.05	.60	.75
2. Sum: P (Popular responses)	.23	.00	1.38	1.54	.14	.03	.26
3. Sum: S (Oppositional responses)	.06	–.08	.52	.01	.01	.77	.01
4. Sum: M, M–, FC / Sum: F (Psychological mindedness)	.20	–.02	–2.02	–1.58	.34	.003	.0004
5. Sum: H, A / Sum: Anat., Obj., Bot., Nat. (Interpersonal orientation)	–.03	–.01	.08	.36	.99	.40	.02
6. Sum: Hd / Sum: Ad (Interpersonal non-defensiveness)	–.15	.24	–.87	–.32	.33	.32	.002
7. Sum: W / Sum: D, Dd, dd, dr (Intellectual integrative capacity)	.10	.12	–2.06	–1.71	.17	.59	.09
8. Sum: FM, FM–, Fm–, m (Propensity for fantasy)	.11	.00	2.13	2.39	.78	.60	.004
9. Sum: CF, C, C′, c, FK, K, k (Experience of affect)	–.03	.02	2.13	2.31	.29	.06	.70
Multivariate *F* and *P* values: (All nine scales together)					$F36/185$ df = 1.18; $P = .24$	$F9/49$ df = 2.44; $P = .02$	$F9/49$ df = 2.78; $P = .01$

which takes into consideration any such intermeasure correlations (see Bock and Haggard [6]).[4]

2. *Age trends.* Since we were interested in (a) the stable differences among the isolation groups—quite apart from age trends—and also (b) whether the correlations of the measures with age differed for the isolation groups as an indication of relative rates of socialization over the 7- to 14-year-age span, the effect of age was removed from each of the measures (and *P* values) by a covariance analysis (see cols. 1 and 2, Table 1)
3. *Differences among the isolation subgroups.* Since the isolates were drawn from five boarding schools, it is possible that these subsamples within the total isolation group would differ on particular measures (see col. 5, scales 1 and 3). Consequently, the effect of any schools within isolation differences was removed in estimating the overall isolation group differences (col. 7)
4. *Sex differences.* Since children of the two sexes may differ on particular measures (cf. col. 6, scales 2, 4, and 9), the effect of any sex differences was removed in estimating the overall isolation group differences (col. 7).

In reading the following tables, the following considerations should be kept in mind. (a) For simplicity of presentation, only the differences between the isolated and the urban control samples will be given. (b) The *P* values indicating isolation versus control group differences are uncontaminated by effects of the children's age, the schools within isolation, or sex differences.[5] (c) The *P* values cited are univariate measures and, although appropriate for the scale in question, they cannot be used to estimate the overall significance of the set of measures in a table (since the measures are not independent). (d) The group means should be read to determine the direction of the findings; the *P* values should be read to determine the statisti-

[4] For example, the inter-measure *r*s among the nine scales in Table 1 range from –.37 (scales 3 vs. 4) to +.51 (scales 4 vs. 7).

[5] If the effects of the schools within isolation and sex group differences were not removed from the measures, the isolation versus control group differences would be biased (i.e., in error) to some unknown degree.

cal significance of the findings.[6] The larger of the two means indicates "more of" whatever the scale designates. For example, in Table 1, cols. 3 and 4, we see that the isolates gave more S ("oppositional") responses and the controls were more "psychologically minded" (since their scores were less negative, hence they were larger).

Findings

It will not be possible in this chapter to consider in detail each of the 50 or so measures which differentiate between the children in the isolated and the urban control samples. Thus, assuming reliance on the data presented in the tables, only the most salient characteristics of the two groups will be discussed.[7]

The findings will be grouped in terms of the following topics: the parents' socialization pressures and practices (Table 2); the children's general interpersonal orientations and social relationships (Table 3); how they relate to their parents (Table 4); their affect life (Table 5); their ego defenses and resources (Table 6); their cognitive abilities and styles (Table 7); and some indices of their orientation to the future. In general, the characteristics of the isolates will be described in somewhat more detail than those of the urban controls.

SOCIALIZATION PRESSURES AND PRACTICES

It should be noted in passing that, for the isolates, the parents (and possibly the grandparents) embody essentially all of the early socializing pressures which help to mold the child. He has no peer group as such, and no escape except into the frightening forest. In contrast, the controls not only have peer groups and other adults to turn to, but later they also have the anonymity of the city, which gives them a temporary escape from the family and the feeling that "They know everything I do." Consequently, the urban children experience a much greater freedom from their parents than do the isolated children.

[6]The group means for the isolates and controls vary, depending on the number of scale units (which range from 3 to 10), whether single or sum scores are used, and whether raw or transformed (e.g., logarithm) scores are presented, as in the case of the Rorschach determinant (R_d) and linguistic (L) scales.

[7]Particular findings will be referred to by the appropriate table and scale number(s), for example, (2:1-3).

The isolated parents (need to) exert few if any socialization pressures on the child (e.g., if he has a temper tantrum, they just ignore it), and they tend not to verbalize, as by homolies, generalizations as to how the child should behave in specific situations. Rather, they appear to rely on the child's learning by imitation and identification as a result of day-to-day observation.[8] In this type of setting, linguistic formulations and generalizations play a minimal role in the regulation of the child's behavior. Urban parents tend much more than isolates to employ rewards for desirable and punishments for undesirable behavior, all heavily spiced with the familiar "shoulds" and "should nots."

Table 2 Parents' Characteristic Socialization Practices

		Group Means		
	Data Source	Isolates	Controls	Difference (*P* value)
Most characteristic of isolated parents:				
1. I sometimes tease and make fun of my child	Q	4.2	2.0	.0005
2. I think children should be taught not to cry at an early age	Q	3.8	2.3	.02
3. I believe physical punishment is the best method of discipline	Q	3.3	2.3	.02
Most characteristic of control parents:				
4. I take my child's preferences into account in planning	Q	4.0	5.5	.001
5. I believe it is important for a child to play outside and get plenty of fresh air	Q	5.2	6.4	.03
6. When I am angry with my child, I let him know it	Q	3.9	4.8	.03

[8]By and large, the child's world is the parents' world; he rises and goes to bed when they do, and during the day he tries to what the (same-sex) parent does. And, perhaps as a compensation for not having a true world of his own (i.e., with play, peers, etc.), he is allowed to enter the adults' world on an almost-equal footing: he takes part in the adults' conversations, and if asked to leave or go to bed, he does not—until they do.

As for the parents' view of how the children should be reared, the isolated parents take a "traditional" (or adult-oriented) and rather harsh stance with respect to the child, emphasizing self-control, suppression of feeling, and obedience (2:1-3), whereas the urban parents are much more "progressive" (or child-oriented) and considerate of the child's needs and his development of autonomy (2:4-6).

THE CHILDREN'S GENERAL INTERPERSONAL ORIENTATIONS AND SOCIAL RELATIONSHIPS

As compared with the urban child, the isolate tends to be more oriented toward the home, but not to engage so much in constructive activity of his own, at least in his fantasy life (3:1,2). With respect to

Table 3 General Orientations and Social Relationships

Scales	Data Source	Group Means		Difference
		Isolates	Controls	(*P* value)
1. Home oriented	B	5.7	4.4	.002
2. Constructive activity	DP	1.9	2.3	.08
3. Sum: H, A / Sum: Anat., Obj., Bot., Nat. (Interpersonal orientation)	R_d	.1	.4	.02
4. Number of peers introduced into stories	B	4.2	6.4	.01
5. Amount of social play	B	4.4	5.9	.001
6. Conflict with peers	B	4.5	5.9	.002
7. Contact with larger society	B	4.6	5.4	.05
8. Use on inclusive > exclusive pronouns (e.g., we > they)	L	1.2	1.3	.01
9. Use of verbal > nonverbal communication terms (e.g., talk > visit)	L	4.0	4.4	.10
10. Use of words implying social-emotional distance (e.g., alone, angry)	L	2.0	2.7	.01

social behavior, we find the expected: the control children show a stronger interpersonal orientation, they introduce more peers into their stories, they engage more frequently in social play (and also come into conflict with their playmates more often), and indicate more contact with society-at-large, than do the isolated children (3:3-7). It seems that for both groups, then, their experiences have proved the grist for the mill of their fantasy life, at least as revealed by their responses to projective tests. This difference in social orientation extends even to the children's linguistic behavior: the controls tend to use relatively more inclusive (than exclusive) pronouns; when they use communication terms, they involve relatively more verbal (than nonverbal) interactions; and they use more words implying tolerance for social-emotional distance than do the isolates in telling stories to the Bear Test (3:8-10).

HOW THE CHILDREN VIEW AND RELATE TO THEIR PARENTS

Given the parents' child-rearing attitudes and practices, it is not surprising that the control children tend to feel more loved and less rejected and, in general, closer emotionally to their parents than do the isolates (4:1-3). As for the children's view of the mother, the primary socializing agent, the controls indicated that they felt both more "let down" and received more "ego support" from the mother, and also felt freer to be aggressive toward her (4:4-6).[9] Although the attitudes of the control children may reflect a realistic appraisal of their mothers' behavior, it also is likely that they can express their opinions, positive or negative, with greater candor than the isolates.

In view of the almost constant proximity of the family members on the isolated farm, and the absence of others, do isolated children relate to parents of the same—and opposite—sex as urban children do? The question bears, of course, on Freud's classic formulation of the child's attraction to the parent of the opposite sex, and his defense against such feelings. From their responses to two situations in

[9] These scales are based on responses to items in the Family Relations Test. Representative items in these scales are: Scale 4 ("Who forgets sometimes that they've promised you something?" and "Who tells a lie now and then?"); Scale 5 ("Who shows you how things should be done?" and "Who wants you to be among the best at school?") and Scale 6 ("Who can you quarrel with?" and "Who can you be mad at?").

Table 4 Feelings and Relations to Parents

Scales	Data Source	Group Means: Isolates	Group Means: Controls	Difference (*P* value)
1. Feels loved by parents	B	.3	.5	.12
2. Feels rejected by parents	B	.7	.5	.02
3. Emotional closeness to parents	B	2.6	3.2	.005
4. Feels "let down" by mother	FR	2.9	3.8	.02
5. Feels ego support from mother	FR	5.8	6.1	.06
6. Feels free to aggress against mother	FR	2.6	3.3	.07
Intolerance of intimacy with:				
7. Same-sex parent	DP	3.6	3.8	.30
8. Opposite-sex parent	DP	3.1	2.4	.05
9. Compliant to wishes of opposite-sex parent	DP	3.5	2.9	.04
10. Total "normal" score: drawings of parents	DP	27.7	30.0	.05
Use of personal > impersonal terms for:				
11. The mother figure	L	1.3	−1.1	.001
12. The father figure	L	1.5	− .8	.001
13. Others (e.g., siblings, etc.)	L	−1.4	−1.4	.80

the Doll Play Test,[10] the groups did not differ particularly when the same-sex parent was involved; they did differ with respect to the opposite-sex parent. In fact, the isolates were not only less able to tolerate intimacy with the opposite-sex parent, they were also more compliant with the wishes of that parent (4:7-9). It seems reasonable

[10] In these two situations, a doll of the child's sex and one of the same (or opposite) sex parent were alone at home; the instructions read: "One day father (mother) and the boy (girl) have a very pleasant time together." . . . "What do they do?" . . . "What happens next?" . . . "Where are the others?" Responses were scored on a five-point scale from: (1) full acceptance of intimacy (e.g., parent participates in something the child likes, direct and open contact without disruption) to (5) nonacceptance (e.g., no communication, they merely work together, anxiety or guilt-ridden story, no contact or immediately interrupted contact).

to infer from these data that the intensity of any Oedipal feelings and conflicts, undiluted by other available "objects," is greater in the isolates than in the controls.

Findings from two other tests bear on the amount of psychological "breathing space" the child has and its effect on his relations with his parents. In one, in which the children drew their parents, the isolates received fewer "normal" scores than the controls (4:10).[11] This finding suggests that the isolates feelings toward their parents are more highly charged with conflict and ambivalence. Finally, in the linguistic analysis of the Bear Test protocols the isolates, in speaking of parental figures, tended to use the personal e.g., "mother" rather than the impersonal (e.g., "the mother") form, as opposed to the urban controls, but did not do so in speaking of their siblings, grandparents, or friends (4:11-13). These findings suggest that the isolated child may be locked into an almost symbiotic relationship with his parents—but not with other persons.

AFFECT AND ITS EXPRESSION

With life on the isolated farm providing so few social-emotional "safety valves," and with a dearth of available and appropriate conflict-free "objects," a basic question is: What happens to the affect-life of the isolated child, as compared with his urban counterpart? Does the isolate show a stronger tendency to repress his affects altogether, or to suppress their expression, or to express them in ways which differ from those of the urban child? The data in Table 5 suggest that the isolate experiences about as many feelings or affects as the urban child (5:1) and, in general, gives vent to them, including the overall expression of aggression—at least in his (fantasy) responses to the Bear Test pictures (5:2-4). With respect to how an affect such as aggression is expressed, however, it is to be expected that the urban child does so much more often indirectly and in socially acceptable ways (5:5-6)[12]

[11] "Normal" scores indicate aspects of the drawings judged to be appropriate, nondeviant, etc. In our samples, the isolated children should not be handicapped by inexperience in drawing, since they frequently are given paper and crayons to relieve boredom.

[12] The isolate is fully able to experience aggressive feelings—but he tries to avoid their arousal and/or expression. For example, when asked what might happen during an interpersonal conflict, adults spoke readily of the possibility of physical fighting and/or the breakup of a marriage.

Table 5 Affect and Its Expression

Scales	Data Source	Group Means		Difference (*P* value)
		Isolates	Controls	
1. Sum: CF, C, C′, c, FK, K, k (Experience of affect)	R_d	2.1	2.3	.70
2. Total positive affect	B	4.5	5.6	.20
3. Total negative affect	B	5.0	5.4	.30
4. Total aggressive themes	B	5.4	5.1	.80
5. Total indirect aggression	B	4.6	5.6	.005
6. Socialized expression of aggression	B	2.8	3.5	.01
7. Open expression of pleasure at parents' return	DP	2.3	3.0	.01
8. Emotional liveliness of drawings	D_f	2.8	4.0	.01
9. Attachment to favorite animal	DP	2.5	3.0	.15
10. Acceptance of loss of animal	DP	2.6	1.9	.10

Since the social isolate tends not to express his feelings or affects openly in his day-today behavior, we thought that he might use other outlets, such as affective involvement with "Nature" or with animals. Consequently, we probed several avenues of affective expression open to the children of both groups, for example, their pleasure at the parents' return after having been away for "a long time"; their affective expressiveness in their free-choice drawings, and their attachment to a favorite animal. In all of these situations, the urban children tended to express more affective involvement than the isolates did (5:7-10). For example, when the returning parents were greeted, a typical response of an urban child was, "I'm glad you're back; I was lonesome while you were gone"; the typical response of an isolate was, "You must be hungry; let us go in and eat now." Likewise, the free-choice drawings of the urban children were "warmer," more lively and engaging, and less static, than those of the isolates. And, with respect to their favorite animal, the isolates tended to express less involvement in their play with the animal and, later when it had to be sold, they brushed the matter off more easily than the urban children.

It appears that the isolated child, with his lack of opportunity to develop sophisticated and flexible modes of interaction and expression, has learned to defend himself against vulnerability to those feelings or experiences which he does not handle easily, for example, aggression, intimacy, attachment and loss. This tendency is seen in the relative infrequency of the isolates' expression of despair or dejection in their stories (5:11) and in their greeting to the returning parents. In dealing with such poignant feelings, the isolated child typically turns to some practical activity, knowing that the others (e.g., the parents) will understand what he dare not quite feel and cannot say.

EGO DEFENSES AND RESOURCES

We have seen that the isolate tends to inhibit the expression of interpersonal aggression and intimacy by engaging in behaviors which communicate his feelings but enable him to avoid experiencing their full impact. In a more general sense, the isolate—much more than the urban child—deals with conflict (intrapsychic or intrapersonal) by such techniques as passivity, avoidance, or flight in his stories to the Bear Test (6:1). Furthermore, on a measure of the degree of ego control,[13] the urban children tended to be scored in the middle range (i.e., flexible, appropriate control), whereas the isolates more often were scored as showing under- or overcontrol ($P = .05$). This difference was not so clear in the younger group, ages 7 to 10 ($P = .25$), but was marked in the older group, ages 11 to 14 ($P = .005$).

A series of ego defenses was also coded from the Rorschach protocols.[14] The isolates more frequently employ simple ego defenses against specific conflicts, whereas the controls tend to employ generalized defenses, which are a part of their character structure (6:2,3). Furthermore, the defenses which occurred at least 30 percent more frequently than one would expect by "chance" in one group or the other were: perseveration, compulsive traits, resignation, and flight into reality, which characterized the isolates ($P = .01$), and withdrawal, acting out, regression, and flight into fantasy, which charac-

[13] The five-point ego control scale, based on all 10 Bear Test stories, ranged from (1) a lack of impulse control (primary process), through (3) flexible, appropriate control, to (5) excessive, brittle, overcontrol.

[14] All together, 9 "simple" and 11 "character" defenses were coded as being either clearly present (or else absent).

Table 6 Ego Defenses and Resources

	Data Source	Group Means: Isolates	Group Means: Controls	Difference (*P* value)
Ego defenses:				
1. Sum passive defenses	B	2.4	1.8	.001
2. Sum simple defenses	R_s	1.8	1.6	.06
3. Sum character defenses	R_s	2.1	2.5	.02
Ego resources:				
4. General ego strength	R_s	3.6	4.4	.0002
5. Integrative control	R_s	3.1	3.6	.01
6. Constructive use of fantasy	R_s	3.0	3.7	.0004
7. Empathy and object relations	R_s	4.0	4.8	.0004
8. Social contact function	B	2.7	3.5	.005
9. Ego resilience	B	3.0	3.6	.02
10. Ability to integrate conflict in fantasy	B	2.6	3.3	.002
11. Reliance on external controls	B	3.2	2.9	.08
12. Richness of fantasy life	B	2.8	3.5	.05
13. Sum: FM, FM–, Fm, m (Propensities for fantasy)	R_d	2.1	2.4	.004
14. Sum: Hd / Sum: Ad (Interpersonal nondefensiveness)	R_d	– .9	–.3	.002
15. Sum: M, M–, FC / Sum: F (Psychological mindedness)	R_d	–2.0	–1.6	.0004

terized the urban children ($P = .10$). A comparison of these two sets of defense suggests that the intrapsychic structures of the isolated children are less differentiated and more inflexible and intolerant of indirect impulse expression, than those of the urban children.

In terms of an impressive array of ego resources and strengths, it is quite apparent that the urban children show up much better than the social isolates (6:4-15). This generalization makes sense, of course, from an urban frame of reference. True, the urban children show a more extensive, richer fantasy life, more psychological insight and better emotional contact with others, and a greater ability to use their resources to integrate adaptively their impulses, their fantasies, and their interpersonal relationships. But the social isolates have had neither the same opportunity to develop, nor the same need for, the kinds of ego structures so necessary for one to function effectively in an urban setting. Consequently, one cannot say categorically that one mode of adaptation is "better" than the other. Rather, it appears that each is appropriate for the type of life in which it was developed, so that one mode of adaptation should serve adequately for the urban child, and the other for the social isolate—assuming that each remains in the subculture in which he was reared.

COGNITIVE ABILITIES AND STYLES

As we have seen from the projective test data, the social isolate tends to be oriented toward behavior in the "real world." This tendency is reflected also in his language in response to the Bear Test in that he, more than the urban child, uses verbs depicting overt behavior rather than subjective experience (7:1). With this orientation, the isolate should be expected to develop those cognitive abilities and skills which involve, for example, accurate perception, memory, and non-fantasy reasoning. The performance of the isolates on the Embedded Figures test, and on the Digit Span and Arithmetic scales of the WISC is, in fact, equivalent to the urban childrens' (7:2-4). However, on the Picture Arrangement and Comprehension scales of the WISC, which involve familiarity with social customs and norms, and the ability to generalize from them, the isolate reveals the extent to which he is "socially (and cognitively) disadvantaged" (7:5,6).

In terms of how the individual perceives, structures, and depicts the world in which he lives, the isolates and controls differ in several respects. The isolate is more insistent on "seeing things his own way," is less proficient at organizing and integrating his perceptions coherently and meaningfully and, in describing persons, places, or events, uses language which is less precise and differentiating than the urban child's (7:7-10). Thus, on unstructured tasks such as the Rorschach he is judged to be les "intelligent" (7:11)[15] However, the differences in cognitive styles may only reflect the urban child's greater range of experiences, which foster the development of cog-

[15]Intelligence, as rated from the Rorschach, correlates .42 with the WISC Total score. And, as one would expect, the overall scores of the controls are higher than the isolates' on both the Verbal ($P = .02$) and Performance ($P = .002$) scales of the WISC.

Table 7 Cognitive Abilities and Styles

Scales	Data Sources	Group Means: Isolates	Group Means: Controls	Difference (*P* Value)
1. Use of overt > covert behavior verbs (i.e., acts > thoughts and feelings)	L	.6	.4	.001
2. Embedded Figures	EF	19.1	19.4	.50
3. Arithmetic	W	10.4	10.8	.80
4. Digit Span	W	10.1	9.3	.50
5. Picture Arrangement	W	7.5	10.4	.0001
6. Comprehension	W	9.0	11.0	.001
7. Sum: S (Oppositional responses)	R_d	.5	.0	.01
8. Sum: W / Sum: D, Dd, dd, dr (Intellectual integrative capacity	R_d	−2.1	−1.7	.09
9. Perceptual organization	R_s	3.2	4.3	.0001
10. Use of modifiers (percent) adjectives and adverbs)	L	6.0	6.3	.05

nitive differentiation and maturity, and the isolate's greater tendency to rely on the structure of the external world to organize his cognitive life.

ORIENTATIONS TO THE FUTURE

A few items derived from the essay "Myself in 15 Years" will serve to illustrate the different ways in which the two groups view their future lives. For example, we find that the social isolates most frequently bring their parents into their future, which is essentially a continuation of their past and present. The urban controls, on the other hand, appear to assume that they will be mobile in both the geographical and socioeconomic senses, and already have fixed upon glamorous and sophisticated occupations, which are often far beyond their current position in life.[16]

[16]Two scales which characterize the isolates are "Continuity with childhood" (*P* = .002) and "Parents brought into essay" (*P* = .05); and two scales which characterize the urban controls are "Leaving the home area" (*P* = .05) and "Occupational aspirations" (*P* = .05).

In view of the decreasing social and economic viability of the isolated farm, and the increasing emphasis on education, technology, communication, and other interpersonal skills, one can only wonder how well the social isolate can manage to make a nondisruptive transition to the future. We owe them, as well as the urban controls, our appreciation for having participated in our research, and hope that what we have learned can be put to some use in helping children of yesterday find a meaningful place in the world of tomorrow.

Concluding Comment

Because of the variety of findings which we have reviewed, it will not be possible here to discuss their theoretical relevance or significance. It would have been interesting to speculate, however, about the isolate's phenomenological world (as indicated by his substantive responses to the projective tests) and its relation to his intrapsychic structures and his behaviors, or how the isolate's character structure serves to protect him against regression in a monotonous and understimulating environment, or whether the members of an isolated family tend to share a common ego, and its implication for the isolate's apparent inability to handle his feelings of intimacy and anger with the other members of his family. And so on. But an overriding conclusion from our findings should be noted, namely, that the two subcultures, the single isolated farm and the urban setting, each promote the development of intrapsychic structures and behavior patterns which are inappropriate to life in that particular subculture. In this sense, our findings support the proposition that the total adaptation of the individal—both his inner life and his behavior—must be considered in terms of the parameters of his environmental context.[17]

Bibliography

1. Barker, R., *Ecological Psychology:* Concepts and methods for studying the environment of human behavior, Stanford University Press, Stanford, California, 1968.

[17] A theoretical model and rationale for the conceptual inseparability of the individual and his environmental context is given in Haggard [8].

2. Bene, E. and J. Anthony, *Manual for the Family Relations Test, An Objective Technique for Exploring Emotional Attitudes in Children,* National Foundation for Educational Research in England and Wales, London, 1957.
3. Block, J., *The Child-Rearing Practices Report,* Institute of Human Development, University of California, Berkeley (Mimeo), 1965.
4. Bock, R. D., *Multivariate statistical methods in behavioral research* (Ch. 9), McGraw-Hill, New York, 1970.
5. Bock, R. D. and E. A. Haggard, with W. H. Holtzman, Anne G. Beck, and S. J. Beck, *A comprehensive psychometric study of the Rorschach and Holtzman inkblot techniques,* The Psychometric Laboratory, University of North Carolina (Mimeo), Chapel Hill, 1963.
6; Bock, R. D. and E. A. Haggard, The use of multivariate analysis of variance in behavioral research, in D. K. Whitla (Ed.), *Handbook of Measurement and Assessment in Behavioral Sciences,* Addison-Wesley Publishing Co., Inc., Reading, Mass., 1968, pp. 100-142.
7. Bronfenbrenner, U., Early deprivation in mammals: A cross-species analysis, in G. Newton and S. Levine (Eds.), *Early Experience and Behavior,* Thomas, Springfield, Ill., 1968, pp. 627-764
8. Haggard, E. A., Isolation and personality change, in P. Worchel and D. Byrne (Eds.), *Personality Change,* Wiley, New York, 1964, pp. 433-469.
9. Hall, E. T., *The Hidden Dimension,* Doubleday, New York, 1966.
10. Harlow, H. F. and M. K. Harlow, Social deprivation in monkeys, *Sci. Amer.,* 207 (1962) 136-144.
11. Karp, S. A. and N. L. Konstadt, *Manual for the Children's Embedded Figures Test,* Cognitive Tests, Brooklyn, 1963.
12. Klopfer, B., M. D. Ainsworth, W. G. Klopfer, R. R. Holt, *Developments in the Rorschach Technique,* Vol. 1, World Book Co., New York, 1954.
13. Lewis, C., *Children of the Cumberland,* Columbia University Press, New York, 1946.
14. Lynn, D. B. and R. Lynn, The structured Doll Play Test as a projective technique for use with children, *J. Proj. Tech.,* 23 (1959), 335-44.
15. Machover, K., *Personality Projections in the Drawing of the Human Figure,* Thomas, Springfield, Ill., 1949.
16. Zyzanski, S. J., A multivariate normal analysis for categorical data, Ph.D. dissertation, Psychology, University of North Carolina, Chapel Hill, N.C., 1968.

Index